ORTHOPAEDICS

PROBLEMS IN PRIMARY CARE

Orthopaedics, problems in primary care.

ISBN 1-878487-33-7

Practice Management Information Corporation
Los Angeles, California 90010

Printed in the United States of America

ORTHOPAEDICS

PROBLEMS IN PRIMARY CARE

Edited by Randall E. Marcus, M.D.
Department of Orthopaedics
Case Western Reserve University
School of Medicine
and University Hospitals
Cleveland, Ohio

Practice Management Information Corporation
Los Angeles, California 90010

Problems in Primary Care

Other books in the series

Anesthesiology, Sanford L. Klein, D.D.S., M.D. and Dennis F. Landers, M.D., Ph.D., 1990. ISBN 0-87489-481-6

Gastroenterology, Sanjiv C. Chopra, M.D. and Daniel Sugarman, M.D., 1990. ISBN 0-87489-460-3

Neurology, James L. Bernat, M.D. and Frederick M. Vincent, M.D., 1987. ISBN 0-87489-407-7

Otolaryngology, edited by D. Thomas Upchurch, M.D., F.A.C.S., 1989. ISBN 0-87489-442-5.

Pulmonary Medicine, edited by Robert D. Brandstetter, M.D., 1989. ISBN 0-87489-468-9

Rheumatology, Matthew H. Liang, M.D., W. Neal Roberts, M.D., Celeste Robb-Nicholson, M.D, and Lori Bannon, M.D., 1990. ISBN 0-87489-421-2

CONTRIBUTORS

MICHAEL J. BOLESTA, M.D.
Department of Orthopaedics
Case Western Reserve University
School of Medicine
and University Hospitals
Cleveland, Ohio

DANIEL R. COOPERMAN, M.D.
Department of Orthopaedics
Case Western Reserve University
School of Medicine
and University Hospitals
Cleveland, Ohio

SANFORD E. EMERY, M.D.
Department of Orthopaedics
Case Western Reserve University
School of Medicine
and University Hospitals
Cleveland, Ohio

HARRY E. FIGGIE, III, M.D.
Department of Orthopaedics
Case Western Reserve University
School of Medicine
and University Hospitals
Cleveland, Ohio

MARK P. FIGGIE, M.D.
Department of Orthopaedics
Cornell University
and The Hospital for Special Surgery
New York, New York

DONALD B. GOODFELLOW, M.D.
Department of Orthopaedics
Case Western Reserve University
School of Medicine
and University Hospitals
Cleveland, Ohio

MATTHEW J. KRAAY, M.D.
Department of Orthopaedics
Case Western Reserve University
School of Medicine
and University Hospitals
Cleveland, Ohio

JOHN T. MAKLEY, M.D.
Department of Orthopaedics
Case Western Reserve University
School of Medicine
and University Hospitals
Cleveland, Ohio

RANDALL E. MARCUS, M.D.
Department of Orthopaedics
Case Western Reserve University
School of Medicine
and University Hospitals
Cleveland, Ohio

JOHN W. SHAFFER, M.D.
Department of Orthopaedics
Case Western Reserve University
School of Medicine
and University Hospitals
Cleveland, Ohio

GEORGE H. THOMPSON, M.D.
Department of Orthopaedics
Case Western Reserve University
School of Medicine
and University Hospitals
Cleveland, Ohio

RONALD P. WILLIAMS, M.D., Ph.D.
Department of Orthopaedic Surgery
University of Texas Health Science Center
San Antonio, Texas

Illustrations
by
Nancy A. Burgard, M.A.

CONTENTS

PREFACE

Complaints related to the musculoskeletal system account for a large portion of the problems seen in primary care. The purpose of this text is to provide a detailed approach for the proper evaluation of orthopaedic problems in these patients. The ten chapters are arranged in a regional manner from the cervical spine to the ankle and foot, including a chapter on pediatric orthopaedics, devoted to the unique problems of children; a chapter on musculoskeletal tumors (lumps and bumps); and a chapter on orthopaedic emergencies. Each chapter discusses not only a plan for the patient evaluation, but gives specific recommendations for treatments by the primary physician and advice on when to make appropriate referral to a specialist.

A thorough understanding of the musculoskeletal problems commonly seen in primary care will provide for prompt relief of a patient's symptoms at the earliest opportunity and make the most efficient use of the health care dollar.

I would like to thank my outstanding group of contributors, each of whom spent a great deal of time and effort organizing and presenting their area of expertise in a manner that would be most useful to the primary care physician. Special thanks to Ora Link and Valerie Schmedlen for their excellent word processing; and my administrative assistant, Christine Mullins and nurse clinician, Patricia Conroy, both of whom helped with this project. I would also like to give thanks to Melanie C. Karaffa and her colleagues at Practice Management Information Corporation for their work on this publication.

Randall E. Marcus, M.D.
Cleveland, Ohio
1991

1

CERVICAL AND THORACIC SPINE
By Sanford E. Emery, M.D.

CERVICAL SPINE

The cervical spine is a common site of pain and disability in the adult population from the young to the elderly. The pain can be traumatic or neoplastic in origin but is usually of a degenerative nature. A careful evaluation of the patient's history and physical examination can go a long way towards accurate diagnosis and appropriate treatment for most patients. Electrical and neuroradiologic studies can help pinpoint a diagnosis in appropriate cases. As in many spinal conditions, knowledge of the natural history of the disorders is essential to avoid undertreatment or overtreatment of patients.

Anatomy

The cervical spine is made up of seven vertebral bodies with intervening discs. The discs are made up of a fibrous outer covering called the annulus and an inner content called the nucleus pulposus. The basis of many of the degenerative conditions of the cervical spine lies in the natural history of disc degeneration. In children the nucleus pulposus is jelly-like in consistency. It begins to desiccate with age and actually undergoes biochemical changes in the proteoglycan structure. This process begins primarily in the second and third decades of life and slowly progresses with age. It should not be considered a disease but, rather, the natural course of aging discs, although for unknown reasons it is more pronounced in some people than others. With loss of elasticity in a disc comes minute fissures and clefts as well as loss of disc height and bulging of the annulus. This altered biomechanical situation prompts the bone to slowly respond with spur (osteophyte) formation. These spurs can occur at the insertion of the ligaments and annulus, in the facet joints, and in the uncovertebral joints along the back edge of the vertebral body near the neural foramen. The loss of disc height and osteophyte formation, called cervical spondylosis, can be seen on plain x-rays (see Figs. 1-1 and 1-2).

Figure 1-1A   Figure 1-1B

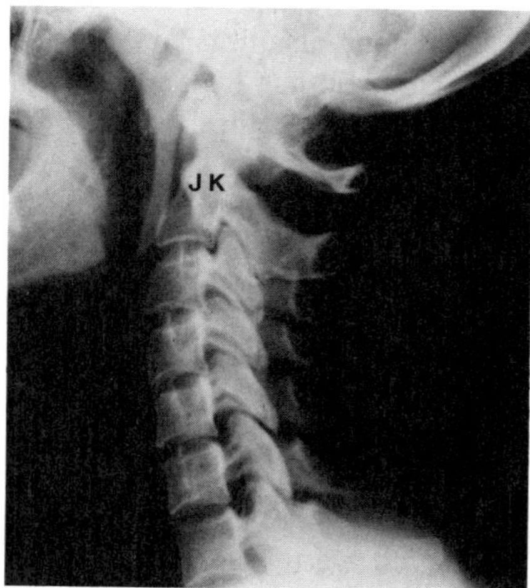

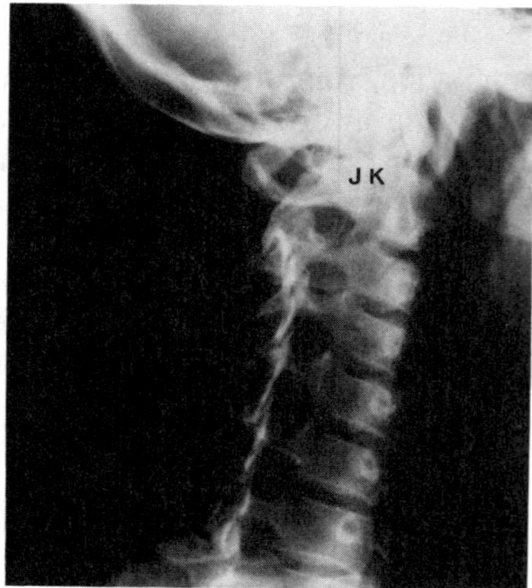

Figure 1-1. This lateral plain film (A) and oblique view (B) show a normal cervical spine in a young woman. The disc space heights are equal and no osteophytes are present on either view. Note the size of the foramen on the oblique x-ray.

Figure 1-2A

Figure 1-2B

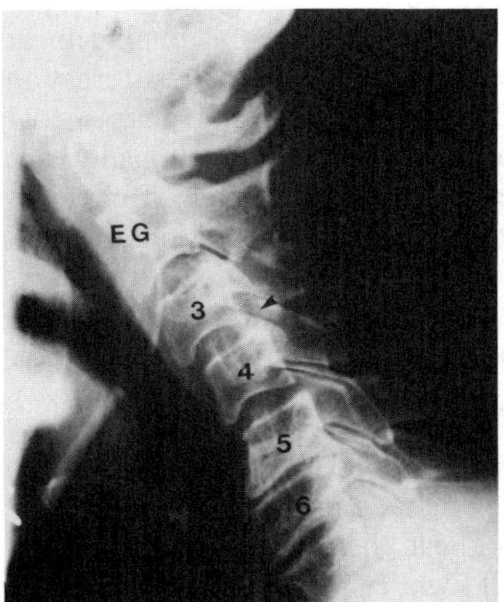

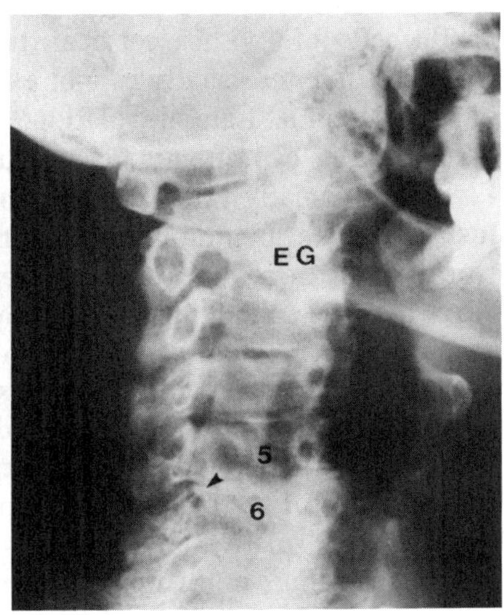

Figure 1-2. This lateral x-ray (A) of a different patient demonstrates cervical spondylosis. Note the severe disc space narrowing at C5-C6 and C6-C7 with posterior osteophytes. One should look for spinal cord compression at C5-C6 because the canal has narrowed to 12mm at this level. Note the compensatory subluxation of C3 on C4 (arrow). This is due to degenerative changes and is frequently seen at levels above stiffer, more spondylitic segments. The oblique view (B) shows how uncovertebral osteophytes can encroach upon the neural foramen, commonly causing radicular symptoms.

Physical Examination

A general examination of the neck looking for masses or other causes of neck symptoms not related to the spine is, of course, important but beyond our focus. The most salient aspects of the physical examination regarding the spine include palpation, range of motion, and, most important, the neurologic examination. People with cervical disc disease may have tenderness posteriorly over the spinous process of the involved area and often have paraspinal muscle tenderness and spasm. The location of tenderness is nonspecific, although patients with C1-C2 arthritis and neck pain will usually have suboccipital tenderness and those with a disc herniation at C5-C6 or C6-C7 will have tenderness in the lower cervical spine. Evaluation of range of motion is diagnostically useful. People with a cervical disc herniation or neural impingement from osteophytes usually cannot extend their necks without exacerbation of their pain. Lateral rotation, with or without some gentle axial compression, can often elicit radicular pain down the symptomatic arm. Flexion is usually fairly comfortable in this subpopulation of patients. Instability due to trauma degenerative or rheumatic conditions is often worse in flexion, and the examiner must allow the patient to actively move their neck under their own power and avoid stressed manipulation.

A good neurologic examination is critical for appropriate evaluation of cervical spine patients. Motor strength (see Table 1-1) and sensory deficits should be carefully tested in the upper extremities and, if suspicion of myelopathy exists, in the lower extremities as well. A careful exam of the hand can help pinpoint a dermatomal distribution of sensory abnormality. Reflex testing can help localize nerve root compression but, more important, will identify patients with significant spinal cord compression and myelopathy. Gait and balance should also be checked to help rule out myelopathy.

Table 1-1. Motor Examination

Muscle Group/Function	Major Root(s)
Shoulder Abduction	C5, C6
Shoulder External Rotation	C5, C6
Biceps	C5
Triceps	C6, C7
Supination	C6
Pronation	C7
Wrist Extension	C6
Wrist Flexion	C7
Finger Flexion	C8
Intrinsics	T1

Clinical Conditions

Acute Cervical Disc Herniation

Acute cervical disc herniations occur more commonly in the younger population, and there may be no associated spondylitic changes on x-ray. A younger disc is softer and better hydrated and more likely to protrude into or even extrude outside of the annular ring. This can cause spinal cord compression if centrally located, however, it is more common to have nerve root compression with a posterolateral disc herniation. These patients usually present with neck and arm pain. Often there is no known antecedent trauma, and patients may simply wake up with a stiff neck that evolves into neck and arm pain, sometimes over a period of days to weeks. Paresthesia into the fingers in a dermatomal distribution may be present, and motor weakness may be detectable on careful examination. A reflex may or may not be decreased in the affected arm. Neck extension and lateral rotation are usually limited and may aggravate the pain or paresthesia. Severity of symptoms may fall anywhere on the spectrum from mild pain to disabling pain with or without significant motor weakness.

Cervical Spondylosis with Radiculopathy

Patients with cervical spondylosis and radiculopathy probably makes up, the greatest number of those seeking medical care for neck and arm pain symptoms. Radiculopathy implies nerve root compression. This is usually from a disc bulge or herniation in association with bony osteophytes producing neural impingement (see Fig. 1-3A,B). The age range of this group is usually older than those with acute soft disc protrusions, but the complaints are similar, with neck and arm pain of varying degrees. The symptoms may have been brought on by minor trauma, although not necessarily so. Physical findings are similar to those described for a disc herniation, i.e., a limitation of neck extension and often rotation, detection of sensory deficits, motor root weakness or hyporeflexia. Bilateral symptoms may occur, but one side is usually significantly worse than the other. As with most neural compression

Figure 1-3A

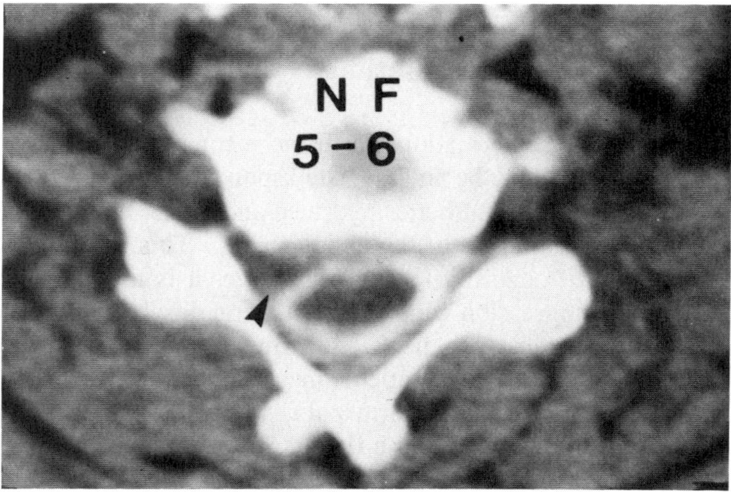

Figure 1-3B

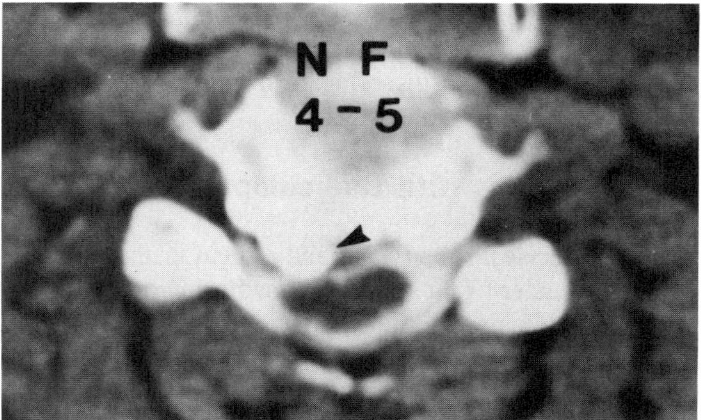

Figure 1-3. This CT myelogram is of a 63-year-old woman with neck and right arm pain. At C5-C6 (A) the dye is abruptly cut off from entering the C6 root sleeve on the right by gray material (**arrow**) suggesting a soft disc protrusion in the usual posterolateral position. At C4-C5 (B) there is similar root impingement with some deformation of the spinal cord as well, but this is from a large bony osteophyte (**arrow**).

problems there are two physiological components: 1) actual mechanical compression, and 2) the host inflammatory response in and around the nerve root. The latter is still relatively poorly understood from a basic science standpoint, but local biochemical inflammatory mediators probably play a major role.

Cervical Spondylosis with Myelopathy

Patients with cervical spondylosis with myelopathy may present with less acute symptoms than patients with acute cervical disc herniation or cervical spondylosis with radiculopathy, yet these patients need to be identified since treatment considerations are important and slightly different. They may have neck pain as well as radicular component in their upper extremities, since myelopathy and radiculopathy can co-exist given the appropriate pathology; however, some of these patients may have no neck pain at all. Their chief complaint may be difficulty with gait or balance or, perhaps, with fine motor control use of their hands. They may notice some numbness in their upper and/or lower extremities and may feel generally weak. Bladder or bowel dysfunction may be present in severe cases. The underlying pathology is spinal cord compression, usually from a combination of disc compression and osteophyte formation. A congenitally narrow spinal canal is considered a predisposing factor in patients who develop cervical myelopathy. The diagnosis can largely be made on physical examination, as these patients will exhibit long tract signs with hyperreflexia and possibly gait abnormality, clonus, a positive Babinski's sign, and/or positive Hoffmann test, depending on the degree and duration of spinal cord compression. Vibration and position sense testing evaluates the posterior columns, and evidence of dysfunction here indicates severe pathology. A less common cause of spinal cord compression in cervical disc disease is subluxation. As segments become stiffer (and may even autofuse) from spondylitic changes, the bodies above a stiff segment can become hypermobile from the increased biomechanical stress. Subluxation, either anteriorly or posteriorly, may occur causing neural impingement. This is termed compensatory subluxation (See Fig. 1-2A). This can easily be identified on flexion/extension lateral cervical spine x-rays.

Neck Pain with Spondylosis

Patients with neck pain with spondylosis do not exhibit radicular symptoms or signs of myelopathy. They may have neck pain of varying degrees, with or without radiation to the shoulder or interscapular area, that is often intermittent and chronic in nature. X-rays often show degenerative disc disease and facet joint arthrosis. The source of the neck pain is "discogenic" in nature, perhaps caused by small microtears in the annulus fibrosis. The facet joints in the posterior elements are synovial joints, like most joints in the body, and certainly are subject to degenerative changes with osteoarthritis. Patients with neck pain may or may not be symptomatic despite obvious roentgenographic findings of arthrosis. Again, a good history and neurologic examination can help distinguish these patients from those with radiculopathy or myelopathy.

Cervical Whiplash

Certainly all patients who have experienced vehicular trauma with the possibility of a cervical spine injury should have a full clinical and radiographic evaluation to rule out any bony, ligamentous, or neurologic injury. Cervical whiplash is so common that we will briefly comment on it here. Usually it results from a rear-end car accident where the patient's head and neck is stretched into extension, which is then often followed by a flexion force. Neck pain may be immediate or may only be noticed a day or so after the injury. Stiffness and pain are present, often with radiation to the shoulders or the interscapular region. In moderate to severe cases, any attempted range of motion, even flexion, is painful. Muscle tenderness and spasm is evident. Radicular symptoms or signs suggest the possibility of a disc herniation as well. Most of these patients will recover with time and conservative measures. It should be stressed to the patient that it takes weeks and often months before their symptoms will abate, and they should not expect to be "normal" a week after their injury. Some patients may have symptoms for longer than a year.

Diagnostic Evaluation

As already emphasized, the history and physical examination is extremely important and helpful in evaluation of cervical spine problems. Radiography is the other cornerstone of patient evaluation. Plain x-rays yield significant information regarding the presence and degree of cervical spondylosis. Less common problems such as bony destruction from tumor or infection can become apparent on plain films. The size of the spinal canal can be directly measured from the lateral view. Osteophytes can be seen in the lateral (see Fig. 1-2A) as well as the oblique views to show foramina encroachment (see Fig. 1-2B). Severe facet arthrosis, with or without subluxation, may also be identified on the oblique views. An anterior-posterior view may show cervical ribs at C7, which may predispose a patient to thoracic outlet syndrome. An open mouth odontoid view can confirm a diagnosis of C1-C2 osteoarthritis. Flexion and extension views may be necessary to rule out subluxation and are especially important in those with rheumatoid disorders.

Magnetic resonance imaging has become an excellent tool for evaluation of all spinal pathology including the cervical spine. Diagnoses of disc herniations, spinal cord or nerve root compression, and/or less common findings of tumor, infection, or syringomyelia can be confirmed through the use of magnetic resonance imaging. It is an expensive examination, however, and should be reserved for patients without a positive diagnosis or those that may potentially require surgical intervention. Although the resolution of magnetic resonance imaging is constantly improving, the best neuroradiologic investigation of the cervical spine is still myelography with water soluble contrast followed by CT-myelography. This gives better definition of the pathology with respect to neural impingement and in most cases is still considered necessary for accurate preoperative planning (see Figs. 1-3A, B).

Electromyography and nerve conduction velocity studies are not necessary in the routine evaluation of a patient with cervical spine problems; however, these studies can be very helpful in differential diagnostic situations, particularly in separating peripheral nerve entrapment syndromes from cervical radiculopathy. Thoracic outlet syndrome, ulnar cubital tunnel and radial tunnel syndrome, as well as carpal tunnel syndrome or ulnar nerve entrapment at the wrist, can present much like cervical root compression. Electrical studies can also suggest a "double crush" syndrome where the nerve may be compressed at two or more points along its path from the spinal cord down to the distal extremity. Peripheral neuropathy, most commonly from diabetes, alcohol use or thyroid disease, also enters into the differential diagnosis and can be suggested by history, physical examination, laboratory values, and electro-diagnostic studies.

Nonoperative Treatment

As already stated, it is important to understand the natural history of cervical disc disease in order to undertake the appropriate therapeutic measures. The large majority of patients presenting with neck and arm pain from an acute cervical disc herniation or cervical spondylosis with radiculopathy can be successfully treated with conservative measures.

The three major modes of treatment include:

1. Soft cervical collar. Immobilization is very helpful in relieving pain and often radicular symptoms by limiting the extremes of motion and thus minimizing the dynamic impingement on a nerve root, decreasing synovial inflammation from facet joint arthrosis, or resting overworked paraspinal muscles in the whiplash patient. Use the small part of the collar (i.e., where the Velcro® strap is) in the front under the patient's chin since the small part is better tolerated than the wider part (which can cause extension of the neck and may aggravate degenerative conditions).

2. Anti-inflammatory agents. Aspirin or nonsteroidal anti-inflammatory drugs can be used with relative safety and efficacy. Mild narcotics or muscle relaxers may be used, but for short periods only. Anti-inflammatory drugs help decrease pain but also probably moderate the local

inflammatory changes around a nerve root, a disc or in a facet joint.

3. Physical therapy modalities. Heat treatments and gentle massage may be useful in alleviating pain associated with muscle spasm. Cervical traction is often helpful for a cervical disc herniation with root compression, particularly in the younger population without significant spondylosis. Home traction kits may be used, but the patient should have instruction from a physician or experienced physical therapist regarding its usage. Neck manipulation can be hazardous in certain instances and generally should be avoided. Transcutaneous electrical nerve stimulation may help the patient with chronic pain, but is recommended only after a thorough diagnostic evaluation.

Using these conservative measures, most patients with cervical disease can be relieved of most, if not all of their symptoms. These conditions can be intermittent in nature, with flare-ups of their symptomatology that can extend over many years with or without new trauma. The severity and frequency of symptomatic episodes will lead the clinician to a more or less vigorous diagnostic and therapeutic work-up and disposition.

The use of nonoperative measures applies to patients with disc herniations, spondylosis and radiculopathy, as well as to patients with neck pain alone or whiplash. Patients with evidence of myelopathy represent a different entity and warrant full evaluation after the diagnosis is suspected. Most of these patients will require surgical intervention to stop the slow progression of their myelopathy. These patients should certainly be referred for evaluation to a neurologist, orthopaedist, or neurosurgeon experienced in treating cervical spine conditions in order to determine the most appropriate course of treatment.

Surgical Intervention

The presence of cervical myelopathy is usually an indication for surgical intervention to relieve the spinal cord compression. Most patients with cervical myelopathy have had chronic compression for a long time and prompt, but not necessarily emergent referral or evaluation, is indicated. Rapidly progressive neurologic deterioration however, would be an urgent situation.

Those patients with radicular signs and symptoms unresponsive to conservative measures make up the largest group of surgical candidates. Most of these patients can be treated conservatively and observed for weeks to even months to see if their symptoms will improve. Only after failing conservative measures should elective surgery be considered. A patient with demonstrable motor root weakness should have a complete evaluation by a neurological or orthopaedic specialist, since significant weakness may require more aggressive treatment to insure the best outcome for the patient.

THORACIC SPINE

Clinical conditions of the thoracic spine are less common than problems in the cervical and lumbar spine. This is largely due to the regional anatomy. The thoracic vertebrae are supported by the rib cage and are much less mobile. They, therefore, are less subject to degenerative disc disease and osteoarthritic conditions than the more mobile cervical and lumbar areas. This is not to say that disc degeneration, facet joint arthrosis, and costovertebral joint changes do not occur and cannot be symptomatic, but the incidence is lower.

Clinical Conditions

Thoracic Disc Herniation

Protrusion of a disc in the thoracic level is becoming more appreciated as a cause of thoracic back pain, with or without a radicular component. Physicians have become more aware of the possibility for this problem, and magnetic resonance imaging has made it much easier to establish the diagnosis. These patients will often have vague, aching back pain that may radiate around the rib cage, usually unilaterally. It can mimic renal disease or cardiac or other medical conditions, and there are anecdotes of cardiac catheterizations and cholecystectomies performed in an attempt to relieve pain that was actually caused by a thoracic disc protrusion. Large disc protrusions may cause spinal cord compression with evidence of myelopathy in the lower extremities. A good neurologic examination is critical in the initial evaluation of these patients. Thoracic disc herniations can be associated with Schmorl's nodes, and these can at times be seen on plain films. Often plain radiographs are normal, however, and magnetic resonance imaging has become the best means of diagnosis. Operative indications include evidence of lower extremity weakness or myelopathy, as well as pain unresponsive to conservative measures. Nonoperative treatment generally consists of anti-inflammatory agents, physical therapy modalities, and a planned exercise program. As with disc herniations anywhere in the spine, thoracic disc herniations are not necessarily symptomatic and must be carefully correlated with the patient's history and exam.

Pathologic Compression Fractures

Pathologic compression fractures are a common cause of thoracic back pain in the elderly, particularly in women where the prevalence of osteoporosis is very high. When the bone becomes weak enough, be it from osteoporosis, tumor, Paget's disease, etc., and cannot support the mechanical loading, a compression fracture may result. These patients often notice the acute onset of pain usually without radiation. The diagnosis can be made by plain radiographs; however, the clinician must always keep in mind the possibility of a neoplastic process as the underlying etiology. If the patient's symptoms have not significantly improved after approximately three months, a tumor work-up is warranted. A bone scan is an excellent screening tool to begin with, as well as baseline laboratory work including a complete blood count, sedimentation rate, serum protein electrophoresis, calcium, phosphorous, alkaline phosphatase, and creatinine. Rarely, what appears to be a simple compression fracture may have a "burst" component with retropulsion of bone into the spinal canal. These patients may have neurologic deficit if the compression is severe enough and full neurologic and neuroradiologic work up is indicated. For simple osteoporotic compression fractures, judicious use of anti-inflammatory drugs and mild narcotics in the acute period are usually sufficient. A lightweight orthosis may be helpful, although this is sometimes not well tolerated and can be expensive. Osteoporosis in and of itself can give rise to backache, probably from microfractures and postural changes. Medical treatment of the metabolic bone disease may improve these patients.

Thoracic Stenosis

Thoracic stenosis is relatively uncommon although diagnosis has increased since radiologic cross-sectional imaging has been available. Patients with thoracic stenosis may have back pain with or without neurologic deficits. They may have vague sensory feelings in their legs or perineum without having any motor symptoms. The basic pathology is that of a small thoracic spinal canal with spinal cord compression. Neurologic examination may reveal evidence of myelopathy in the lower extremities. The diagnosis would be confirmed with computed tomography scanning or magnetic resonance imaging. As with patients who have a thoracic disc, those with thoracic stenosis should be evaluated by orthopaedic or neurosurgical consultants experienced in care and treatment of the spine.

Bibliography

Bohlman H.H. and Zdeblick T.A.: Anterior Excision of Herniated Thoracic Discs. <u>Journal of Bone and Joint Surgery</u>, 1988; 70-A:1038.

Emery S.E. and Bohlman H.H.: Osteoarthritis of the Cervical Spine. In Moskowitz R.W., Howell D.S., Goldberg V.M., Mankin H.J. eds. <u>Osteoarthritis: Diagnosis and Management</u>, 2nd edition. Philadelphia: W.B. Saunders Co., 1991.

Emery S.E. and Bohlman H.H.: The Pathophysiology of Cervical Spondylosis and Myelopathy. <u>Spine</u>, 1988; 7:843.

Hohl M.: Soft Tissue Neck Injuries. In The Cervical Spine Research Society's eds. <u>The Cervical Spine</u>, 2nd edition. Philadelphia: J.B. Lippincott Co., 1989, pp. 436-441.

Hoppenfeld S.: <u>Orthopaedic Neurology</u>. Philadelphia: J.B. Lippincott Co., 1977.

2

THE SHOULDER AND ELBOW

By Randall E. Marcus, M.D.
Harry E. Figgie, III, M.D.
Mark P. Figgie, M.D.

Increasing interest in sports activities, as well as common degenerative conditions, produce many complaints related to the shoulder and elbow areas. Many problems related to the shoulder and elbow can be successfully diagnosed and treated by the primary care physician who is familiar and comfortable with the anatomy, biomechanics, and evaluation of these regions. Appropriate referrals to specialists can then be made for the more complex problems requiring further treatment.

This chapter will discuss the evaluation and treatment of problems in the shoulder and elbow with particular emphasis on the common complaints seen in primary care.

THE SHOULDER

In order to diagnose and treat disorders of the shoulder region one must understand the complex relationships of the bony-anatomy, muscular-anatomy, and neuroanatomy. Common sources of shoulder pain include: tendinitis and lesions of the rotator cuff and biceps, adhesive capsulitis, arthritis involving the glenohumeral and acromioclavicular joints, and fractures and dislocations.

Anatomy

The shoulder joint consists of the humeral head located within the glenoid fossa of the scapula (see Fig. 2-1). The superior portion of the joint is the acromion, which connects to the clavicle at the acromioclavicular joint. The clavicle attaches to the sternum at the sternoclavicular joint, which is the only bony attachment of the shoulder girdle to the trunk.

Strong ligamentous attachments are found at both the sternoclavicular and acromioclavicular joints in order to resist the high forces that are transmitted through these areas. Injuries that disrupt these ligaments result in instability and dislocation of these joints. Rupture of the

Figure 2-1. Shoulder Bone Structures: Anterior View

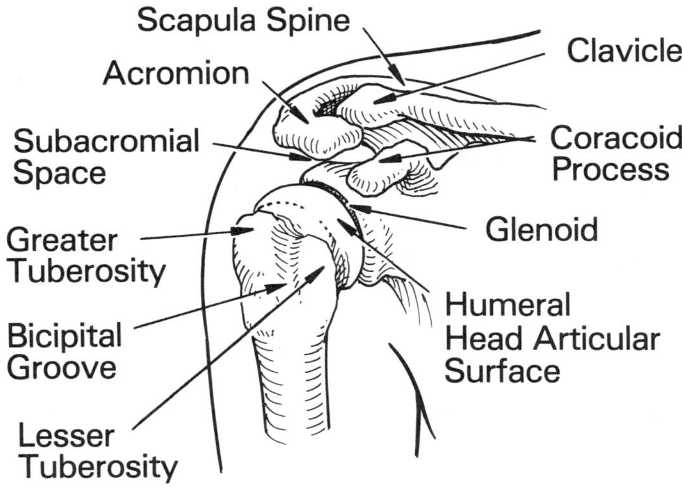

acromioclavicular ligaments and the ligaments connecting the clavicle to the anterior scapular process (coracoid) produce a "shoulder separation" with a relative prominence of the distal clavicle due to loss of support to the scapula and arm.

The acromion is the extension of the scapula ridge and is the site of attachment, along with the lateral clavicle, for the deltoid muscle. The deltoid is a large, fan-shaped muscle that is responsible for most of the power with abduction and forward flexion of the shoulder. The rotator cuff (see Fig. 2-2), consisting of the subscapularis, supraspinatus, infraspinatus, and teres minor, constitutes the major muscular support to the shoulder. These muscles are vital in stabilizing the shoulder and allowing for the deltoid to abduct and forward flex the shoulder. The subscapularis is a major internal rotator of the shoulder, while the supraspinatus acts in abduction and the infraspinatus and teres minor act in external rotation. Since the shoulder is a relatively unconstrained

Figure 2-2. Rotator Cuff Musculature Posterior View

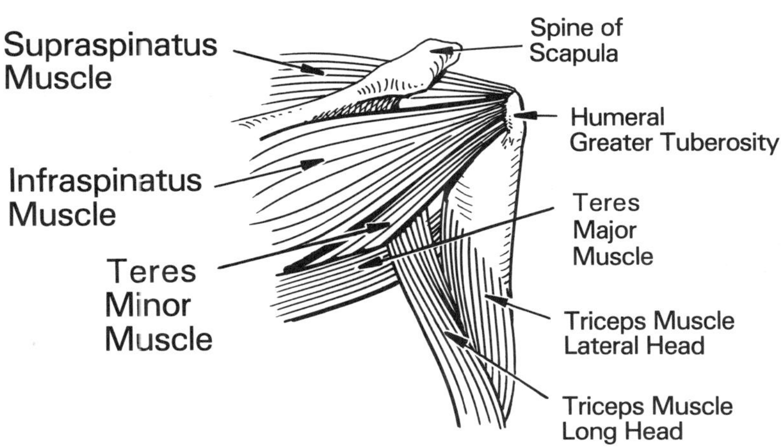

joint, the rotator cuff acts to stabilize the joint. Disorders of the rotator cuff result in loss of function due to an interruption to these complex muscular relationships. The tendon to the long head of the biceps is intra-articular in its initial portion. Its attachment is at the superior portion of the glenoid and is intra-articular before transversing the bicipital groove. This relationship helps the biceps tendon act as a humeral head depressor.

The glenohumeral joint is essentially unconstrained. The surface of the glenoid is a shallow dish providing no inherent bony stability or constraint and allows full abduction, flexion, and rotation. A cartilaginous band, the glenoid labrum roughly doubles the depth of the glenoid socket, thus providing more stability.

Biomechanics

The shoulder is usually not considered to be a weight-bearing joint; however, mechanical studies have shown that one body weight worth of force can be generated simply by raising the extended arm. The amount of force generated is roughly 25% to 50% more when the arm is elevated with the elbow extended than when the arm is elevated with the elbow flexed. The act of initiating abduction generates a joint reaction force that is directed in an upward plane at the superior edge of the glenoid.

As the arm abducts, there is motion at the glenohumeral joint as well as scapulothoracic motion. The relationship of relative motion of the glenohumeral joint to the scapulothoracic motion is in a ratio of 2 to 1.

History and Physical Examination

A careful history must be obtained with specific reference to previous injury and onset and quality of pain. For example, gradual onset of pain in the subacromial region that is worse with overhead activities is often associated with impingement problems. Severe disabling pain that awakens the patient at night accompanied with loss of motion of the shoulder is almost always diagnostic of adhesive capsulitis.

Most patients with degenerative rotator cuff tears will not remember an inciting incident and will only state that they woke up one morning and could not fully elevate their arm.

Careful physical examination must be performed, including a neurologic examination and evaluation of the cervical spine. In addition, apical lesions in the lung may also produce shoulder pain, as will gallbladder disease. Passive and active range of motion of the shoulder should be measured, including forward flexion, abduction, internal rotation, and external rotation. This should be compared with the range of motion in the opposite shoulder. In degenerative conditions, internal rotation is usually the first motion to be lost, resulting in an inability of the patient to place their hand behind their back. Palpation of the shoulder girdle should be performed, beginning with the sternoclavicular joint and the acromioclavicular joint. Palpation of the greater tuberosity for lesions of the rotator cuff and of the biceps tendon for bicipital tendinitis should be performed. The biceps muscles should also be evaluated, as biceps ruptures (long head) will result in displacement of the biceps muscle more distally along the arm.

Pulses can be palpated at the cubital fossa and wrist particularly if there is concern regarding a vascular lesion. Patients with thoracic outlet syndrome presenting as pain and numbness in the upper extremity can have unilateral dampening of the radial pulse with elevation, abduction, and external rotation of their arm when they rotate their neck towards and away from the extremity. Thoracic outlet syndrome is evaluated by these Adson's maneuvers and by noninvasive vascular testing. While a significant number of asymptomatic patients will be able to obliterate their radial pulse in these positions, unilateral dampening of the pulse on the symptomatic side may be significant.

Impingement of the rotator cuff and the undersurface of the acromion can be checked with a maneuver described by Dr. Charles Neer and called the impingement sign. This involves passive forward elevation of the humerus to 70 degrees. Further flexion will produce pain at the anterior acromion in patients with impingement problems. Injection of local anesthetic beneath the anterior acromion will immediately relieve the pain in these patients which confirms the diagnosis of impingement. This maneuver helps separate impingement lesions from other causes of shoulder pain.

The drop arm test should be performed as a test for a rotator cuff tear. The shoulder is passively abducted to 90 degrees with the elbow in full extension. An inability to hold the shoulder abducted and gradually lower the arm, is a drop arm sign and is considered to be associated with a large rotator cuff tear. However, a patient may still have a negative drop arm sign with a rotator cuff tear.

External rotation power against resistance should also be examined as loss of power or the production of shoulder pain is consistent with a rotator cuff injury.

Stability of the shoulder should also be checked, and this is usually performed with the arm in abduction and external rotation. A positive apprehension sign will cause the patient to guard the shoulder in this position and feel as if the shoulder will dislocate. Anterior and posterior motion can be checked in this position to feel if there is any subluxation of the joint. In addition, with the arm in abduction, internal and external rotation can be performed to feel if there is subacromial crepitus and catching consistent with rotator cuff disease. In a young patient, instability may produce impingement symptoms whereas in an older patient, large rotator cuff tears may produce instability.

Diagnostic Studies

After careful physical examination and history, several diagnostic studies may be indicated. The most common is plain radiographs consisting of the anterior-posterior view of the shoulder, a trans-scapular view, and often an axillary view. The anterior-posterior view will give a good view of the glenohumeral joint and often the acromioclavicular joint. The trans-scapular view will give an outlet view of the acromion and allow for evaluation of any osteophytes under the acromion. An axillary view gives a better view of the glenoid and the articular surfaces. On the anterior-posterior view, any superior subluxation of the humeral head out of the glenoid is often indicative of significant rotator cuff pathology.

Other diagnostic studies useful in determining soft tissue anatomy include arthrography with or without computed tomography scanning, magnetic resonance imaging, and ultrasound of the shoulder.

Arthrography is helpful in diagnosing full-thickness rotator cuff lesions. When arthrography is combined with computed tomography scanning, an excellent evaluation of the glenoid labrum is obtained. The arthrogram is also helpful in diagnosing adhesive capsulitis as the loss of the inferior intracapsular recess is well-demonstrated. Magnetic resonance imaging is useful in rotator cuff lesions, as partial-thickness tears can be identified. In addition, irritation of the rotator cuff can often be identified due to the intratendonous edema seen. Thus, earlier diagnosis of problems may be possible. Furthermore, magnetic resonance imaging is the procedure of choice for identification of osteonecrosis of the humeral head. Ultrasound of the shoulder has been attempted in order to diagnose rotator cuff tears, but this technique is extremely dependent upon the experience of the radiologist performing and reading the ultrasound. Bone scan may be helpful in identifying septic or degenerative changes but may not be as sensitive as magnetic resonance imaging in the diagnosis of avascular necrosis of the humeral head.

Clinical Conditions

Subacromial Impingement, Biceps Tendinitis, and Rotator Cuff Lesions

Probably the most frequent cause of shoulder pain is due to anterior impingement of the rotator cuff under the acromion. The site of this impingement can be an osteophyte at the anterior acromion, impingement under the coracoacromial ligament, or degenerative spurs at the acromioclavicular joint. Any narrowing of the outlet for the supraspinatus tendon may result in subacromial bursitis, edema, and inflammation of the tendon. The congenital size of the outlet due to the shape of the acromion may also affect the rotator cuff impingement. Although the supraspinatus tendon is most frequently involved in an impingement syndrome, inflammation may cause a cleft or rupture to develop between the supraspinatus and infraspinatus tendons. In addition, the infraspinatus may be involved and, with more severe lesions, the biceps tendon will be frayed at its insertion into the bicipital groove.

Rupture of the long head of the biceps may occur with long-standing impingement lesions.

The diagnosis of impingement has been described earlier with the reproduction of pain with passive elevation of the shoulder. This impingement sign is usually quite accurate. In addition, palpation of the greater tuberosity may reproduce pain at the site of the insertion of the supraspinatus. Abducting the arm with internal and external rotation will also bring the glenoid tuberosity under the acromion and will reproduce pain.

Three stages of impingement syndrome have been described, including stage I, edema and hemorrhage; stage II, fibrosis and tendinitis; and stage III, rotator cuff tears, biceps rupture, and secondary bone changes. Stage I lesions usually occur in active individuals younger than 25 years who engage in activities requiring excessive overhead motion, including pitchers and quarterbacks. It may also occur in "weekend warriors" who have intermittent high-peak stress loads placed on their untrained shoulder. In this stage, treatment is conservative and the patient usually responds to rest, nonsteroidal anti-inflammatory agents, physical therapy, and the occasional subacromial corticosteroid injection. In stage II lesions, fibrosis and tendinitis are a biologic response to thickening caused by repeated episodes of impingement. This is often seen in active individuals between 25 and 50 years of age. Calcification can sometimes be seen about the rotator cuff on plain radiographs. One must also remember that this lesion in patients under 40 years of age may be associated with shoulder instability. Thus, in the young patient with impingement syndrome, a careful examination of shoulder stability should be performed, since the impingement may be secondary to anterior and posterior subluxation. In stage III, patients have developed complete tears of the rotator cuff and/or biceps rupture. Secondary bone changes may occur at the subacromial region or at the glenoid tuberosity. In stage III, the supraspinatus is often completely torn or degenerated due to repeated trauma and this may result in marked weakness of abduction and external rotation. In addition, biceps tendon ruptures will produce a weakness of forward flexion and elbow flexion and supination.

Treatment

The initial treatment of an impingement syndrome should involve symptomatic treatment including rest, moist heat, and nonsteroidal anti-inflammatory medications. This should be followed by a physical therapy program including initial stretching, followed by strengthening exercises. If the patient does not get relief of pain or cannot tolerate physical therapy, then subacromial corticosteroid injections may be beneficial. This is usually performed through a posterior injection below the acromion. Repeated steroid injections are not recommended, since steroid injections may produce softening and further rupture of the tendon.

Patients who do not respond to conservative treatment should be considered for surgical decompression. An arthrogram or MRI study may be useful in order to document the presence of partial or complete rotator cuff lesions. The presence of a rotator cuff lesion is not an absolute indication for surgery, since many patients with rotator cuff tears will respond to conservative treatment and therapy. However, most rotator cuff tears will not completely heal and reconstitute, as the tears tend to occur in an avascular portion of the supraspinatus tendon.

Those patients that have failed conservative treatment may be candidates for referral and surgical treatment. With straightforward impingement problems, subacromial decompression is required. This involves identifying the site of impingement and removing any structures that decrease the supraspinatus outlet. The basis of surgical therapy includes anterior acromioplasty with coracoacromial ligament release and occasionally requires acromioclavicular joint resection. This subacromial decompression can be performed either as an open procedure or arthroscopically. If a rotator cuff tear is documented, the surgery should be performed as an open procedure. An incision is made near the anterior acromion that splits the deltoid muscle. The split may be made between the anterior and middle thirds of the deltoid but should not be extended more than 5 cm, otherwise injury of the axillary nerve with denervation of the anterior deltoid may occur. The coracoacromial ligament is excised, and the anterior undersurface of the acromion is removed. The subacromial bursa is excised, and the rotator cuff is inspected for any tears. If any tears are identified, these can be repaired by excising the tear and repairing longitudinal tears directly. Tears that are retracted off the glenoid greater tuberosity will require creation of a trough of bone and suturing the retracted tendon into the trough. Patients begin therapy within three to four days of surgery with pendulum exercises and active assisted motion. Active motion is delayed until 10 to 14 days after surgery. In patients with rotator cuff repairs, active abduction is avoided for a six-week period.

The advantage of arthroscopic subacromial decompression is avoidance of violating the deltoid muscle. Subacromial arthroscopic decompression is usually performed as outpatient surgery, thus avoiding hospital stays. Coracoacromial ligament surgery and anterior acromioplasty can be performed with this approach. Because the deltoid is not violated, the chance of weakness in forward flexion is avoided and rehabilitation may begin immediately. However, the rotator cuff and unrecognized instabilities cannot be repaired during this procedure. Patients with arthroscopic acromioplasties begin therapy on the first postoperative day and can begin active forward flexion at that time. Results of acromioplasty have been encouraging. Ellman reported 88% good to excellent results with arthroscopic subacromial decompression and Hawkins reported 87% satisfactory results with open acromioplasty. In addition, Bigliani reported 80% good to excellent results in subacromial decompression in patients younger than 40 years of age.

Patients with massive rotator cuff tears may develop rotator cuff tear arthropathy due to superior subluxation of the shoulder and alterations of the biomechanics of the joint, resulting in stresses along the superior glenoid and degeneration of the cartilage with subchondral cyst formation. Cuff tear arthropathy may produce significant pain and functional disability in the patient. Often conservative treatment will not help, and the patient has significant night pain and loss of rotary motion as well as flexion and abduction. Surgical repair of the rotator cuff alone is not indicated, as secondary changes at the glenohumeral joint will result in continued pain. In addition, it is difficult to achieve repair in these massive cuff tears. Often, total shoulder replacement or hemiarthroplasty is required. Although an inadequate rotator cuff cannot be repaired, pain relief can be obtained and improvement in rotary motions can be achieved so that the patient does improve in function.

Bicipital tendinitis may frequently occur in impingement problems and rotator cuff lesions. The intra-articular portion of the biceps tendon may become frayed at its insertion into the bicipital groove. In addition, there may be some subluxation in and out of the groove, further fraying or irritating the tendon. Often, subacromial decompression will relieve the symptoms of bicipital tendinitis. If the patient has shoulder instability, restoring or correcting the instability will also improve the impingement and bicipital irritation. Treatment of bicipital tendinitis should focus on treating the cause of the impingement. This often involves subacromial decompression. Direct injections of corticosteroid in the biceps tendon should be avoided, since steroid injections may soften the tendon and cause it to rupture. Symptomatic treatment-- including rest, nonsteroidal anti-inflammatory agents and moist heat--may be indicated. Tenodesis of the biceps tendon in the groove with a resection of the proximal portion of the tendon should be avoided unless performed in conjunction with a decompression and acromioplasty, as the tendon acts as a humeral head stabilizer. In fact, in patients with bicipital tendinitis secondary to impingement, tenodesing the tendon may actually cause the impingement to worsen, since it allows for slight superior subluxation of the humeral head.

Rupture of the long head of the biceps tendon is not uncommon effect of minimal trauma. Patients present with transient pain and ecchymosis at the biceps muscle. There is an easily palpated lump in the proximal biceps. Except in the high-performance athlete, rupture of the long head rarely needs surgical repair. Patients usually respond quickly to local symptomatic treatment and gradual resumption of full activities.

Arthritis of the Glenohumeral Joint

Arthritis of the glenohumeral joint can occur from primary osteoarthritis, gout, alkaptonuria, septic arthritis, hemophilia, rheumatoid arthritis, and juvenile rheumatoid arthritis. Posttraumatic arthritis may occur secondary to recurrent dislocation of the shoulder or fractures of the head of the humerus. Fractures of the glenoid are rare but may result in secondary changes. Avascular necrosis may also result in secondary osteoarthritis and may be due to sickle cell disease, lupus erythematosus, Gaucher's disease, steroid-induced avascular necrosis, or idiopathic avascular necrosis. Charcot arthropathy may also occur at the shoulder as a result of neuropathic conditions such as stroke, syringomyelia, or brachial plexus palsy. In addition, large tears of the rotator cuff produce alterations of the shoulder joint mechanics, resulting in secondary osteoarthritis. Ankylosing spondylitis also has a high incidence of shoulder joint involvement, often with heterotopic ossification resulting in severe restrictions of motion at the shoulder.

Fortunately, arthritis of the weight-bearing joints, including the hip and knee, is a more serious clinical problem than arthritis of the shoulder. However, patients with shoulder arthritis often present with pain in the shoulder, and particularly, loss of internal rotation. Abduction may be limited with large osteophytic changes as the inferior recess is stretched across the osteophytes. The initial treatment should be symptomatic relief including anti-inflammatory medication, moist heat, and physical therapy. The patient may not be able to tolerate strengthening exercises, but the rotator cuff should be rehabilitated isometrically. Intra-articular steroid injections may not be of benefit in this instance unless there is a marked intra-articular synovitis. For those patients who fail conservative treatment, referral for consideration of surgery is indicated. Surgical options include implant arthroplasty or arthrodesis. In the older patient or in the younger patient with multiple joint arthritis or with lower use demands, total shoulder arthroplasty may be an excellent treatment. However, in younger patients with high use demands, such as laborers, shoulder arthrodesis may be the better option. Total shoulder replacement has met with good results, especially in those patients with intact rotator cuffs.

Rehabilitation after total shoulder replacement includes pendulum exercises immediately following surgery, followed by passive range of motion exercises and active assisted exercises soon after. Forward flexion is encouraged as this is the most important motion to obtain to improve function. External rotation is usually limited for the first six weeks while the subscapularis muscle is healing. At four to six weeks postoperatively, the patient begins resisted exercises and strengthening exercises. Because the deltoid muscle and rotator cuff are intact, rehabilitation is usually more successful in patients with osteoarthritis than in patients with rheumatoid arthritis. Infection rates in total shoulder replacements are low, and complications such as wound sloughs and nerve palsies are infrequent. The most common neurologic complications are traction injuries to the musculocutaneous nerve, which courses near the coracoid process, and the axillary nerve, which is near the inferior edge of the capsule. Durability of shoulder replacements with intact rotator cuffs is usually good; however, when failure occurs it is usually due to glenoid component problems.

The other surgical option for young, active patients with arthritis is fusion. In patients with good ipsilateral extremity joints, including the elbow, wrist, and hand, arthrodesis in a functional position may bring satisfactory pain relief and a good result. This is especially true in patients with high use demands such as laborers. Arthrodesis may also be indicated in patients who have not had successful rotator cuff repairs or shoulder replacements. Complications are frequent with shoulder arthrodesis, including pseudarthrosis and continued pain. In a series of 17 shoulder arthrodeses, nine had moderate to severe residual pain. Functional deficits including an inability to work with the arms overhead or abducted were also noted. Shoulder arthrodesis is not recommended in patients with rheumatoid arthritis because increased stress is placed on the ipsilateral upper extremity joints, which may be involved with rheumatoid arthritis.

Problems of the Acromioclavicular Joint

The most common injury seen to the acromioclavicular joint is shoulder separation which can be divided into three basic groups. A grade I injury is a sprain of the ligaments between the acromion and the clavicle producing minimal deformity and pain at the joint; a grade II injury is a tear of the acromioclavicular ligaments and a sprain of the strong ligaments between the clavicle and the coracoid process. This produces a slight elevation of the distal clavicle and pain at the joint. A grade III separation is a complete tear of both the acromioclavicular and coracoclavicular ligaments. This produces severe pain at the joint with pronounced upward displacement of the distal clavicle.

Diagnosis can be confirmed with a plain anterior-posterior radiograph of the acromioclavicular joint (a weight-bearing stress view is rarely indicated).

Treatment consists of cold packs for 48 hours followed by heat. A sling and figure-of-eight dressing are used for comfort. A Kenny-Howard brace may be used to attempt to reduce the articular surfaces of the joint. As pain symptoms resolve, range of motion exercises should begin.

Surgical intervention is rarely indicated for the acute injury and is reserved for high-performance athletic patients whose range of motion includes over-the-head activities. For those patients who develop late arthritis symptoms of the acromioclavicular joint, resection of the joint and distal clavicle gives a satisfactory result. Patients with grade I sprains can be treated by the primary care physician. They should avoid contact sports for six weeks to reduce the risk of converting the separation to a grade II or III injury. Patients with grade II and III injuries should be evaluated by an orthopaedic surgeon.

Fracture and Dislocation

Fractures involving the proximal humerus may be seen by the primary care physician. Most of these fractures can be treated with nonsurgical procedures. Unless these injuries are non-displaced, they should be referred to an orthopaedic surgeon. Most fractures of the clavicle without neurovascular or skin problems can be treated with a sling and figure-of-eight dressing. Fractures of the scapula are usually the result of high-energy trauma and should be seen by an orthopaedic surgeon. These patients are at a potentially high risk for pulmonary problems including pneumothorax. Dislocations of the shoulder are an orthopaedic emergency and are discussed in chapter 10.

THE ELBOW

Disorders of the elbow joint may be related to muscular, ligamentous, bony, or articular pathology. Frequently the symptoms are due to an over-use condition and most problems about the elbow can be managed successfully using nonsurgical procedures. Prior to considering the pathological status of the elbow, one must understand the anatomy and biomechanics of this joint.

Anatomy

The elbow joint consists of an articulation between the distal humerus, proximal ulna, and proximal radius (see Fig. 2-3). The distal humerus has two articular surfaces: the trochlea which articulates with the ulna, and the capitellum which articulates with the radius. The ulnotrochlear articulation functions as a pure hinge joint with degrees of freedom only in flexion and extension. The radiocapitellar and proximal radioulnar joint allows for axial rotation with pronation and supination (see Fig. 2-4).

Figure 2-3. Elbow Anterior View

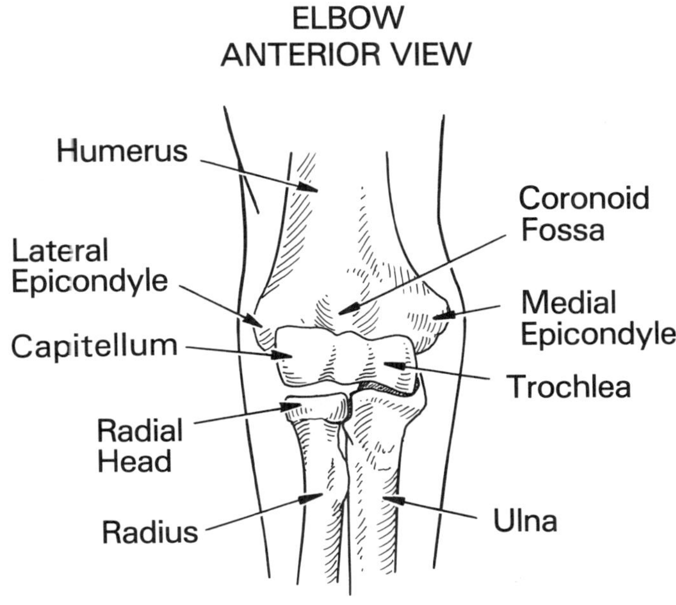

The trochlea itself is bicondylar and saddle-shaped in nature with an asymmetry between the medial and lateral condyles. It is covered with hyaline cartilage over its articulation.

The capitellum is spheroidal in shape and articulates with the concave aspects of the proximal radius. The depression of the radial head and the articulation with the ulna is covered by hyaline cartilage. This allows for approximately 90 degrees each of pronation and supination.

The proximal ulna consists of the olecranon, which is the site of the attachment for the triceps tendon. The olecranon bursa lies dorsally over the triceps insertion on the olecranon. The greater sigmoid notch articulates with the trochlea at the humerus. The distal humerus has three recesses or sulci that allow for increased range of motion of the elbow. The coronoid fossa accommodates the coronoid process while the radial fossa, which is above the surface of the capitellum, accommodates the radial head in positions of elbow flexion. The olecranon fossa accommodates the tip of the olecranon in full extension.

Figure 2-4. Elbow Lateral View

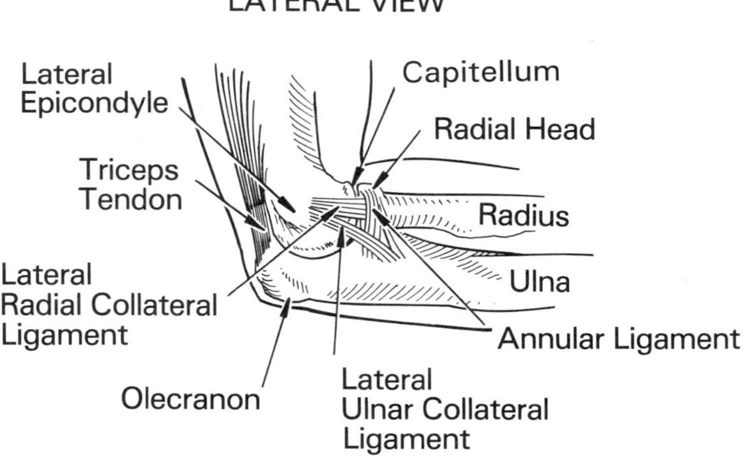

The elbow is supported by the medial collateral and the lateral collateral ligament complexes. The medial collateral ligament is more discrete and provides the majority of the resistance to varus stress of the elbow.

Biomechanics

The normal elbow has an arc of 160 degrees of flexion from full extension, 80 degrees of pronation, and 85 degrees of supination. However, as shown by Morrey and colleagues in 1981, the majority of activities of daily living can be performed with an arc of flexion from 30 to 130 degrees and an arc of rotation of 100 degrees divided equally between pronation and supination. Primary functions of the elbow include positioning the hand in space, providing a stable axis for the forearm, and functioning as a weightbearing joint in patients who require assisting devices including crutches and canes for walking.

Rotational stresses may also be high, which is important when discussing total elbow replacement surgery. The stability of the elbow joint is provided by the joint surface congruity, static soft tissue stabilizers including the medial and lateral collateral ligament complexes, and the dynamic stabilizers including the flexor and extensor muscle masses that attach to the epicondyles.

Evaluation of the Elbow

A meticulous history of the elbow problem should be obtained. The location of the pain, the chronology of the problem, and factors that increase or decrease the symptoms should be noted. The mechanism of injury can also be important in diagnosing the problem.

Physical examination including inspection of the upper extremity for erythema, swelling, or deformity is performed. Palpation of the distal humerus, radial head, and proximal ulna is important in locating the pathology. Finally, placing the joint through a complete range of motion at both the radiocapitellar (supination-pronation) and ulnotrochlear (flexion-extension) joints is performed. Crepitus and/or loss of motion or pain is noted.

Diagnostic Testing

Diagnostic studies to further evaluate the elbow may include plain radiographs including anterior-posterior and lateral films. Small abnormalities such as loose bodies may sometimes be identified, but they can be difficult to see due to the contours of the elbow. Further evaluation may require arthrogram of the elbow combined with computed tomography scanning or lateral tomograms of the elbow. These are especially helpful in cases of contracture where there is heterotopic bone formation. Bone scanning and MRI scanning of the elbow may be very helpful in cases of avascular necrosis or osteochondritis dissecans. Patients with ligamentous instability should be evaluated with varus and valgus stress radiographs.

Clinical Conditions

Olecranon Bursitis

Inflammation producing pain and swelling of the olecranon bursa is a common elbow problem seen by primary care physicians. The inflammation may occur from acute or chronic trauma. The problem is often seen in architects and draftsmen who often lean on their elbow while working at their desks. Gout and other inflammatory conditions can cause bursitis at the olecranon. Finally, infection can be a primary or secondary etiology of the inflammation.

The patient typically presents with a swollen bursa with varying degrees of pain and erythema. Radiologic evaluation is usually normal. Diagnosis is confirmed with aspiration of the bursa. Laboratory examination of the fluid for cell count, crystals, and bacteria is performed. Appropriate treatment with oral anti-inflammatory medication and/or antibiotics is usually successful in acute cases. Local steroid injection into the bursa is also often helpful in treating sterile bursitis. The patient should also rest the area and protect the bursa from trauma by using a pad.

Recurrent olecranon bursitis should be referred for surgical evaluation and possible excision.

Tennis Elbow/Epicondylitis

The term "tennis elbow" is used to designate conditions that result from repetitive stress and cause pain and tenderness in the epicondyle. The tenderness is caused by single or multiple small tears within the common tendon of origin of the extensor muscles laterally and the common flexor tendon medially.

The pathology is extra-articular in the common tendon aponeurosis and the triangular subaponeurotic space.

Rest, ice, and isometric exercise are the cornerstone of initial management. Local injection with corticosteroids into the tendinous insertion at the epicondyle is performed when symptoms persist. Elimination of the abnormal forces causing the problem (late backhand racket stroke with wrist extension, poor or oversized grip) is important to prevent recurrence of symptoms.

Resistant tennis elbow is rare and requires referral to a surgeon for possible surgical release and realignment of the impaired tendon.

Elbow Instabilities

The elbow may become unstable following dislocation, radial head fracture with ligament rupture, or repetitive valgus stresses. The most common sites of instability are at the medial collateral ligament, olecranon fossa, and radiocapitellar joint. Depending on the degree of instability and direction of applied force, symptoms will present in different ways. With a primary lateral overload, osteochondritis dissecans will develop in a child or adolescent ("little league elbow"). Plain radiographs will confirm the diagnosis. In children the management is rest, with surgical repair only if the piece is large or detached. In the adult, loose bodies are managed surgically. Posterior elbow pain and/or medial collateral ligament pain is managed by splinting and bracing. If this fails to minimize symptoms, reconstruction of the ligament may be necessary. If osteophytes exist in the olecranon fossa, a partial olecranon excision can be performed simultaneously. Occasionally, patients with marked medial instability may even present with ulnar nerve symptoms due to stretching of the nerve at the cubital tunnel.

Elbow Arthritis

Arthritis of the elbow can be caused by rheumatoid arthritis, juvenile rheumatoid arthritis, osteoarthritis, ankylosing spondylitis, or hemophilia. Repetitive trauma has been associated with primarily lateral compartment arthritis. Major trauma may also be a contributing factor, especially in patients who have had elbow dislocation combined with radial head fractures, which cause valgus instability. Intracondylar fractures of the distal humerus may also result in joint incongruity and secondary degenerative changes. Avascular necrosis of the elbow is much less frequent than avascular necrosis of the shoulder but can occur in patients on high-dose steroids or in those with lupus. Osteochondritis dissecans is a common disease of the capitellum in younger patients and may result in degenerative changes at the radiocapitellar joint. Patients may also develop Charcot changes at the elbow, which is more prominent in patients with brachial plexus injuries, quadriplegia, diabetes, and syringomyelia.

Patients with arthritic changes of the elbow frequently present with pain and loss of motion. Commonly, the patients have lost terminal extension due to the amount of force required to obtain the last 30 degrees of extension. Pronation and supination and resisted valgus stresses may also be painful in patients with radiocapitellar disease. Patients may have difficulty performing the common activities of daily living, including feeding themselves, lifting with the arm extended, combing their hair, attending to personal hygiene, and turning a doorknob. Arthritis of the elbow can be distinguished from the more common problem of lateral epicondylitis by both physical and radiologic examination.

Initial treatment for osteoarthritis of the elbow may include symptomatic therapy consisting of rest, anti-inflammatory medication, moist heat, and physical therapy including stretching and strengthening exercises. Resting static splints are especially useful in preventing contractures. Dynamic splinting is contraindicated. However, once contractures have developed they do not usually improve with therapy alone. Intra-articular cortisone injections may also be useful, especially in episodes of severe pain.

Surgical treatment may be indicated in more advanced cases of osteoarthritis, including patients with loose bodies, marginal osteophytes, and marked joint destruction. Surgical options include loose body excision either arthroscopically or with an open incision, radial head resection for radiocapitellar disease, excisional arthroplasty, fascial arthroplasty, distraction arthroplasty, or total elbow replacement for more advanced cases. Arthrodesis of the elbow is also a surgical consideration but is considered a salvage procedure only, and its use is rarely indicated as it produces a marked functional deficit.

Loose bodies occur in the elbow joint with a frequency second only to their occurrence in the knee. These loose fragments may occur due to calcification of loose cartilage fragments and may cause destruction of the cartilage when entrapped in the articulating surfaces. Open excision may be necessary to remove them but, preferably, they may be removed arthroscopically. Loose bodies most commonly originate from the radial head and capitellum. Symptoms are, most frequently, pain, stiffness, and clicking with supination and pronation. Secondary contractures of the anterior joint capsule further limit flexion and extension. In such cases, radial head resection with anterior capsulectomy may be indicated.

In summary, patients with arthritis of the elbow may require surgical treatment if they fail conservative therapy. For young patients or those with high use demands, distraction arthroplasty with anterior capsulectomy is recommended. Total elbow arthroplasty should be reserved for elderly patients or the young patient with low use demands, multiple joint arthritis and/or systemic arthritis where no other procedure is available. In patients with satisfactory bone stock, the durability of the implant appears excellent. However, in patients with loss of distal humerus, custom-fit devices are required in order to optimize outcomes.

Fractures and Dislocations

Fractures and suspected fractures about the elbow should be referred to an orthopaedic specialist. Routine radiologic examination of the injured elbow may be quite difficult to interpret and minimally displaced fractures may not be seen. The presence of the "fat pad sign" on lateral radiograph should alert the physician to the likelihood of an elbow joint fracture. The fat pad sign is a radiolucency posterior to the distal humerus. This is not visible on the lateral views of a normal elbow. Hemarthrosis or joint effusion displaces the normal fat pad posterior to the humerus to produce the radiolucency. An anterior fat pad sign may be seen in normal elbows.

Dislocations about the elbow are an orthopaedic emergency and are discussed in Chapter 10.

Bibliography

Bigliani L.U., D'Alessandro D.F., Duralde X.A., et al.: Anterior Acromioplasty for Subacromial Impingement in Patients Younger than 40 Years of Age. <u>Clin. Orthop.</u>, 1989; 246:111-116.

Ellman H.: Arthroscopic Subacromial Decompression: Analysis of One-to-Three-Year Results. <u>Arthroscopy</u>, 1987; 3:173-181.

Ellman H., Hanker G., and Bayer M.: Repair of the Rotator Cuff: End-Result Study of Factors Influencing Reconstruction. <u>J. Bone Joint Surg.</u>, 1986; 68A:1136-1144.

Figgie H.E., III, Inglis A.E., Goldberg V.M., et al.: An Analysis of Factors Affecting the Long-Term Follow-Up of Total Shoulder Arthroplasty in Inflammatory Arthritis. J. Arthroplasty, 1988; 3:123-130.

Froimson A.I., Silva J.E., and Richey D.: Cutis Arthroplasty of the Elbow. <u>J. Bone Joint Surg.</u>, 1976; 58A:863.

Goodfellow J.W. and Bullough P.G.: The Pattern of Aging of the Articular Cartilage of the Elbow Joint. <u>J. Bone Joint Surg.</u>, 1967;49B:175-181.

Gurd F.B.: The Treatment of Complete Dislocation of the Outer End of the Clavicle. <u>Ann. Surg.</u>,1941; 113:1094-1098.

Hawkins R.J., Brock R.M., Abrams J.S., et al.: Acromioplasty for Impingement with an Intact Rotator Cuff. <u>J. Bone Joint Surg.</u>, 1988; 70B:795-797.

Hawkins R.J., Misamore G.W., and Hobeika P.E.: Surgery for Full-Thickness Rotator-Cuff Tears. <u>J. Bone Joint Surg.</u>, 1985;67A:1349-1355.

Hawkins R.J. and Neer C.S. II: A Functional Analysis of Shoulder Fusions. <u>Clin. Orthop.</u>,1987; 223:65-76.

Kumar V.P., Satku K., and Balasubramaniam P.: The Role of the Long Head of Biceps Brachii in the Stabilization of the Head of the Humerus. <u>Clin. Orthop.</u>, 1989; 244:172-175.

London J.T.: Kinematics of the Elbow. <u>J. Bone Joint</u>,1981; 63A:529.

Morrey B.F.: Post-Traumatic Contracture of the Elbow: Operative Treatment Including Distraction Arthroplasty. <u>J. Bone Joint Surg.</u>, 1990; 72A:601.

Morrey B.F., Askew L.J., An K.N., and Chao E.Y.: A Biomechanical Study of Normal Functional Elbow Motion. <u>J. Bone Joint Surg.</u>, 1981; 63A:872-877.

Morrey B.F., Askew L.J., and Chao E.Y.: Silastic Prosthetic Replacement of the Radial Head. <u>J. Bone Joint Surg.</u>, 1981; 63A:454-458.

Mumford E.B.: Acromioclavicular Dislocation. <u>J. Bone Joint Surg.</u>, 1941; 23:799-802.

Neer C.S. II: Anterior Acromioplasty for the Chronic Impingement Syndrome in the Shoulder. <u>J. Bone Joint Surg.</u>, 1972; 54:41-50.

Neer C.S. II, Craig E.V., and Fukada H.: Cuff Tear Arthropathy. <u>J. Bone Joint Surg.</u>, 1983; 65A: 1232-1244.

Neer C.S. II, Flatow E.L., and Lech O.: Tears of the Rotator Cuff: Long-Term Results of Anterior Acromioplasty and Repair. <u>Orthop. Trans.</u>, 1988; 12:673-674.

Poppen N.K. and Walker P.S.: Forces at the Gleno-Humeral Joint in Abduction. <u>Clin. Orthop.</u>, 1978; 135:165.

Swanson A.B., Jaeger S.H., and LaRochelle D.: Comminuted Fractures of the Radial Head. <u>J. Bone Joint Surg.</u>, 1981; 63A:1039-1049.

Worcester J.N. and Green D.P.: Osteoarthritis of the Acromioclavicular Joint. <u>Clin. Orthop.</u>, 1968; 58:69-73.

42

3

WRIST AND HAND

By John W. Shaffer, M.D.

Hand and wrist problems are extremely common and include injury, deformity, and disease. Treatment of patients with hand disabilities has been provided by hand surgery subspecialists who number a few hundred, but thousands of emergency care physicians, family practitioners, surgeons, and allied health personnel often provide definitive first-hand treatment. This chapter has been written for primary care physicians of various backgrounds who will commonly be the first to see the patients prior to referral to a hand surgeon specialist. When evaluating patients with hand and wrist problems, the primary care physician must decide whether the patient can be given definitive immediate care, or should the patient be referred for urgent treatment by a hand specialist, or can definitive treatment for the patient's problem be safely referred for later care by the consultant.

HISTORY

A complete history is important in evaluating patients with hand problems. The presence of diabetes, hypertension, heart disease, liver disease, bleeding disorders with coagulopathy, and pulmonary disorders may pose problems for comprehensive management. It is important to document the medications patients are already taking, especially anticoagulant drugs. Patients who may require immediate surgery should be asked about their last ingestion of food or drink and they should be told not to eat or drink until a decision about surgery has been reached.

A history of allergies should be documented. It is important to know the status of tetanus immunization. If the patient has an animal bite, one must consider the possibility of rabies. When patients present with hand injuries, it is important to concentrate on the mechanism of current injury. Specific questions such as how was the injury sustained, was there a tool involved, was it a power tool, etc., provide important documentation for the record both for immediate treatment and for subsequent medical-legal review. It is important also to record whether there is a history of previous hand injuries.

PHYSICAL EXAMINATION

After the patient has been made comfortable, it is important to observe the hand in its resting position. Patients with obvious tendon injury will demonstrate the loss of normal hand resting position where each digit is slightly flexed (see Fig. 3-1). The hand should be examined for active function by having the patient actively flex and extend the digits and wrist through a full range of motion (see Figs. 3-2,3-3). It is important to palpate the hand and wrist in all areas to elicit focal tenderness and areas of swelling. Sensibility can be evaluated by stroking the area of potential loss with a cotton wisp or a very fine sterile needle, comparing the feeling in the area with that of the adjacent normal area or opposite hand. When a wound is present, one must determine whether the injury is serious enough to require immediate surgery. If surgery is required, probing the wound is unnecessary in the emergency room and may contaminate the open wound. With a deep laceration, it is important to evaluate the function of the anatomic structures lying distal to the wound. If there is a fracture with malalignment, sometimes simple traction will restore the hand alignment to a satisfactory position pending definitive care.

Figure 3-1. This patient demonstrates an obvious tendon injury with inability to flex the tip of the ring finger to the distal palmar crease comparable to the adjacent digits.

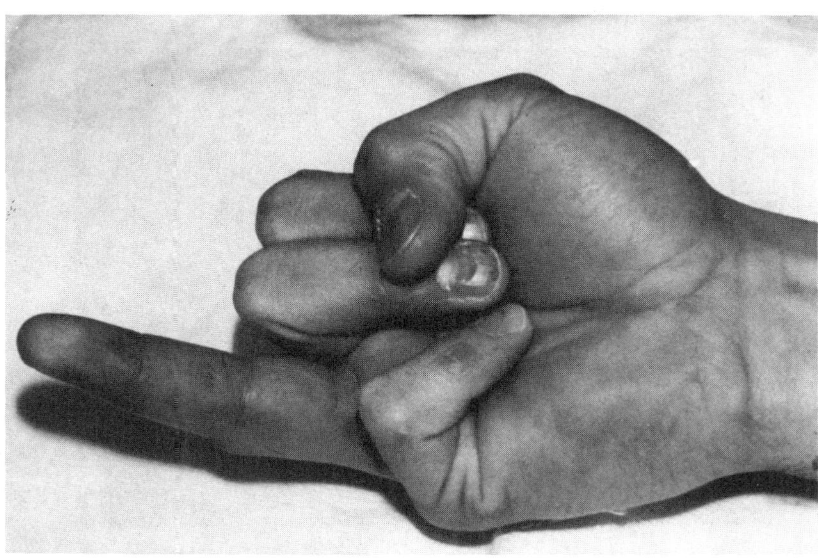

Figure 3-2. This patient demonstrates an inability to completely extend the proximal interphalangeal join of the involved finger following closed injury. The distal interphalangeal joint is hyperextended while the proximal interphalangeal joint is slightly flexed. This boutoniere finger deformity is related to a posttraumatic disruption of the central slip of the extensor tendon at the proximal interphalangeal joint.

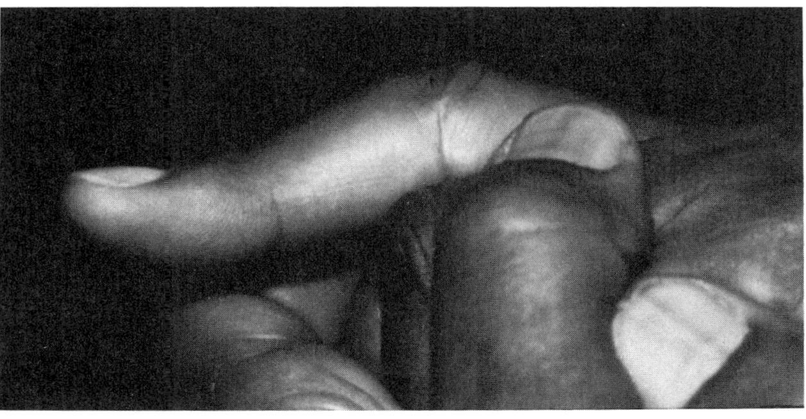

Figure 3-3. This patient demonstrates an inability to extend the distal interphalangeal joint of the small finger following a gunshot wound. The extensor tendon has been disrupted from its insertion onto the distal phalanx of the small fingertip, producing a mallet finger deformity.

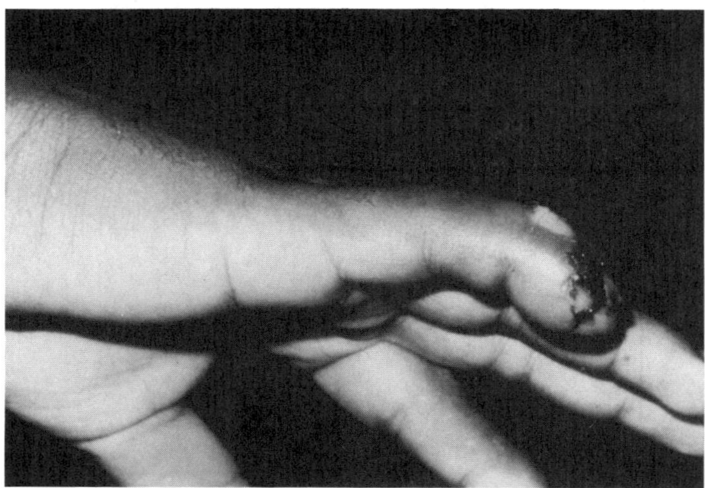

Skin

Small, open wounds typically can be managed by local wound care, irrigation, and closure. However, sometimes small innocuous-appearing wounds can be associated with significant underlying damage, including the presence of a foreign body (see Fig. 3-4).

Vascular System

It is important to check for arterial insufficiency, including lack of pulse, pallor, pain, paresthesias, and paralysis. An Allen test can be used to evaluate major vessel patency at the wrist. This test is performed by compressing both the radial and ulnar artery. With exsanguination of the hand by elevation and then sequential release of the ulnar artery and then the radial artery, one can evaluate how the fingertips perfuse through each isolated vessel. It is normal for recirculation to occur within three to five seconds of release of the artery being tested.

Figure 3-4. An innoculous, small puncture wound on the radial aspect of the index finger near the metacarpophalangeal joint resulting from a foreign body. The patient suspected that foreign material was retained within the digit.

(A) Appearance of the puncture wound.

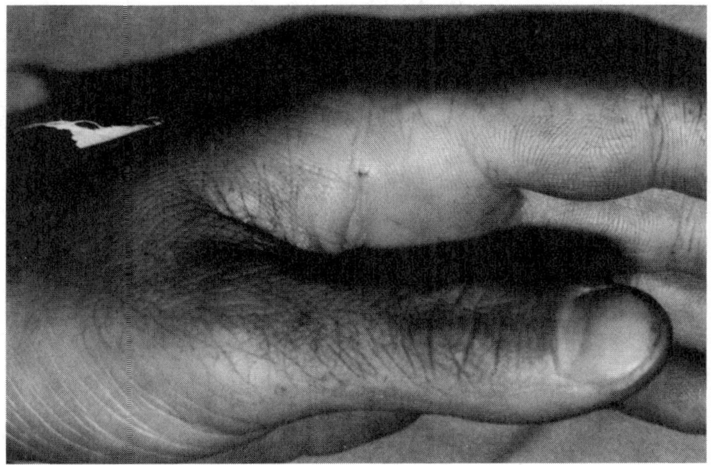

(B) Radiographic appearance of the foreign body seen at the metacarpophalangeal joint line of the index finger.

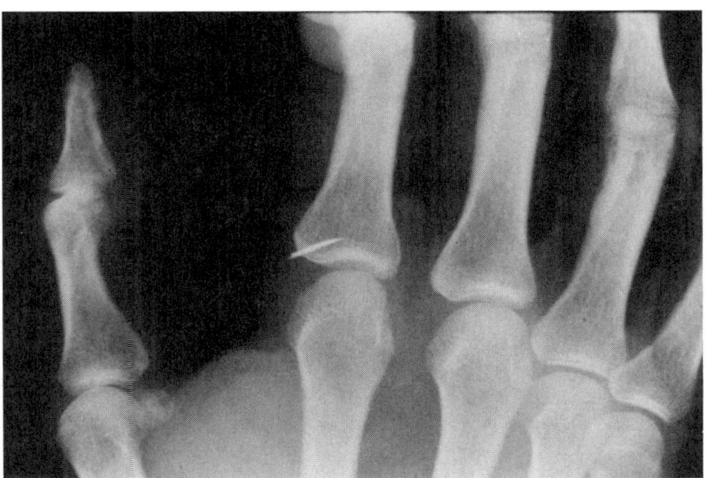

(C) Operative exploration of the digit.

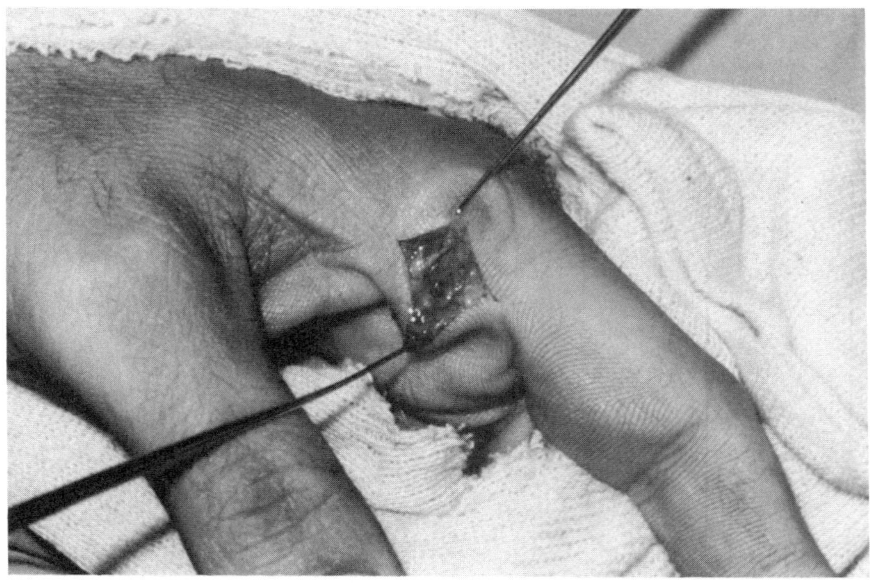

(D) Appearance of the foreign body removed from the digit.

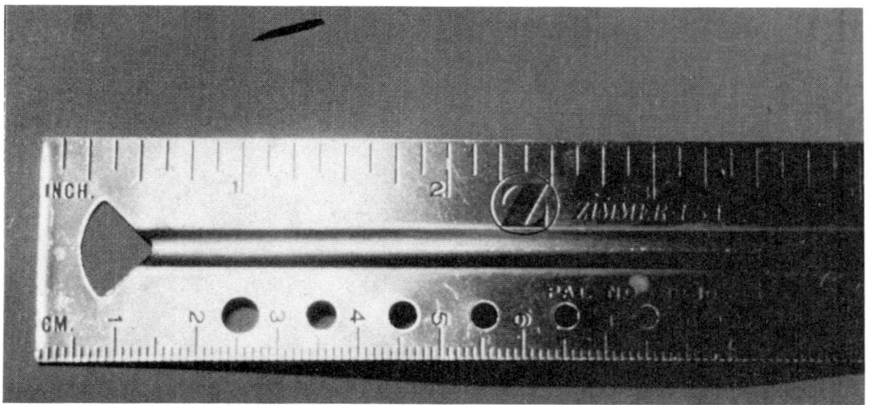

Tendons

The attitude in the hand and fingers helps to determine if tendon laceration of flexor or extensor tendons has occurred. In partial tendon lacerations, the attitude of the tendons may appear normal and active function may appear normal as well. Only on direct inspection of the open wound can one sometimes determine if a partial tendon laceration is large enough to require definitive tendon repair. Flexor tendon lacerations greater than 50% should be referred to a hand surgeon, while similar injuries to extensor tendons often can be repaired by a figure-of-eight or horizontal mattress suture at the time of wound closure in the emergency room.

Nerves

One has to assume that any nerve in the area of a wound has been damaged unless testing proves that the nerve is functional. Nerve testing can be accomplished by comparing sensibility of the injured part to the adjacent portion of the hand or the opposite hand. This can be done with smooth metal objects, such as a ballpoint pen barrel or paper clip, and/or cotton wisps to make a determination of sensibility impairment. When a patient is seen in follow-up after a suspected nerve injury, the lack of sweating distal to the site of injury is a characteristic sign of sensory nerve injury.

Skeletal System

Fractures and dislocations produce obvious deformity. Non-displaced fractures and injuries to ligaments do not often produce deformity, but on direct palpation will produce localized tenderness. Sometimes it is necessary to do gentle stress testing at joints for instability or subluxation, though often patients experience so much pain with this manipulation maneuver that the actual test requires local infiltrate.

Special Tests

Radiologic Evaluation

Radiologic examination is the most common diagnostic modality utilized for hand and wrist problems. An x-ray is always indicated if there is a suspicion of skeletal injury, whether new or old, or if there is concern about the presence of a foreign body. It is important to view the x-rays yourself rather than to trust a phone or written report. In general, the x-rays are done in an anterior-posterior and lateral projection, although special views are often necessary for complete evaluation. For example, in evaluating a possible wrist ligament injury, one should include a clenched-fist supine anterior-posterior wrist radiograph. Xeroradiographs should be used for ruling out the presence of non-radiopaque foreign bodies. For wrist injuries with tenderness on the palmar surface, a carpal tunnel view will often be done to rule out possible hook-of-the-hamate or pisiform fracture. Oblique views are included in evaluating scaphoid fractures. In children and in patients with obscure wrist injuries, comparison views often can reveal an injury by contrasting the injured with the uninjured hand and wrist. Stress views of a joint such as in gamekeeper's thumb injury can help to diagnose ligamentous injury.

Wound Culture

Wounds that present after six to eight hours, human and animal bites, and grossly contaminated wounds should be cultured. Gram stains should be obtained and examined. It is important to consider the possibility of unusual organisms such as microbacteria and fungi.

Routine Diagnostic Laboratory Tests

It is important to obtain the appropriate diagnostic tests, especially if the patient history reveals special problems including diabetes mellitus, renal disease, liver disease, etc. In addition, blood clotting studies and a sickle cell preparation are indicated when careful history provides appropriate reasons to be concerned.

HAND PROBLEMS REQUIRING URGENT TREATMENT

Major hand injuries are best handled by hand surgeons. However, in an acute situation these patients will require initial care by any physician who accepts responsibility for emergency care. Consequently, an overview of five major hand injuries is provided here.

Lacerations with Serious Hemorrhage

Hand and wrist lacerations rarely involve life-threatening hemorrhage; however, partially lacerated arterial and venous injuries can produce heavy bleeding. An arterial injury produces bright red pulsatile bleeding from the wound, while a partially lacerated vein will produce a steady ooze. It is usually not necessary to perform blind clamping into a bloody wound. In fact, this heroic attempt to control bleeding often can damage nerves traveling in association with vessels, so this technique should be avoided. The preferred technique is direct pressure on the area of bleeding. One should apply a bulky semi-compressible sterile bandage and hold it in place with an Ace bandage or alternative elastic wrap. Pressure should be applied tight enough to control the bleeding, but if the compression dressing is applied too tightly, it will function like a tourniquet. Neurovascular status distal to a compression bandage must be monitored carefully. An alternative technique to control serious hemorrhage is to apply a tourniquet, although this technique is usually unnecessary. Sometimes patients will arrive in the emergency room with a tourniquet in place. These tourniquets should be removed in favor of a compression dressing. If heavy bleeding returns in spite of a bulky compression bandage, the arm tourniquet should then be applied. A pneumatic tourniquet allows quantitative compression and is preferred, although a blood pressure cuff will suffice. It should be applied 100 mm above systolic pressure and should be held in place with a clamp to the tube to maintain inflation pressure. Once a tourniquet is put in place, prompt transfer and definitive surgery should be initiated immediately, since a tourniquet becomes intolerably painful after 30 minutes.

Amputations with Replantable Parts

Microvascular surgery has become refined to the extent that serious amputation injuries to digits including complete hand and complete wrist level amputations now can be reattached. Replantation is not always in the patient's best interest; however, function as well as cosmesis can be outstanding following successful replantation surgery. The following principles should be followed in determining which patients are replantation candidates. Replantation is worth considering in sharp amputations; crush and avulsion amputations have a less favorable prognosis for limb survival and function. The level of injury is an important consideration. An amputation of a finger through the proximal phalanx can be successfully accomplished, but usually the finger function is poor because of severe scar formation and adhesions within the flexor tendon sheath. In contrast, a sharp wrist-level amputation can be done with a high probability of replant survival and excellent function as the expected result. In general, children do better than adults when considering replantation outcome.

The indications for replantation include injury to multiple digits, amputations of the thumb especially if the amputation level is proximal to the interphalangeal joint, amputations in children, and clean amputations of the hand, wrist, or distal forearm. Contraindications include amputations due to severe crush or avulsion, single-digit amputations in adults especially if the amputation level is between the metacarpophalangeal joint and the proximal interphalangeal joint, heavily contaminated amputations, and patients with a significant history of smoking. There are some absolute contraindications, which include severe associated medical problems or injuries, severe multi-level injury of the amputated parts, refusal by the patient to agree to avoid cigarette smoking after the replantation and, finally, a psychotic patient who has deliberately amputated a body part.

The emergency management includes obtaining x-rays of both the amputated part as well as the hand itself. These radiographs should be transported with the patient if the patient becomes a candidate for replantation and is to be referred to a replantation center. The patient is treated by one thorough evaluation while the amputated part is treated independently in another full evaluation. After the evaluating physician has obtained the patient's history and physical examination, the open wound should be cleansed and dressed with sterile gauze saturated in normal saline. It is best to place an intravenous line into the patient for hydration and administration of medications. Tetanus prophylaxis should be provided and prophylactic antibiotics given, usually a cephalosporin, penicillinase-resistant penicillin, or erythromycin. The patient should be given nothing by mouth pending definitive evaluation by the hand surgeon. Analgesics are given as necessary for pain management, but not in excess where the patient would be unable to communicate with the replant surgeon.

The amputated part should also be gently cleansed and placed in a sterile bandage (See Fig. 3-5). The amputated part should not be perfused. The amputated part wrapped in saline-saturated gauze should be placed in a watertight container. This container then should be placed in a larger container containing ice water. The ideal temperature for cold protection is 4° C. degrees. It is _inappropriate_ to freeze the amputated part by placing ice directly on the amputated part.

Mangling Injuries

Industrial and farming injuries involved machines such as punch presses, milling machines, rolling bars, conveyor belts, and power saws. Sometimes injuries at home from power lawn mowers and snow blowers can also cause mangling injuries. Emergency care lays the groundwork for definitive management to salvage all viable and useful tissue. Initial wound care involves careful evaluation of the extent of hand injury, radiographs, and preparation for definitive surgery. In the operating room, adequate debridement of all devitalized tissue is essential, including the removal of all foreign bodies and grossly contaminated tissue. Initially it is better to leave wounds open. A second look recheck

Figure 3-5. Amputation of a child's thumb from a lawn mower injury.

(A) The appearance of the hand with the thumb amputation and incomplete amputation of the adjacent index and long finger.

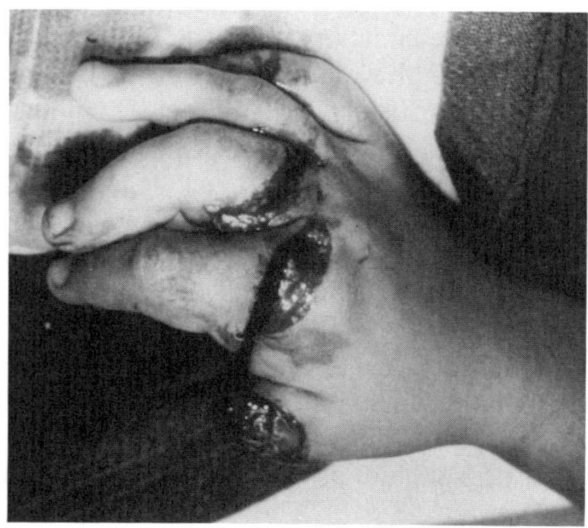

(B) Close-up view of the incompletely amputated index finger and long finger, with the index finger demonstrating cyanosis and significant circulatory insufficiency. Both the amputated thumb and the incompletely amputated index finger must be revascularized as an emergency.

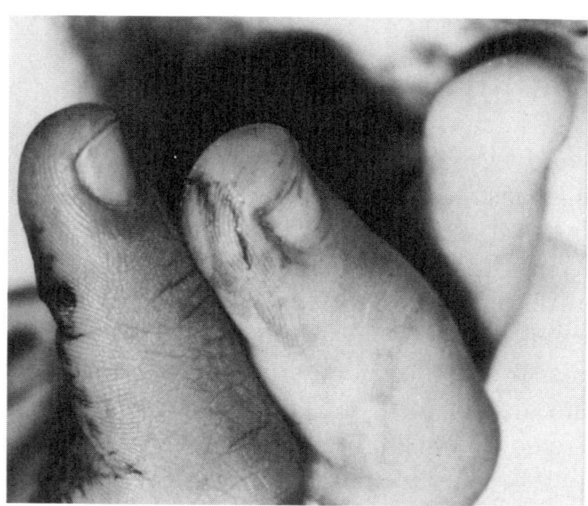

in surgery two to three days later is helpful in determining whether tissue demarcation is better defined. An anesthetic at this second surgery is necessary so that additional debridement, possible delayed closure, and possible skin grafting can be provided as necessary. The injured extremity should be elevated to help prevent swelling following debridement. Skeletal alignment can be provided by simple external splints, but often placement of Kirschner wires are needed to provide stable fixation for fracture care.

Compartment Syndromes

Compartment syndromes are serious injuries that may well be more subtle in their initial appearance than frankly bleeding open injuries or mangled hands. The magnitude of these injuries may not be apparent on initial examination. The problem evolves due to the accumulation of subfascial pressure from ongoing bleeding or vascular compromise to deep structures. If untreated, the end result--namely, Volkmann's ischemic contracture, results in loss of sensibility and limited motor function. Closed injuries, such as prolonged pressure on an extremity from an unconscious patient or after drug overdose; severe crush from industrial hydraulic roller injuries or a too-tight cast; stab or puncture wounds, hemophiliac bleeding, and oozing following arterial puncture, provide a spectrum of injury circumstances that can result in compartment syndrome. The common mechanism of injury, though, is fluid exudation at the capillary level within a tightly constrained fascial compartment. It is important to have a high index of suspicion to avoid the late sequelae of compartment syndrome.

In the development of this syndrome, patients will often complain of severe hand and wrist pain intensified by passive stretch of the involved muscles. The injury most commonly involves the digital flexors in the forearm and passive extension of the digits will cause severe pain. However, it can also occur in the extensor musculature or intrinsic muscles of the hand. To test the intrinsic compartment syndrome musculature, one holds the metacarpophalangeal joints in full extension and then passively flexes the interphalangeal joints of the fingers. The measurement of subfascial pressure in a suspected compartment syndrome patient can be obtained using commercially available pressure measuring systems. A needle or a Wick catheter can be placed into the involved compartment to determine whether compartment pressure is greater than 30 mm of mercury. This elevated pressure is considered to be dangerously high when it is maintained for periods greater than eight hours. Definitive treatment of compartment syndrome is surgery, and it is felt to be an urgent surgical indication. The constricting fascial compartment must be widely opened and left open. On delayed closure, often a skin graft is necessary for wound closure because of the amount of wound swelling three to five days after the definitive fasciotomy.

High Pressure Injection Injuries

Substances such as plastics, paints, sealants, and lubricants can be accidentally injected into the fingertips with pressures up to several hundred to a few thousand pounds per square inch. Workers typically discharge a spray gun with these toxic substances while wiping the tip of the spray gun with one of their fingertips (see Fig. 3-6). On initial inspection of the wound, the digit itself can appear minimally injured. Unfortunately, after several hours pass, the patients experience intense pain and tenderness that may well course into the palm. Usually the discomfort extends the entire length the foreign material has traveled within the digit and hand. Sometimes the foreign material can be visualized on x-ray.

The definitive treatment is to take the patient to the operating room for generous surgical incision, exposure of the foreign material, and removal. The debridement may be quite tedious and take considerable time to accomplish. Often it is necessary to do a second-look recheck in surgery two to three days following primary debridement. It is extremely important to remember that with both compartment syndromes and injection injuries, the hand and wrist may appear quite normal at the time of initial evaluation. One must take a careful history and have a high index of suspicion for accurate diagnosis.

Figure 3-6. Spray-gun injury to index finger tip.

(A) Appearance of the hand on presentation in the emergency room.

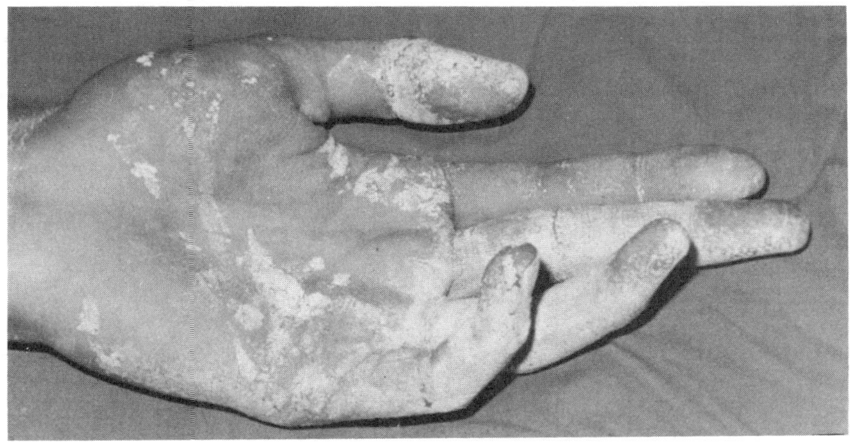

(B) Radiographic appearance demonstrating paint within the pulp of the involved index finger.

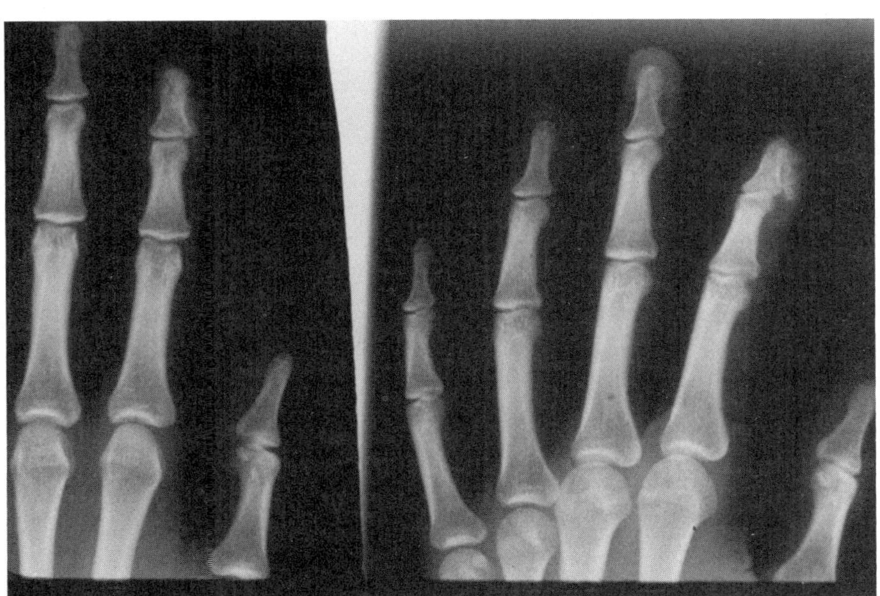

(C) Index finger after removal of paint from the index finger using Neosporin ointment.

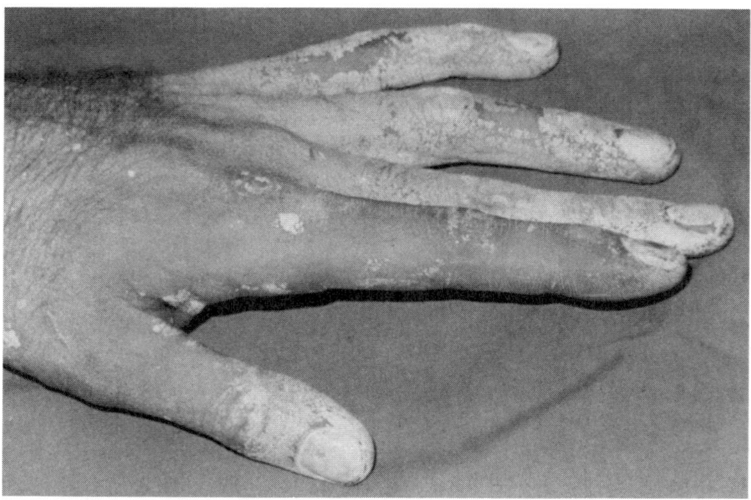

(D) Surgical incision exposing paint debris within the pulp surface of the index finger.

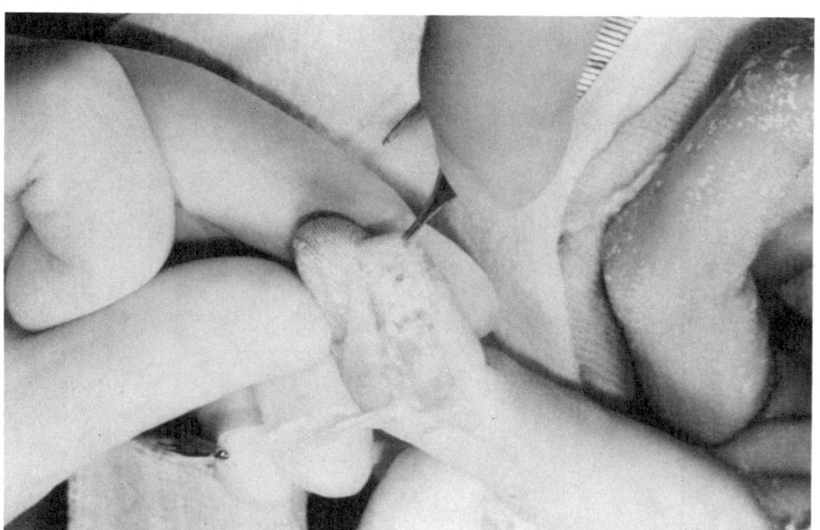

(E) Appearance of the removed paint particles from the pulp surface of the index finger.

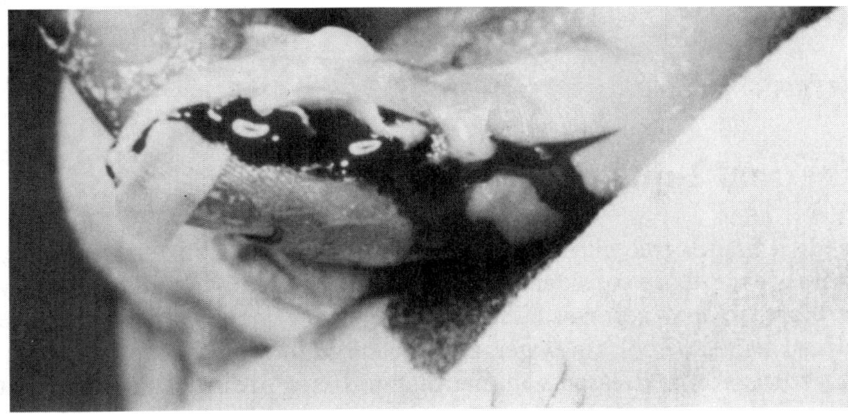

(F) Appearance of the index finger two weeks following debridement surgery.

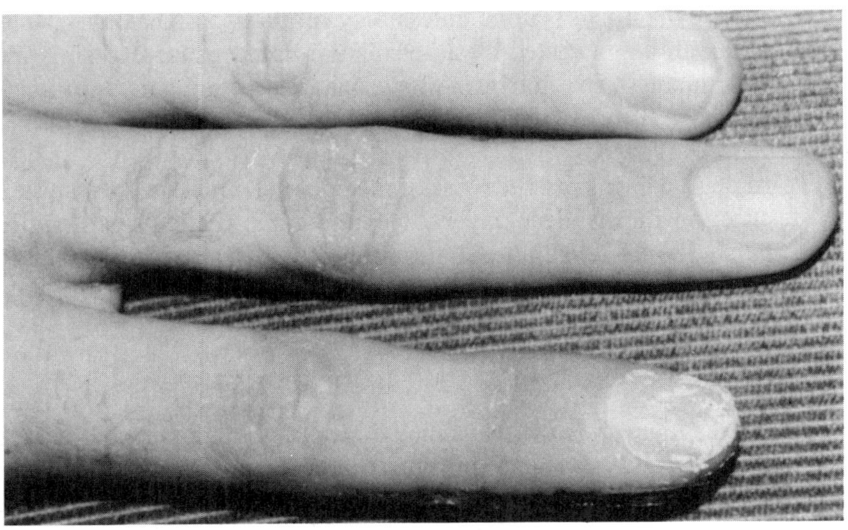

HAND PROBLEMS REQUIRING EARLY TREATMENT

Burns

Thermal Injuries

In a first-degree burn, there is erythema and some blister formation. Patients experience considerable pain in these injuries, though fortunately they are seldom serious. Initial management includes cleansing the injured hand in cool tap water and rinsing with a mild soapy solution. The burns can be dressed with petrolatum-based dressings and wrapped in surgical gauze.

Second-degree burns produce injury involving the outer portion of the dermis. Patients experience deep erythema and extensive blistering. It will take longer for healing of a second-degree burn and there is a greater likelihood of associated edema, infection, and scarring. It is better to leave the blisters alone unless they rupture spontaneously. The burned area can be protected by a petrolatum-based gauze dressing and splints producing an intrinsic-plus hand position to minimize arthrofibrosis. Topical treatment commonly used includes 1% silver sulfadiazine (Silvadene).

Third degree burns produce loss of the complete thickness of the skin and destruction of the deep layer of epithelium. Patients with third degree burns should be admitted into the hospital, and usually the burn eschar will be excised, and the open area covered by skin grafting.

Chemical Burns

Initial treatment should always include copious water irrigation using cold tap water, however, the appropriate lavage following cold water irrigation should be: dilute ascetic acid for an alkali burn and dilute sodium bicarbonate for an acid burn. Phenol is best neutralized by ethyl alcohol.

Electrical Injury

Serious electrical injuries allow the passage of high voltage electrical current through living tissue. Current travels through tissue planes of least resistance, including blood vessels and nerves. Unfortunately, soft tissue damage can be extensive both at the site of current entry into the patient and exit. Patients should be admitted into the hospital and observed quite closely for evidence of soft tissue necrosis. Multiple debridements may be necessary and sometimes soft tissue injury is so severe that amputation of involved parts becomes necessary.

Cold Injury

In determining the extent of cold injury, the duration of exposure as well as the temperature involved are important considerations. The injuries may be indolent and patients may be unaware of the magnitude of the problem as the frostbite is evolving. Early symptoms include burning and erythema. Patients may develop blisters. The immediate treatment is prompt rewarming of the injured extremity in water 40°C to 42°C. If there is a soft tissue irreparable injury, it is most appropriate to allow the demarcation zone of viable versus necrotic tissue to develop prior to planning elective amputation of the irreparably damaged tissue; in other words, early debridement has usually not been necessary.

Infections

Many infections of the hand can be treated in the office or emergency room including paronychia, felon, infected wounds, abscesses, cellulitis, and herpes.

Paronychia

A paronychia is an infection of the periungual tissue of the base of the nail. A common organism is <u>Staphylococcus aureus</u>. Sometimes early paronychia presents with regional cellulitis without abscess formation (see Fig. 3-7). With early treatment including soaks, an abscess may present that requires incision and drainage. Chronic paronychias occur in people continuously exposed to water, usually in their employment (see Fig. 3-8), such as kitchen personnel. One must also consider an indolent fungal infection in addition to pyogenic bacteria. Topical treatment that may be effective includes a mixture of antifungal ointments such as 3% iodochlorhydroxyquin (Vioform) mixed with a second topical Nystatin-Neomycin sulfate-gramicidin-triamcinolone acetonide (Mycolog). The medicine may need to be applied for several weeks.

Felon

Felon is a deep infection of the fingertip pulp often associated with a history of penetrating injury. A very common organism is <u>Staphylococcus aureus</u>. Patients often present with intense throbbing pain of their fingertip with considerable local swelling and tenderness. Surgical options include a unilateral longitudinal incision near the nail-skin margin. Sometimes the abscess presents with mid-pad pain, swelling, and tenderness. In that case, it is possible to do a simple incision and drainage at the point where the abscess is pointing. The exudate is cultured and antibiotic treatment based on culture and sensitivity provided. Usually the wound is initially packed open until drainage stops. The initial empirical antibiotic is usually a penicillinase-resistant penicillin or a cephalosporin. A felon may be complicated by osteomyelitis of the distal phalanx if it is not treated appropriately initially. If osteomyelitis presents in the fingertip, the appropriate course usually is hospitalization for operative debridement and curettage of the infected bone. Often antibiotics must be used for at least a two week duration.

Abscess and Infected Wounds

When patients present with abscesses and infected wounds from a prior injury with sutures, the sutures should be removed so that any purulent material can be drained. Sometimes it is necessary to take a sterile clamp and spread the wound apart to allow easy drainage of

Figure 3-7. Finger paronychia at an early stage presenting with local cellulitis but without abscess formation.

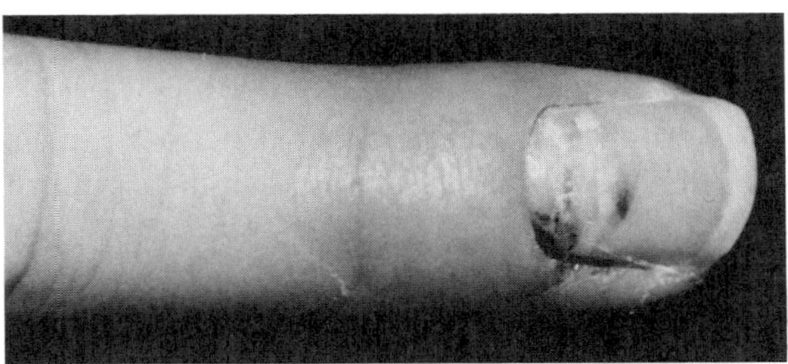

Figure 3-8. Chronic paronychia demonstrating nail bed abnormalities and thickening of the nail fold.

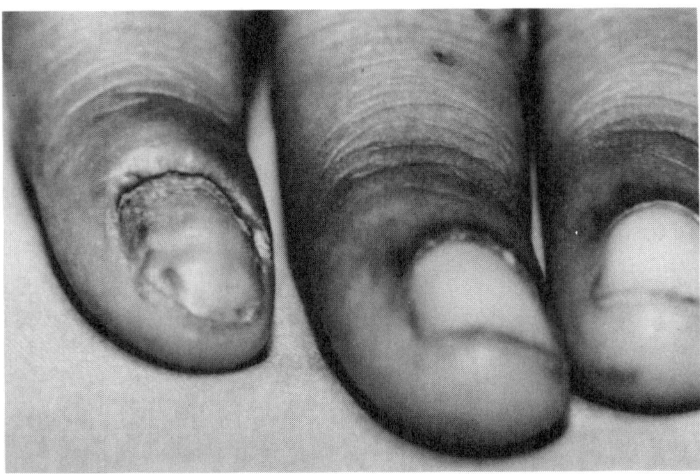

purulent material. Wounds typically should be packed open for continuing treatment. Antibiotics used are determined on the basis of culture and sensitivity reporting of the purulent exudate. To assist in keeping the open wound spread for drainage of the infection, one can use a rubber drain or apply topically zinc oxide ointment.

Cellulitis

Cellulitis in the hand is often produced by streptococcus and patients present with erythema, swelling, tenderness, and sometimes a red streak extending into the proximal forearm along the lymphatic channels. There usually is no abscess formation, and patients present with fever and prostration. Fairly typically, their illness can be controlled promptly with penicillin administration.

Herpes Infections

Patients presenting with herpes infection involving their fingers and thumb will complain of considerable pain. Usually their hands were exposed to herpes infection through their jobs. This group of patients includes dental personnel, medical personnel working in intensive care units, operating room anesthesia teams, and coronary care unit personnel. Often one will see painful vesicles around the pulp and the nail fold (see Fig. 3-9). These lesions may recur. The definitive diagnosis can be made using fluorescent antibody studies of fluid expressed from a vesicle. Symptomatic treatment including topical steroid ointment may help reduce symptoms, although the natural course for this disease is two to three weeks. Surgical management is contraindicated.

Infections Requiring Hospitalization

Severe infections of the hand should be treated by prompt hospitalization for definitive care.

Suppurative Tenosynovitis

Patients with suppurative tenosynovitis may have infected tendon sheaths on the volar surface of the wrist and in the palm extending all the way out to the distal portion of the finger overlying the middle phalanx. These infections of the flexor tendon sheath are not uncommon. Patients

Figure 3-9. Herpes simplex infection of the index fingertip in a nurse anesthesist.

(A) Vesicles around the nail fold.

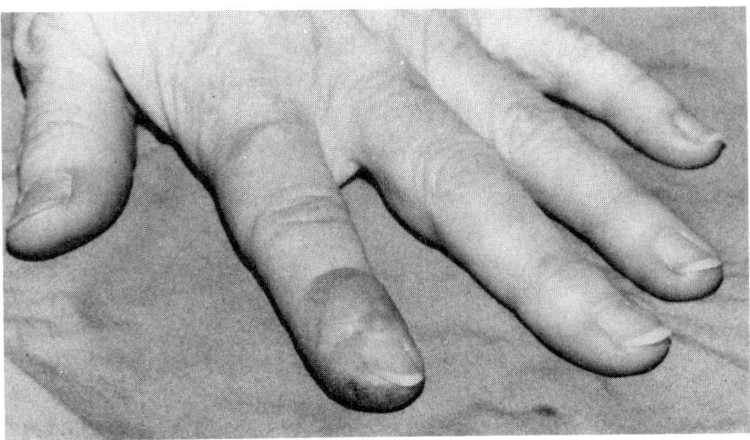

(B) Vesicles around the pulp.

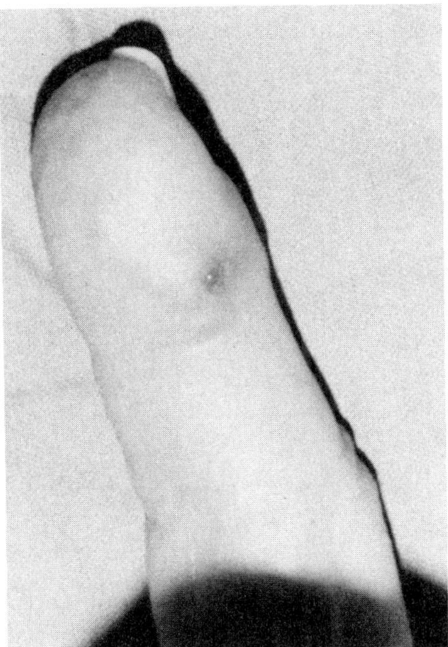

complain of severe pain, swelling of the finger, and difficulty moving the finger without accentuating their pain. Four classic signs of suppurative tenosynovitis are symmetrical swelling along the flexor tendon sheath from the distal palmar crease to the profundus insertion into the distal phalanx, tenderness and erythema along the flexor tendon sheath, partial flexion posture of the involved digit, and, most important, severe pain on passive extension of the digit. Suppurative tenosynovitis should be treated by surgical incision and drainage of the flexor tendon sheath. This should be performed in the operating room and followed with appropriate parenteral antibiotic administration.

Deep Space Infection

A mid-palmar and thenar space infection may occur after penetrating trauma. The mid-palmar space lies between the flexor tendons and the metacarpals of the long, ring, and small finger. The thenar space lies between the flexor tendons of the index and adductor pollicis muscle. In both infections, patients present with pain in the affected area. When diagnosed, the infection should be treated by surgical incision and drainage. One must do the procedure in the operating room under controlled circumstances using a tourniquet application to allow visualization of the neurovascular structures. Postoperatively, antibiotics should be administered.

Septic Arthritis

Intra-articular infection may occur following penetrating injuries or by hematogenous spread. It is most notorious after human bite injuries from altercations. The involved patient may strike another person and suffer a metacarpal neck fracture in conjunction with direct inoculation of human bite material from a tooth puncture wound. If untreated, normal mouth flora organisms can incubate and infect the subcutaneous tissue overlying the metacarpophalangeal joint as well as the metacarpophalangeal joint itself. X-rays of the metacarpophalangeal joint should be obtained. If an infection is confirmed on needle aspirate for culture and sensitivity and gram stain, operative debridement of the joint infection should be performed. The wound should be packed open, and a drain should be used to maintain the open drainage. Bacterial cultures often grow both gram-positive and gram-negative organisms, and often for effective management one needs to use a penicillinase-resistant penicillin analog and aminoglycoside parenterally.

Tendon Injuries

The principal aim of the primary care physician is to diagnose tendon injuries accurately, provide initial care, and arrange surgical consultation. Flexor tendon injuries should be repaired by hand surgeons in the operating room. Often flexor tendon injuries are associated with injuries to adjacent nerves. When to repair flexor tendon injuries is the subject of much discussion. Some hand surgeons feel that flexor tendon injuries should be repaired within a few hours of injury, while other hand surgeons feel that comparable successful management of these injuries can be accomplished one to three weeks after the injury without adversely affecting the results. Immediate treatment includes accurate diagnosis, open wound irrigation, closure with sutures, bulky bandage, prophylactic antibiotic therapy, and rehabilitation to regain full function.

Extensor tendon injuries can be repaired by the primary care physician unless the tendon has retracted. In that case, the patient should be referred to a hand surgeon for definitive tendon management in the operating room. Partial tendon lacerations often can be left alone, though a tendon laceration greater than 50% of the tendon diameter is best treated by suture placement.

Nerve Injuries

Just as described in flexor tendon injuries, the primary care physician should establish an early accurate diagnosis and provide meticulous wound care to lay the groundwork for surgical repair by a hand surgeon using microsurgical nerve repair techniques under regional or general anesthesia. A primary care physician should know the surgical anatomy of the nerves in the hand and know what the nerve function is for muscle groups. Sensory assessment is best provided by a paper clip to allow two-point discrimination to be assessed. For normal nerve function one would expect two points to be perceived when spread apart five to six millimeters. In addition to two-point discrimination, one can use a cotton wisp for light touch assessment and a small needle for pinprick assessment. In children, a helpful technique is to soak the hand and then to observe the hand for normal wrinkles of maceration that occur when the hand has been soaked in water. If the nerve has been injured, the cutaneous distribution of the injured nerve will not show intact wrinkling following soaking. The initial treatment of a nerve laceration includes wound care. The wound should be irrigated, skin margins debrided if they are irregular, and skin edges sutured. This primary care reduces the chance of infection and, on referral, hand surgeons can schedule patients for nerve repair in the operating room under ideal conditions. Nerve repair is best done by surgeons who use magnifying loupes or an operating microscope to provide accurate alignment of nerve fascicles. Nerve repair should be performed within the first few weeks of injury. Nerves that are not repaired in a timely manner may retract, producing nerve gaps that cannot be mobilized satisfactorily. In that case, nerve grafts may be necessary for definitive nerve repair.

Bone and Joint Injuries

The most important consideration for bone and joint injuries is accurate diagnosis. The patient's history often provides information that suggests the likelihood of fracture or dislocation. Abnormal swelling, ecchymosis, and tenderness further suggest the diagnosis of a bone and joint injury. Biplanar x-rays of the entire bone suspected of injury should be taken, including the joints at each end of the bone. In the wrist, the scaphoid is the most common carpal bone fractured and for accurate diagnosis often a third scaphoid view (oblique position) is necessary for visualization of the fracture. Once fractures are diagnosed, one must determine whether these injuries are displaced or anatomic in their bony configuration. If the injuries are displaced, an immediate consultation with a hand specialist may be necessary. However, stable fractures without displacement may be immobilized for later referral to the specialist using simple finger splints or gutter splints crossing the wrist using plaster materials. These provide satisfactory, safe immobilization for pain management and prevent further injury of the soft tissue structures around the area of fracture.

Digital dislocations are quite rare at the metacarpophalangeal joint but quite common at the proximal interphalangeal joint. Often, once diagnosis is established by x-ray, digital dislocations can be treated by a traction reduction maneuver. If indeed the digit reduces itself anatomically, and post-reduction radiographs show satisfactory alignment, a finger splint can be applied with the digit in slight flexion for the first few days after injury. When the patient is seen in follow-up by the treating hand surgeon, early range of motion will usually be initiated if the joint is stable.

Fingertip Injuries

Fingertip injuries include crush injuries to the fingertips with resultant hemorrhage under the nail producing a subungual hematoma (see Fig. 3-10). The patient complains of severe throbbing pain and on examination one will usually see blood beneath the nail. Immediate management usually includes a "heat" puncture of the nail with a red-hot paper clip to allow the subungual hematoma to be drained.

Finger pad injuries often can be treated with nylon sutures for skin approximation. However, in crush injuries that produce fracture of the distal phalanx, avulsion of the nail, and laceration of the nail bed, the patient should be referred to a hand surgery specialist for definitive treatment of the injury. Often this will include digital block with local anesthetic, debridement, irrigation, and reapproximation of the skin and nail bed with suture (see Fig. 3-11). The finger should be immobilized in a finger splint, and careful postoperative wound checks will be necessary for monitoring of healing.

When there is tissue loss to the tip of the finger, the patient usually will require attention by a hand surgeon. Treatment options include debridement, management by open technique where the wounds will close by marginal epithelialization, or grafting techniques. Each case must be individually assessed, but it is appropriate for patients with fingertip amputation to be referred to the hand surgeon for immediate management.

Foreign Bodies

Puncture wounds and lacerations in the hand may allow introduction of foreign material into the hand. The foreign material may not be seen during inspection of the puncture wound and on plain radiographs. These injuries may require additional special radiographs by xeroradiogram technique.   This technique provides better definition of soft tissue contours and may allow visualization of the foreign body. It is wrong to probe blindly for foreign bodies in puncture wounds.   If they are

Figure 3-10. Crush injury to the fingertip producing hemorrhage under the nail. (A) The subungual hematoma has been decompressed by puncture of the nail with a red-hot paper clip to allow the subungual hematoma to be drained. (B) The nail has fallen off and there has been minimal regrowth of the replacement nail proximally at 10 weeks.

Figure 3-10A   Figure 3-10B

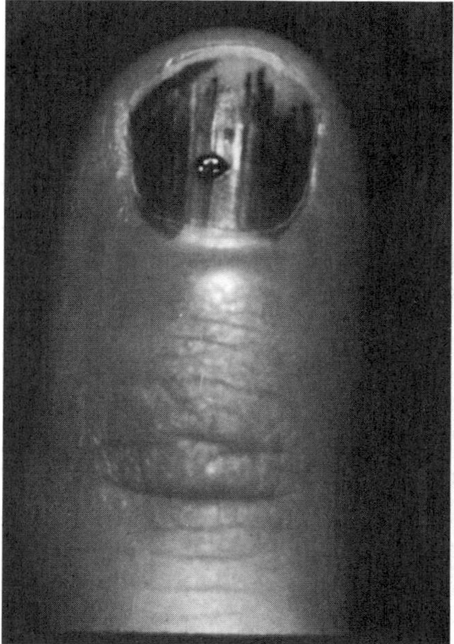 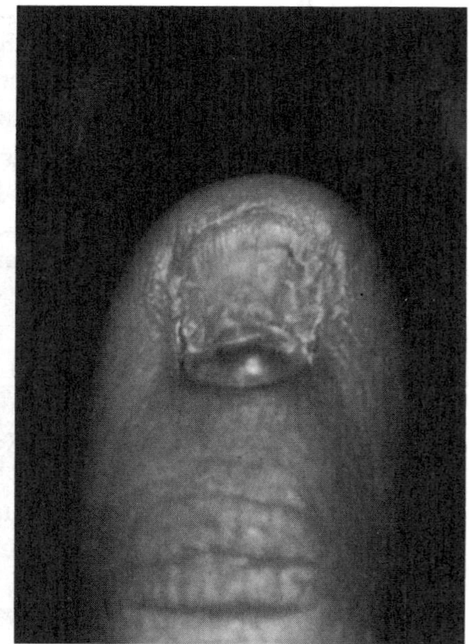

(C) The appearance of the nail regrowth at seven months. (D) The appearance of the nail at one year with no apparent abnormality.

Figure 3-10C   Figure 3-10D

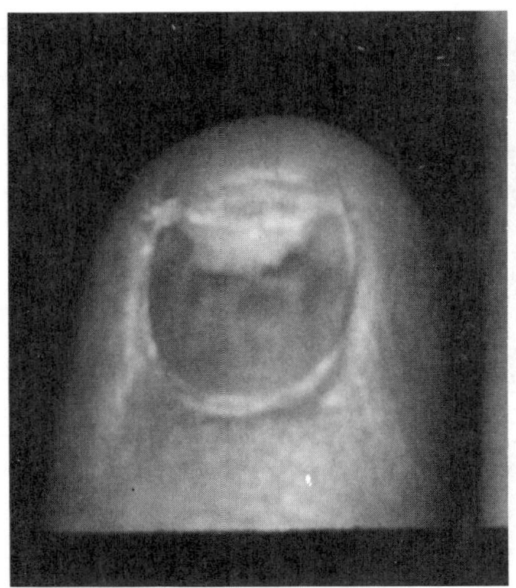 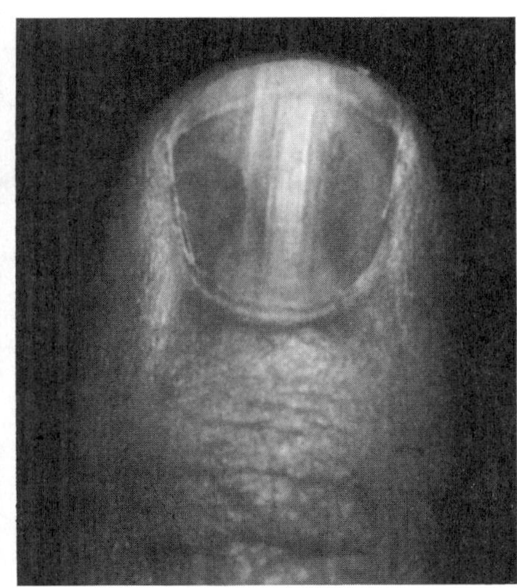

Figure 3-11. Fingertip injury producing nail avulsion.

(A) Appearance of the nail avulsion prior to surgery.

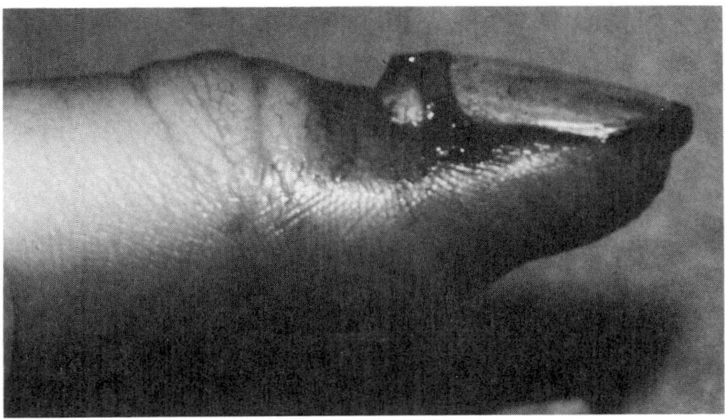

(B) Appearance after the nail has been removed to allow visualization of the laceration of the nail bed to be seen.

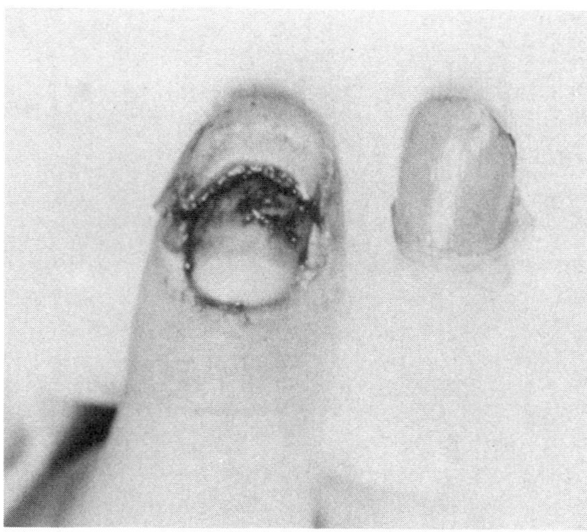

(C) The appearance of the nail following recovery, with nail regrowth at six months.

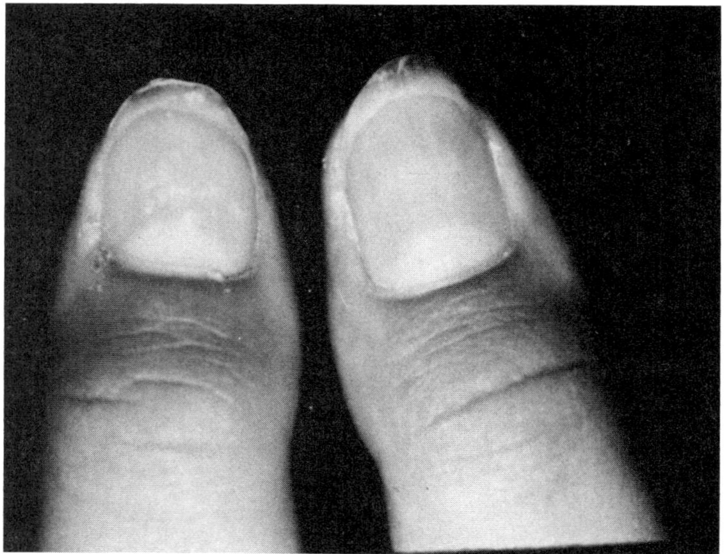

treated in the emergency room, usually it is necessary to apply a tourniquet and of course obtain appropriate anesthesia. The puncture wound should be incised, the wound should be cleansed, and following spread of the skin margins to allow visualization of the deep bed, a foreign body, if present, should become apparent. If brief exploration of the wound in the emergency room does not yield a foreign body, but one is strongly suspected, the patient should be referred to a hand surgeon, and follow-up exploration performed in the operating room.

Bites and Stings

Animal bites may include the threat of rabies. If there is any question in this regard, a consultation should be requested of the local health department. Wounds should be cultured by both aerobic and anaerobic means. Radiographs are typically taken to rule out fracture and the presence of foreign bodies. Following copious irrigation of the puncture wounds, skin margins should be approximated but left open to allow egress of serum or purulent material that may accumulate. Antibiotics are usually started that include oral cephalosporins administered every six hours.

Cat scratch fever is thought to be from a virus that usually is self-limiting and does not require definitive care, although secondary infection may occur that requires antibiotics for treatment.

The brown recluse spider produces the most common spider bite of concern in the United States, occurring in particular in the central and southeastern regions of the country. The brown recluse spider is identified by a characteristic fiddle shape on its upper thorax. Often the bite is felt to be just a sting of minimal consequence, but after several hours' time, the site of the spider bite becomes red and tender and often blisters form. The inflammation progresses such that by 24 to 48 hours after the bite there is an associated macular rash that is seen over the entire body. The appropriate local treatment for these spider bites includes incision, drainage of the bite material, and total excision of the bite site skin margins. When cutaneous necrosis develops, it is necessary to debride the skin margins.

COMMONLY SEEN OFFICE PROBLEMS

Sprains

Each joint in the hand is stabilized by several ligaments. With trauma, incomplete tears of these ligaments can produce local pain, swelling, and tenderness to manipulation and direct palpation. Usually injuries that are stable can be treated by ice application for the first 24 to 48 hours followed by gentle range of motion exercises and anti-inflammatory medication. In chronic sprains, one may need to apply warm compresses several times a day and perform gentle range of motion exercises. Sometimes patients with chronic sprains benefit by a referral to a hand therapist for more sophisticated therapy including ultrasound, general passive and active motion exercises, edema management, and intermittent splinting.

Trigger Thumb and Fingers

Triggering of digits is related to stenosis of tendons within the flexor tendon tunnels of the hand. It most commonly occurs on the flexor surface of the ring and long finger, but it also is quite common in the thumb. Patients complain of a catching sensation, snapping, locking, or jumping of the affected digit. Often they feel that the problem is located dorsal to the proximal interphalangeal or distal interphalangeal joint, but more commonly, the point of stenosis is on the palmar surface near the proximal end of the pulley system just proximal to the metacarpophalangeal joint. Often a nodule is palpated at this pulley location. Patients will describe considerable pain and will be reluctant to fully flex and extend the digit. They often complain that symptoms are particularly pronounced upon awakening but reduce as the day progresses. The immediate treatment of the stenosing tenosynovitis is a steroid injection within the pulley of a mixture of topical anesthetic and low concentration steroid. A combination that often is effective is triamcinolone 10 mg (1 cc) combined with 1 cc of 2% plain lidocaine. Patients must be advised that following the injection they may experience numbness that will pass after several hours. A repeat injection is sometimes necessary within three weeks of the initial injection. Surgery is occasionally necessary for persistent symptoms.

de Quervain's Disease

The stenosing tenosynovitis known as de Quervain's disease is an inflammatory condition that involves the tendons of the first extensor compartment of the dorsum of the wrist including the abductor pollicis longus and extensor pollicis brevis. Patients may describe a triggering sensation over the first extensor compartment as these tendons pass under the first extensor compartment retinaculum on the radial side of the wrist. Palpation over the first compartment reveals thickening and tenderness while the Finkelstein's test usually is positive. This test is performed by having the patient flex the thumb grasping it with his other fingers, and then actively ulnar deviating the wrist. Patients will experience sharp pain near the radial styloid. A trigger point injection into the first extensor compartment of a mixture of triamcinolone 10 mg (1 cc) and lidocaine 2% (1 cc) will usually provide symptomatic relief, though it may be necessary to perform an additional injection within three weeks for maximum benefit. Occasionally it is necessary to surgically release the first extensor compartment retinaculum for definitive management of a chronic problem.

Ganglion Cysts

Ganglion cysts occur in four locations: the dorsal wrist near the scaphoid-lunate-capitate articulation; on the volar wrist near the radial artery and the flexor carpi radialis tendon originating from the scaphoid articulations; over the flexor tendon sheath in the distal palm arising within the pulley system of the flexor tendons; and on the dorsum of the distal interphalangeal joint associated with distal interphalangeal joint osteoarthritis. Primary treatment usually consists of making the diagnosis and reassuring the patient that the lesion is benign. Symptomatic ganglions sometimes are best treated by aspiration, though patients need to be advised that there may be recurrence of the cysts. If patients remain symptomatic following aspiration, occasionally it is necessary to excise a dorsal wrist ganglion. Flexor tendon ganglions that are symptomatic on the volar wrist or base of the finger usually are treated by excision. In a similar way, symptomatic ganglions associated with distal interphalangeal joint arthritis often are treated by ganglion excision and debridement of the dorsal osteophyte at the distal interphalangeal joint.

Dupuytren's Contracture

Dupuytren's contracture is a soft tissue lesion in the palmar fascia of the hand that occurs most frequently in middle-aged persons (see Fig. 3-12). It is seven times more common in men than in women. It is felt to be associated with alcoholism, although it may also be familial. In the early phase, patients may present with a palm nodule that is mildly painful. After time, which can be years, patients may develop progressive contracture of their digits. Most commonly, contracture involves the ring finger. When contracture progresses, the only effective treatment is surgical excision of the pathologic fascial band. Following excision the lesion may recur.

Nerve Entrapment Syndromes

Carpal Tunnel Syndrome

The most common nerve entrapment involves entrapment of the median nerve within the carpal canal at the wrist. Patients complain of hand tingling especially at night. They describe numbness and pain in the median nerve distribution (namely, pulp surface of thumb, index, long, and radial side of ring fingers). Sometimes they experience pain referred more proximally into the upper extremity between the elbow and shoulder. Symptoms may be aggravated by repetitive use of the

Figure 3-12. Dupuytren's contracture involving the palm and the ring and small finger.

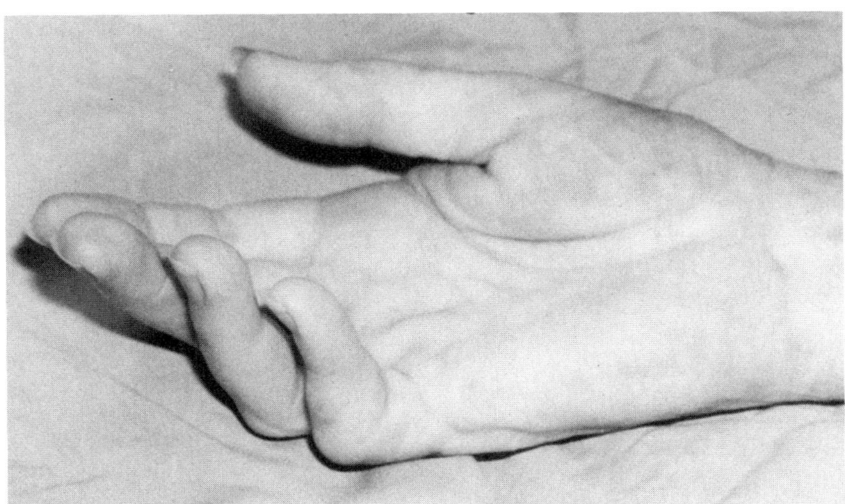

hand. Symptoms are often bilateral, though the dominant, more active extremity is usually most symptomatic. Additional associations include rheumatoid arthritis, Colles' fracture, pregnancy, and diabetes mellitus, although the largest group of patients is the idiopathic category. It would appear that the most common explanation for the syndrome is non-specific flexor tenosynovitis. Advanced carpal tunnel disease will produce wasting of the thenar intrinsic muscles, the notable atrophic muscle is the abductor pollicis brevis (see Fig. 3-13). In addition to atrophy in long-standing entrapments, the patients will have a Tinel's sign elicited by light percussion over the carpal canal producing an electric shock-like sensation locally and sometimes radiating to the tips of the thumb, index, and long finger. The most useful clinical test is the Phalen's test where the wrist is put in full flexion. In the full-flexion position, the median nerve is compressed additionally, producing numbness and paresthesias in the median nerve distribution within 60 seconds. The differential diagnosis includes cervical radiculitis, thoracic outlet syndrome, and other peripheral neuropathies. Neurodiagnostic studies done in the EMG laboratory assist the physician in establishing an accurate diagnosis. Non-surgical treatment includes night splinting

Figure 3-13. Advanced carpal tunnel disease demonstrating thenar wasting.

(A) Attempted palmar abduction demonstrating atrophy of the abductor pollicis brevis intrinsic muscle.

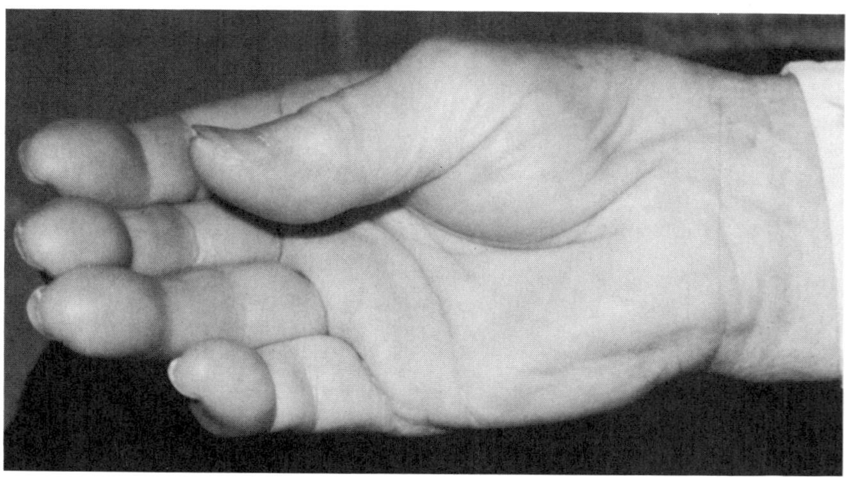

(B) Inability to completely palmar abduct the thumb secondary to advanced thenar wasting of the abductor pollicis brevis.

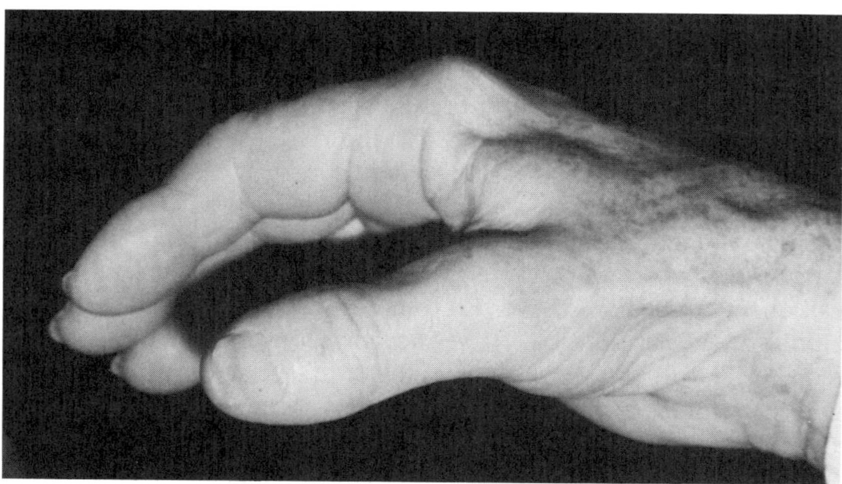

with the wrist in neutral position, and careful injection of a steroid-lidocaine combination into the carpal canal (taking great care to avoid injection into the nerve), and nonsteroidal anti-inflammatory medications. In patients who have intractable symptoms and evidence of conduction delay on EMG, the definitive treatment is surgical decompression of the carpal tunnel. This is done usually in ambulatory surgery with regional upper extremity anesthesia.

High Median Nerve Compression

The median nerve may also be compressed more proximal in the forearm. In long-standing cases, the patient may present with weakness of the anterior interosseous-innervated muscles including the flexor pollicis longus and flexor digitorum profundus to the index finger. Since the anterior interosseous nerve is a pure motor nerve, patients more commonly present with weakness but no sensory loss.

Ulnar Nerve Compression

Ulnar nerve compression is much less common at the wrist, but is seen fairly often at the elbow as the ulnar nerve travels through the cubital tunnel. At the wrist level, the ulnar nerve travels through Guyon's canal bordered by both the hamate and the pisiform as well as the pisohamate ligament. This nerve may be compressed by either a thrombosis or aneurysm of the ulnar artery or repetitive trauma such as that seen in workers using a jackhammer (hypothenar hammer syndrome). In addition, mass lesions such as lipoma or ganglion arising from the pisohamate joint may compress the ulnar nerve in Guyon's canal necessitating surgical treatment.

At the elbow, the cubital tunnel syndrome is produced by entrapment of the ulnar nerve as it courses underneath the medial epicondyle within the cubital tunnel. It may also be triggered by direct trauma to the medial aspect of the elbow or chronic mild compression. Patients complain of numbness in the ulnar portion of the ring finger and the entire small finger on both the palmar and dorsal surface. Long-standing entrapment can produce weakness of the hand intrinsics including the interosseous muscles, adductor pollicis muscle, flexor carpi ulnaris, and flexor digitorum profundi to the ring and small finger. Patients with cubital tunnel syndrome often respond to simple treatment such as padding the elbow to avoid aggravating compression of the nerve. When symptoms persist in spite of this simple treatment, the surgical procedure of choice is decompression of the ulnar nerve in the cubital tunnel by surgical neurolysis performed under regional or general anesthesia.

Radial Nerve Compression

The radial nerve may be compressed at mid-humeral level by prolonged pressure resulting in a neurapraxia. Patients will be unable to extend their wrist or fingers at the metacarpophalangeal joint. The so-called "Saturday night palsy" is produced by the patient compressing the radial nerve on the posterior aspect of the mid-humeral level. It is seen in patients who are intoxicated to the extent that they are nearly comatose. Because of prolonged pressure, the radial nerve suffers a first-degree injury that may well take several weeks for spontaneous recovery. Another location for radial nerve entrapment is on the lateral aspect of the elbow as the nerve courses into the supinator tunnel and travels along the shaft of the radius covered by the supinator muscle. This nerve entrapment may produce motor paresis of the posterior interosseous nerve, resulting in inability to extend the fingers and thumb, yet allowing normal wrist extension because of the intact radial nerve function more proximal to the supinator tunnel.

Arthritis

Both rheumatoid arthritis and osteoarthritis are commonly seen in the hand. In rheumatoid arthritis, proliferative synovial pannus initially will present with joint swelling. Patients will complain of stiffness, swelling, and pain relieved by gentle range of motion. The patients may complain of trigger fingers, wrist tenosynovitis, and, in long-standing cases, attrition extensor and flexor tendon ruptures. The flexor tenosynovitis may be associated with carpal tunnel syndrome. Differential diagnosis of rheumatoid arthritis includes: infection, gout, pseudogout, and acute calcific tendinitis. Initially, treatment is non-surgical to relieve symptoms, including splinting, hand therapy, education regarding hand protection, and various medications. Since this is a systemic disease, it is best treated in a team approach by an interested primary care physician, internist, or rheumatologist acting as the quarterback. Surgical treatment includes attention to the intractable synovitis if unresponsive to medical means to control the synovitis. Simple synovectomy may well be indicated. However, if the disease progresses with hand deformity, reconstructive surgery including arthroplasties and arthrodesis may be indicated for control (see Fig. 3-14).

In osteoarthritis, degenerative change is commonly seen at the basal joint of the thumb (trapezio-metacarpal) joint. However, degenerative change is also seen at the proximal interphalangeal joints and, to a lesser extent, at the distal interphalangeal joints where Heberden's nodes are commonly seen. Wrists may become arthritic and adversely affect the hand activities used in daily living. For end-stage arthritic conditions, surgical reconstruction including various arthroplasty and arthrodesis techniques have been indicated to allow patients to have pain relief and to maintain satisfactory hand function.

Figure 3-14. Advanced rheumatoid arthritis producing bilateral hand deformities.

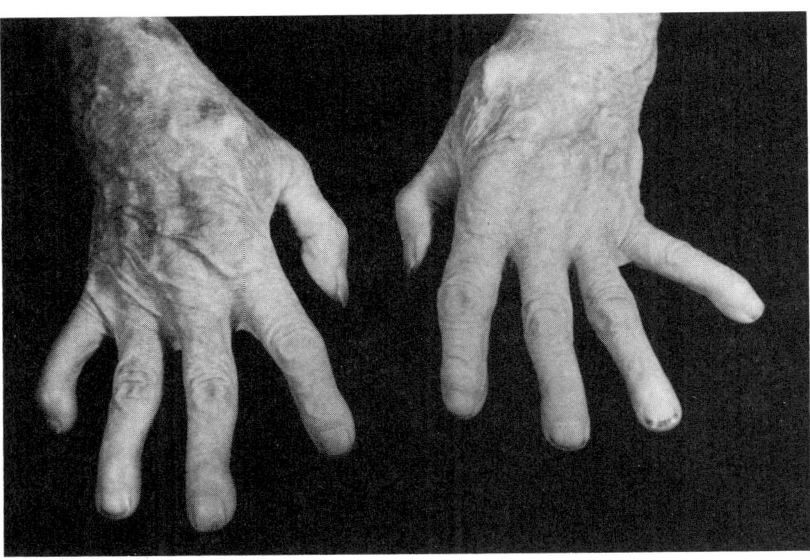

HAND THERAPY TO MAINTAIN OR IMPROVE HAND FUNCTION

For any hand injury or hand impairment from disease, preservation of function is the ultimate goal. Following medical and/or surgical treatment, a compromised hand may produce a scar that can adversely affect hand flexibility. The combination of immobilization, edema, and scar formation can result in stiffness. Even minor illnesses and injuries that are followed by prolonged immobilization can result in impaired hand function.

With trauma, one would anticipate edema as a normal response to injury. If the hand is kept dependent and if the joints are not actively moved, the hand may become chronically swollen. The natural cycle is for this edema to result in scar contraction with joint stiffness, fixation, and deformity. Resulting in a non-functional hand. The goal of hand therapy is to avoid this result by utilizing therapy techniques to maximize hand function. Qualified hand therapists can work with patients with injured and diseased hands to maintain range of motion, and can also assist in the proper immobilization for comfort. Short arm splints can be fabricated, allowing proper positioning at the metacarpophalangeal joints (45 to 70 degrees flexion), wrist extension (30 to 35 degrees), and slight interphalangeal flexion (10 degrees). Normally the thumb-index finger web is kept open. This intrinsic plus position helps to keep the soft tissue structures stretched, yet allows patients a comfortable rest position during healing (see Fig. 3-15). Therapists advise the patient regarding the importance of elevation, exercise, and hand hygiene, including washing and soaking. Most important, therapists can assist patients in becoming actively involved in their own rehabilitation. Following hand injury and disease, treatment is not complete until maximum functional recovery has been achieved.

Figure 3-15. Diffuse polyneuropathy resulting in claw deformities of the fingers and thumb. In contrast to the intrinsic plus position producing full metacarpophalangeal joint flexion and interphalangeal joint extension, the intrinsic minus position of advanced neuropathy produces the opposite deformity. The metacarpophalangeal joints are postured in full hyperextension and the proximal interphalangeal joints are postured in full flexion.

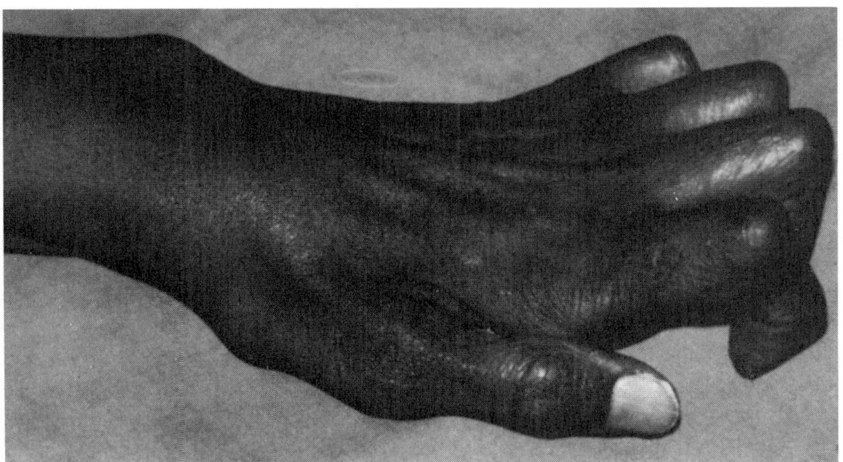

Bibliography

Carter P.R.:   Common Hand Injuries and Infections, a Practical Approach to the Early Treatment. Philadelphia: W.B. Saunders Co., 1983.

Flatt A.E.: The Care of Minor Hand Injuries, Third Edition. St. Louis, C.V. Mosby Co, 1972.

Green D.T. :   Operative Hand Surgery. New York: Churchill Livingstone Co., 1988.

Lampe E.W.:   Surgical Anatomy of the Hand. CIBA Clinical Symposium. Summit, New Jersey: CIBA-Geigy Pharmaceutical Co., 1969.

Newmeyer W.L.: Primary Care of Hand Injuries. Philadelphia: Lea and Febiger Co., 1979.

4

THE LUMBAR SPINE

By Michael J.Bolesta, M.D.

HISTORY

Low back pain is among the most frequent complaints encountered by the physician. In their lifetime, between 60% and 90% of all adults will have at least one episode of back or back related leg pain sufficient to preclude normal activities for a period of time. Back complaints comprise 20% of all workers compensation claims. In many cases, the exact etiology is elusive, defying even the most sophisticated evaluation. Fortunately, the vast majority of adults with their first episode of back pain will enjoy a self-limited course regardless of treatment. The challenge for the primary care physician is to determine which patients need simple assurance and supportive measures and which require more vigorous evaluation and treatment.

The differential diagnosis of back pain is extensive (see Table 4-1). The most important step, as in many areas of medicine, is a careful, detailed history. The physician should elicit the patient's account of pain and its location, intensity, and quality (e.g., dull, sharp, aching, burning). Often the patient will volunteer any relationship to an accident, activity, or other illness. For other individuals, such information must be sought with questions about change in occupational or recreational activities. It is useful to know whether the symptoms began abruptly or insidiously. The occurrence of pain that is more prominent at night and interferes with sleep, in the appropriate symptom complex, may raise suspicion of a neoplastic process.

The location and distribution of the pain should be described as best as possible. Pain in the lower extremities, particularly below the level of the knee, suggests irritation of the inferior lumbar or first sacral nerve roots. Observant patients may describe a pattern of discomfort that fits a specific dermatome. Beside characterizing the quality of the pain, patients should be questioned concerning associated perceptions of paresthesias, numbness, and hypersensitivity, which again suggest nerve lesions, compression, or inflammation. One should ask patients if they perceived any weakness in the extremity and, if so, in what muscle groups and with what activities. An attempt should be made to correlate symptoms or their relief with activities such as sitting, standing, walking, and recumbency. If ambulation is limited, it should be ascertained if it is because of pain, weakness, or a combination of factors. Patients should describe how the symptoms interfere with activities of daily living.

It is well known that the Valsalva maneuver will raise intrathecal pressure and may aggravate back or leg pain.

The physician should ask about coughing, sneezing, and defecation. The physician also could inquire as to the presence of bladder or bowel dysfunction. Loss of rectal or bladder sensation, inability to initiate

Table 4-1. Differential Diagnosis of Low Back Pain

Trauma
Nonspecific back pain
Disc herniation
Degenerative disc disease
Lumbar stenosis
Infection
Deformity
Neoplasm
Aortic and peripheral vascular disease
Retroperitoneal tumor
Renal disorders
Pancreatic disorders
Neural tumors
Arteriovenous malformation
Rheumatologic disorders

evacuation, or incontinence should lead to prompt evaluation, as this suggests significant cauda equina or conus medullaris lesions. It is generally felt that prompt intervention, when feasible, offers the best chance of bladder and bowel recovery. The patient's vocation and recreational activities may provide important clues as to etiology, amount of disability, and prognosis. The history of previous back pain, the usual course of such episodes, and how the current symptoms compare with past episodes should be elicited.

Past medical and surgical history can often provide leads such as a history of a primary neoplasm known to metastasize to bone. A review of systems may also guide the physical examination and subsequent work-up.

PHYSICAL EXAMINATION

During the history, physician should observe mannerisms to gauge the amount of discomfort the patient is experiencing in the office. Depending on the duration of symptoms, one may observe pain behavior such as grimacing, moaning, and grunting. Such behavior must be weighed against the individuals social, cultural, and educational background and within the context of objective findings.

The entire lumbar region should be examined with the patient in the erect position. Skin is inspected for scars and cutaneous lesions that may suggest spinal pathology. Café-au-lait spots may suggest neurofibromatosis. Hairy patches in the lumbosacral region may be associated with dysraphism.

The shape of the lumbar region should be inspected. Normally there is lumbar lordosis, which may be exaggerated in obese individuals. Loss of this lordosis or flattening of the low back is observed when pain is present and may be associated with spasm of the paralumbar musculature. If the pain or spasm is unilateral, there may be a list to one side, producing the appearance of a scoliosis. The examiner should place her or his hands on the tops of the iliac crest to see if the pelvis is level; a limb length inequality can produce the appearance of a scoliosis.

The patient should indicate where they perceive the pain to be. The physician then should gently palpate the lumbar region, systematically covering the mid to lower thoracic region, as pathology in this area can be referred to the lumbar spine. Both the midline and flank should be palpated for areas of tenderness. Deep palpation over the buttock in the region of the sciatic notches will often produce local discomfort and occasionally radiating pain when there is lower lumbar root irritation. Similarly, gentle palpation of the popliteal fossa may reveal tenderness. When upper lumbar root (L2, L3, and L4) pathology is suspected, palpation along the femoral nerve may also elicit tenderness.

Later, when the patient is recumbent, one can examine the patient in the prone or lateral decubitus position, repeating observation and palpation, asking the individual to relax as much as possible. The relationship of the spinous processes and the presence of muscle spasms may be easier to observe in these positions. When the patient is supine and relaxed, the physician can gently internally and externally rotate the lower extremity, much as one would roll a log. Even with acute back pain, this should not cause discomfort in the spine. It is a good test of hip pathology, which can sometimes be referred to the lumbar region.

The physician then will gently flex the hip while keeping the knee extended. It should be noted at what point this produces back or leg pain. The angle formed by the extremity relative to the horizontal is noted. Straight leg raising is considered positive when there is pain radiating into the lower extremity, which reproduces the patient's symptoms. The severity of root irritation is inversely proportional to the angle that reproduces the symptoms. With true root irritation, the pain is aggravated by dorsiflexing the ankle (Lasègue's sign) and relieved by flexing the knee. It is particularly significant when straight leg raising of the uninvolved limb produces contralateral radicular pain. In the appropriate setting, this is highly suggestive of a large lumbar disc herniation.

All the findings must be interpreted with caution, since individuals who have had several episodes of back pain and have consulted numerous physicians, may unknowingly contribute to an inaccurate diagnosis. To counteract this bias sometime during the evaluation, the physician should extend the patients knee while they are in the sitting position, for example, while testing motor function. If this does not also reproduce the leg pain, the physician may need to discount the supine straight leg raising test. The straight leg raising test is also limited to detecting irritation of the L4, L5, and S1, and occasionally the L3 nerve roots. Irritation of the upper lumbar roots (L2, L3, and L4) may be manifest by the less well-known femoral stretch test. The patient is placed in the lateral decubitus position and the hip is extended while keeping the knee extended. Just as the straight leg raise places the sciatic nerve under tension, this test stretches the femoral nerve. This is most accurate in testing for acute inflammation of the L2 and L3 nerve roots.

Another nerve root tension sign is the bowstring test. In the supine position, the hip and the knee are both flexed to 90 degrees. Maintaining the hip in this position, the knee is slowly extended. As extension is approached, tension is applied to the lower lumbar nerve roots, which may recreate radicular pain.

Lumbar motion is complex and involves multiple segmental articulations, making quantification difficult. Nonetheless, useful information may be garnered despite these limitations. The patient should bend forward as much as possible, within the limits of comfort, keeping the knees extended. The angle formed by the upper body relative to the vertical is the amount of flexion. When there is significant pain and muscle spasm, most of the motion will take place at the hips. If the patient is moving in the lumbar spine, there should be reversal of the normal lumbar lordosis to a gentle kyphosis. If lordosis is maintained, this should be noted. How the patient returns to the upright position can also be informative. Use of the upper extremities to push on the thighs, assisting extension, may denote significant pain or, in other contexts, learned pain behavior. Extension is measured by asking the individual to bend backward as much as possible. The angle formed by the trunk and the vertical is recorded. Similarly, lateral bending is measured by asking the individual to bend to either side. The asymmetry is noted as well as the report of pain.

Chest expansion should be determined in individuals expected of having or known to have a spondyloarthropathy. The tape measure is placed circumferentially at the level of the nipples. The circumference at maximal exhalation is subtracted from that at maximum expiration. A difference of less than five centimeters is indicative of reduced chest wall motion.

Examination is completed with a careful neurologic examination. Each muscle group in the lower extremity is tested for strength, tone, and size of the muscle. One may also look for spontaneous fasciculations. Light touch can be tested by brushing the skin lightly with the fingers or with a cotton swab. Pinprick test is useful since this modality is mediated by separate nerve fibers and pathways. One should use a pin or a pinwheel rather than a needle to avoid cutting the patient. Proprioception and vibratory sensation should be tested in the lower extremities if a peripheral neuropathy or myelopathy is in the differential diagnosis. Diabetes is a common cause of peripheral neuropathy. Deep tendon reflexes are tested and graded. The quadriceps reflex is generally considered to reflect the integrity of the L4 nerve root but could be diminished by lesions of L2 or L3. The Achilles reflex is predominantly S1, and possibly S2. Although not present in all individuals, a reflex of the L5 root is the tibialis posterior. With the patient relaxed, the foot is slightly dorsiflexed and everted. The tibialis posterior tendon is tapped just proximal to its insertion into the navicular. A positive response is plantar flexion and inversion of the foot. Hyperactivity of all the reflexes may be seen in systemic conditions such as thyrotoxicosis or upper motor neuron lesions. Problems at the lower motor neuron level will result in diminution or loss of a reflex. Reflexes may be useful in localization when there is asymmetry. The examiner should look for pathologic findings such as Babinski's reflex and clonus.

A neurologic examination also includes observation of gait. One should look for a limp and, if present, try to determine if this is due to pain or weakness. A painful limp is characterized by shortening the amount of time that weight is borne on that extremity during the gait cycle. The individual should be asked to walk on their heels and toes as this may reveal subtle weakness in the leg muscles that may not be apparent on manual testing. Tandem walking will test strength, coordination, and balance.

In the middle-aged and older individual, peripheral pulses should also be palpated, as vascular disease can produce back or leg pain. Abdominal and pelvic examinations may be performed when there is suspicion that the back pain is of visceral origin.

SPECIAL TESTS

Radiographic Evaluation

Plain radiographs of the lumbar spine are not necessary in every episode of back pain. In a young, active individual with a clear-cut precipitating event, acute pain can often be managed symptomatically. Films are obtained if the symptoms do not subside as expected. If there is more significant trauma involved, films are indicated to look for fractures and dislocations. In older individuals in whom the history suggest neoplastic process, plain films are obtained early as a screening tool. As elsewhere in the body, it should be remembered that approximately 50% destruction of bone is necessary before it becomes evident on plain films.

Along with the radiologist, the clinician should examine the plain films for alignment and symmetry. The presence of degenerative changes such as disc narrowing, sclerosis, and osteophyte formation must be tempered with the fact that such changes are common in the asymptomatic general population, and their incidence increases with age. Abnormalities such as spondylolysis or pars defect, with or without the slip (spondylolisthesis), are present in 6% to 9% of the adult population. Hence, this may or may not be the cause of the individual's pain, and must be correlated with the symptoms and physical findings. Other anomalies that may be asymptomatic include transitional vertebra (lumbarization of S1 or sacralization of L5), spina bifida occulta, and assimilation joints (an articulation between the transverse process of L5 and the sacral ala).

Despite these limitations, plain radiographs can be diagnostic. This is particularly true for inflammatory conditions such as the spondyloarthropathies and infections, neoplastic processes, and metabolic disorders.

Osteopenia, which is the loss of radiographic density of the bone, may be due to several processes, not just osteoporosis. Osteomalacia can produce similar radiographic findings as can marrow processes such as multiple myeloma.

Laboratory Evaluation

In cases of persistent back pain, certain elements of the history may prompt laboratory evaluation. Complete blood count, electrolytes, creatinine, blood urea nitrogen, calcium, phosphorus, alkaline phosphatase, erythrocyte sedimentation rate, and urinalysis provide initial information. The patient's presentation, other medical problems, and the results of these studies may prompt a more specialized test, such as electrophoresis and immunoelectrophoresis of serum or urine, acid phosphatase, HLA-B27, and parathyroid hormone.

Other Tests

Electromyography and nerve conduction studies can identify neuropathies and denervation. It should be kept in mind that electromyography will not show abnormalities until several weeks after an acute process.

Excluding benign self-limited back pain, the specific diagnosis can often be made with modern imaging modalities such as computerized tomography, with and without intrathecal contrast, and magnetic resonance imaging (MRI). These modalities yield excellent anatomic data. They are expensive and probably should be limited to cases in which there is reasonable suspicion of a lesion mandating significant interventions such as surgery, radiation therapy, or chemotherapy. In those cases, it is generally most expeditious to consult with a physician trained in the management of spinal disorders.

SPECIFIC PROBLEMS

Trauma

The history of trauma is generally self-evident. The forces involved to produce fracture or dislocation in the lumbar spine are great and are generally associated with concomitant injuries to other parts of the body.

These should be managed at trauma centers by traumatologists and spine surgeons.

Lesser and more common forms of trauma involve much less energy. These may result from direct blows that contuse the skin and subcutaneous tissue and muscle contusion resulting in muscle spasm, pain, and stiffness. On examination, there may be ecchymosis and tenderness. Vigorous activity, particularly without prior conditioning, can often result in back pain. Generally this is nonfocal. If there is radiation, it tends to be to the buttock and proximal thigh. There may or may not be tenderness and reduced range of motion. Neurologic examination is normal. This could be termed a back strain.

In these soft tissue injuries, treatment is generally supportive as discussed in the treatment section.

Nonspecific Back Pain

Nonspecific back pain overlaps with the back strain described above. This may occur with overuse or may arise spontaneously. It can occur episodically and tends to be modulated by activities. There may be referred pain to the proximal lower extremities, which may be affected by the Valsalva maneuver, but there should be no sphincter dysfunction or other neurologic deficit. Radiographs are often normal but may show disc narrowing or other degenerative changes.

Disc Herniation

Disc herniation commonly occurs in the third to fifth decades but can occur at any age. There may or may not be back pain, but there is almost always lower extremity pain, which is described as sharp and lancinating, often with paresthesias in the same distribution. The pain tends to follow a dermatomal pattern. There can be a history of injury but herniation may occur spontaneously, probably from the cumulative trauma of daily activities. The Valsalva maneuver will often exacerbate symptoms. Sitting is uncomfortable, as it increases the interdiscal pressure. Severity of symptoms tends to be proportional to the size of the herniation. If it is large enough, the patient may not be able to find

Figure 4-1. Sagittal MRI demonstrating a large L5-S1 disc herniation that displaces the thecal sac dorsally.

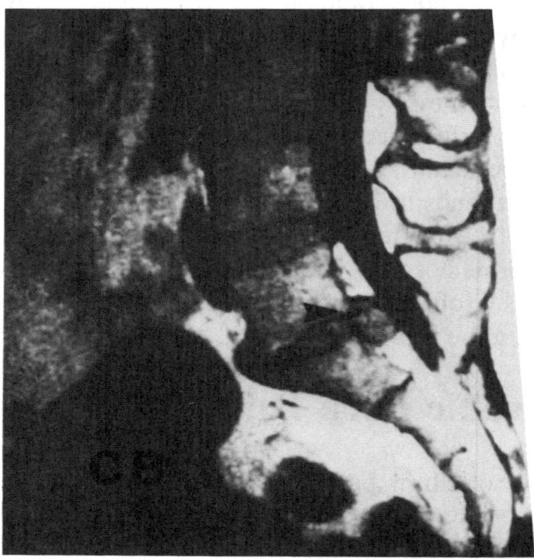

Figure 4-2. Transverse lumbar MRI of the same patient as Figure 4-1 demonstrating large disc herniation (arrowheads). The S1 nerve roots are seen on either side of the herniation. The thecal sac is dorsal to the disc herniation and has a lower signal intensity. This patient required discectomy.

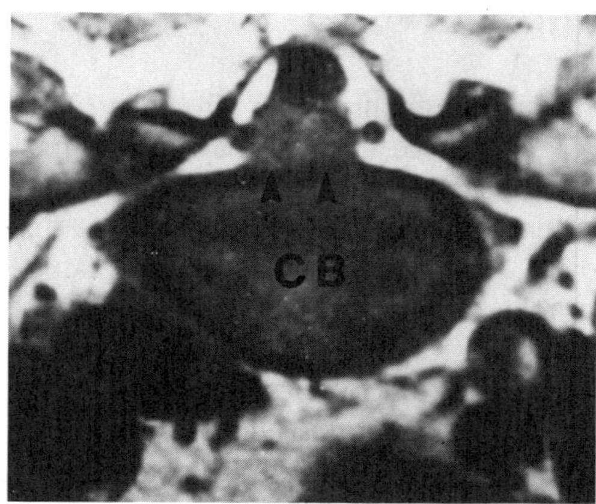

a comfortable position (see Figs. 4-1 and 4-2). The symptoms are probably due to both mechanical effect of the herniation as well as an inflammatory response to the herniated material. Neurologic deficit in the form of weakness, numbness, or altered deep tendon reflexes tends to correlate with the size of the herniation. Prognosis in most cases is good. 60% of individuals will note significant reduction in symptoms over a six to 12 week period. Persistent disabling pain after this amount of time should prompt a referral to a spine surgeon. Referral should be made in the acute period if there is impaired bladder or bowel function, progressive motor weakness, or severe unremitting pain refractory to bed rest. More recent evidence has shown that bed rest of a few days duration is as efficacious as two or more weeks; in fact, it is superior since it avoids deconditioning. Surgical evaluation should also be considered when there are recurring episodes of incapacitating sciatica.

Cauda equina syndrome can be caused by a massive midline disc herniation that compresses multiple roots in the cauda equina, including the lower sacral nerves. It can also be caused by intraspinal tumors, epidural hematoma, and epidural abscess. The patient will often complain of bilateral lower extremity pain, anesthesia in a saddle distribution (possibly including buttocks and posterior thighs), decreased rectal and bladder sensation, incontinence, or difficulty voiding. On examination, rectal sensation and tone are diminished or absent. There is hypesthesia in the perianal and perineal regions. There may or may not be deficits involving proximal nerve roots. Cauda equina syndromes should prompt immediate diagnostic imaging such as MRI or myelography followed by computerized tomography with urgent surgical consultation.

Degenerative Spondylosis

Individuals with degenerative spondylosis often give a history of chronic intermittent back pain of many years' duration and tend to be middle-aged. Like non-specific back pain, discomfort tends to be in the lower lumbar region with little extremity pain except for buttock or posterior thigh. Lumbar motion may be mildly restricted, but muscle spasm and nerve retention signs are usually absent. Neurologic examination is normal. Radiographs show disc narrowing, facet hypertrophy, and osteophyte formation.

Most of these people do not need sophisticated imaging; when it is done, degenerative changes are obvious but do not show narrowing of the spinal canal or neural compression.

Diffuse idiopathic skeletal hyperostosis (DISH syndrome or Forestier disease) has traditionally been viewed as a variant of degenerative arthritis. More recent evidence suggests that it is a metabolic disorder. While DISH syndrome tends to begin in the thoracic spine and creep proximally, the large anterior osteophytes can involve the lumbar spine as well. This represents ossification of the anterior longitudinal ligament, which is radiographically distinct from the bamboo spine seen in ankylosing spondylitis.

Lumbar Spinal Stenosis

In many cases, lumbar spinal stenosis represents progression of degenerative spondylosis. It refers to diminution in the size of the spinal canal, resulting in cauda equina or nerve root compression, depending on where the narrowing occurs. With this broad definition, disc herniation can be thought of as a form of acute spinal stenosis. The symptoms usually begin insidiously. Classically, the patient will complain of aching or vague weakness in their legs, which correlates to activities, particularly walking. In older individuals, this claudication may suggest vascular disease. It may be possible to differentiate neurogenic claudication from vascular disease by detailed inquiry. Vascular claudication tends to occur after a uniform distance, whereas neurogenic claudication is more variable. The discomfort of vascular insufficiency will subside if the patient stands still, allowing the muscle ischemia to resolve. With spinal stenosis, standing itself may aggravate the symptoms; patients will often state that they must sit down or bend forward to obtain relief. This maneuver functionally increases the size of the neural canal. Patients may complain that they walk with a stooped posture. In more severe cases, standing upright without walking may precipitate symptoms.

Such symptoms may occur in young individuals who have congenital or developmentally narrow spinal canals. In the third and fourth decade, these individuals will present either with acute radiculopathy or with neurogenic claudication. The diagnostic work-up will show a small central canal with small disc herniations or bulging discs that would cause only mild transient symptoms in people with normal canals. In mid-life, they present more with neurogenic claudication and only mild to moderate degenerative changes, but these superimposed upon their small canal result in symptoms in the fifth and sixth decades.

More commonly, spinal stenosis is caused by degenerative disease, particularly involving the facet joints. This will narrow the lateral recesses and neural foramina and present with the clinical picture described.

Infection

Unless there is a history of penetrating trauma or surgery, infection in the lumbar spine occurs by hematogenous seeding. Acute back pain in an individual with a known previous infection obviously prompts an evaluation. Depending on the severity of the infection, the host response, and the virulence of the organism, there may or may not be the systemic signs such as fever, chills, diaphoresis, and malaise. There is usually focal tenderness and muscle spasm. The infection tends to begin in the subchondral portion of the disc, spread to involve the disc itself, and then erode through the end plates on either side to involve the vertebral bodies.

Early in the course of a pyogenic infection, radiographs may be normal. The white blood cell counts may also be normal or only mildly elevated. The sedimentation rate is almost always elevated. Bone scan will show increased uptake in the region of the affected disc. MRI is often diagnostic, even before there are radiographic changes. Blood cultures as well as cultures of fluids from potential originating foci such as urine should be obtained. Early surgical consultation is advised.

Deformity

When there is abnormal curvature to the spine, such as scoliosis or kyphosis, there is abnormal loading of the joints and soft tissues resulting in aching. With more severe deformity or with spondylolisthesis, there can be neural compression. In mild cases, treatment may consist of activity modification, non-narcotic medication, bracing, and exercise. Refractory symptoms or documented progression of the deformity generally requires surgical intervention.

Neoplasms

The most common neoplasm to bone is metastatic disease. The most common tumors occur in the breast, lungs, prostate, thyroid, and kidney. The most common primary tumor in the spine is multiple myeloma. Other primary tumors are uncommon but include such lesions as osteoid osteoma, osteoblastoma, aneurysmal bone cyst, and chordoma. Primary lesions in individuals under the age of 20 tend to be benign whereas primary lesions in individuals older than 20 years tend to be malignant. The history, examination, and plain radiographs will guide the staging and diagnostic work-up. The patient's age, the appearance of the lesion, and its location (anterior versus posterior elements) will narrow the differential diagnosis. When focal metastatic disease is suspected, a survey for the primary lesion should be undertaken. Bone scintigraphy may reveal other lesions consistent with widespread metastases. Multiple myeloma may not be apparent on bone scanning and may be picked up with a skeletal survey. Advanced anatomic studies such as MRI and computed tomography will help find the extent of destruction, the presence of neural compression, and the presence of associated soft tissue mass. Ultimately, a tissue diagnosis should be established by a biopsy.

Inflammatory Disorders

Rheumatoid arthritis can involve the lumbar spine, but this is rare, especially when compared with the incidence of cervical involvement.

More common are the spondyloarthropathies such as ankylosing spondylitis, psoriatic arthritis, and spondyloarthropathy associated with inflammatory bowel disease. Ankylosing spondylitis generally presents in early adulthood, more frequently in men. There is usually history of morning stiffness and there may be a positive family history. Lumbar radiographs may initially be normal. Films of the sacroiliac joint should be obtained to look for the characteristic early changes. In most instances the treatment includes physical therapy with an emphasis on correct posture and the use of non-steroidal anti-inflammatory drugs. In long-standing cases of spondyloarthropathy, kyphotic deformity may develop in the thoracolumbar and lumbar regions, which may result from poor posture during the earlier phases of the disease, repeated stress fractures, or acute fracture through the ankylosed spine. In severe cases, this may require surgical intervention.

Neural Lesions

Intrinsic nerve root tumors such as neurofibroma, neurolemma and lipoma of the filum terminale are uncommon and may present with back or leg pain indistinguishable from conditions such as disc herniation. Sophisticated imaging techniques will narrow the differential diagnosis preoperatively. With neurofibroma, there may be a stigmata of systemic neurofibromatosis. If the lesion is large, the neural foramen may be enlarged. With lipoma of the filum, the distance between the pedicles on the anteroposterior radiograph may be increased and there may also be malformation of the posterior elements.

Pain Referred to the Back

Occasionally, a lesion in the thoracic spine will be perceived in the lumbar region. For example, a thoracic disc herniation, particularly in the lower thoracic region, can produce low back pain that mimics the more common lumbar disc herniation. Subtle bladder and bowel dysfunction, or difficulty with balance may raise the question of actual location of the cause of pain. During the physical examination the lower thoracic region should also be palpated in the midline. This should be non-tender; if pain is encountered, attention should be directed to this region, especially if there is corroborating evidence of a thoracic spine lesion.

Neural compression in the thoracic region will often produce a hyperreflexia and possibly pathologic reflexes (e.g., positive Babinski's sign) or ankle clonus. This is opposite the expected diminution of reflexes seen with root or cauda equina compression. In addition, there may be increased tone in the lower extremities. For a more complete discussion of myelopathy, refer to chapter 1.

Hip disease can also produce pain about the pelvis, buttocks, and thighs that may be confused with lumbar pathology. In some patients, there will be radiographic evidence of both degenerative disc disease and osteoarthritis of the hip. In such patients, it may be difficult, if not impossible, to distinguish which symptoms are due to lumbar stenosis and which are secondary to coxarthritis. On examination, restriction of hip motion and reproduction of complaints by attempted hip motion may clarify the issue.

As discussed earlier, peripheral vascular disease can produce activity-related extremity pain that mimics neurogenic claudication of lumbar stenosis. The differentiation was reviewed in that subsection.

The dissecting or rupturing abdominal aortic aneurysm can produce severe lumbar pain. It should be suspected when there is the abrupt onset of severe pain in an older individual, particularly when there are other stigmata of vascular disease. If the patient gives a history of previous back pain, often they will state that this pain is of a different, tearing quality. Because of associated calcification, the aneurysm may have been identified prior to symptoms when lumbar radiographs or a KUB was obtained for other reasons. When painful, an aneurysm requires prompt evaluation by a vascular surgeon.

Arteriovenous malformations may produce back or leg pain, depending on the size. There may be sphincter dysfunction if the conus medullaris is involved. Meningismus may be present if there is hemorrhage into the subarachnoid space. In such cases the spinal fluid will be xanthochromic. The appearances on myelopathy, enhanced computed tomography, and magnetic resonance imaging are characteristic. Urolithiasis produces severe cramping of flank pain that could be confused with lumbar pathology but is unilateral and usually recognized for what it is. Hematuria will help direct the investigation along appropriate channels.

Retroperitoneal and intrapelvic pathology such as neoplasm can also present with varying degrees of back pain. If there is involvement of the lumbosacral plexus, lower extremity symptoms may also be produced.

TREATMENT

Medications

Non-steroidal anti-inflammatory drugs are the cornerstone of treatment of many spine related disorders. Inflammation is invoked as the final mediator of pain in a number of disorders. These medications are non-addictive and, except in certain sensitive individuals, do not affect cognitive function. They can have significant side effects, however, most commonly involving the gastrointestinal system.

Acetaminophen has no anti-inflammatory properties but is a very useful mild analgesic that can be used in patients with benign chronic pain who do not tolerate nonsteroidal anti-inflammatory drugs or who could not tolerate an increased dosage.

Corticosteroids have a limited role in the treatment of lumbar spine problems. Systemic steroids are powerful anti-inflammatory drugs but are associated with significant side effects including immunosuppression, water retention, and avascular necrosis. Epidural steroids have been used in a variety of painful conditions including chronic pain and stenosis. Reports in the literature are conflicting. Their use should probably be limited to individuals who fail other modalities and are not surgical candidates. Although the medication is delivered to the desired site, systemic side effects are still seen, particularly if administered several times.

Muscle relaxants such as methocarbamol (Robaxin), cyclobenzaprine (Flexeril), diazepam (Valium), and carisoprodol (Soma), can be useful in acute pain. They are said to reduce muscle spasm, but their effect may be more one of sedation. They have little use in chronic pain.

Narcotic analgesics are very useful for acute pain such as the severe radiculopathy and herniated disc. Because of their effect on the sensorium, their tendency to induce tolerance, and the problem of addiction in certain individuals, their use should be restricted to short periods with the exception of terminal malignancy. They have no role in the management of chronic pain.

Management of chronic pain is a difficult problem. Anti-inflammatory drugs are used. Several anti-depressant and anti-convulsant drugs could have been used successfully although they do have side effects. Some of these drugs are amitriptyline (Elavil and others), doxepin (Sinequan), fluoxetine (Prozac) among the anti-depressant drugs and carbamazepine (Tegretol) and pheytoin (Dilantin) among the anti-convulsant drugs.

Bracing

It is difficult to totally immobilize the lumbar spine by external means. Even in a body cast that includes one thigh in order to control the pelvis, there is some motion. Anything less than this will allow more motion, so orthotics should be viewed more as a form of support rather than immobilization. They may also provide relief by retaining body heat, serving to remind the patient of their condition, and forcing them to substitute other joint motions to carry out activities.

Braces are most useful in the transition from the acute phase through the subacute phase as the individual increases activities. Long-term use should probably be discouraged in favor of reconditioning the patient with an exercise program. There are patients who will not exercise and who will use bracing long-term with some benefit.

The most popular, least restrictive, and least expensive orthosis is a lumbar or lumbosacral corset, generally equipped with rigid stays.

Therapy and Exercise

A physical therapist will use a variety of modalities to deliver heat or cold to the lumbar region. Combined with massage, this can give significant temporary relief.

Several exercise programs have been developed; the most widely known and used are the Williams flexion exercises and the McKinsey extension exercises. Conceptually, the extension exercises should be most effective in individuals with disc herniations, bulges, and degenerative disc disease, as this should unload those structures. Similarly, flexion exercises would seem more desirable for individuals with facet arthritis and spinal stenosis where flexion will unload the joints and functionally increase the space for the neural elements. The astute therapist will tailor the exercise program to the patient. The goals of the exercise program are to improve flexibility and increase strength of the supporting muscles.

More recently, aggressive rehabilitation programs have been used to increase the chances of resuming employment activities, especially among laborers. This has included trunk strengthening exercises with exercise machines.

Another promising concept is the emphasis on aerobic activity. For those who are still in acute and subacute pain phases, this can still be accomplished by partially unloading the spine in a swimming pool. This could be conventional swimming or walking in a pool, which supplies resistance as well as partial unloading of the spine by buoyancy. In the chronic phase, a whole spectrum of aerobic activity is available, including walking, running, rowing, and bicycling. Regular aerobic activity has many salubrious effects, one of which is to diminish the intensity and perception of pain.

For recalcitrant chronic pain, there are pain programs that utilize a multidisciplinary approach combining several different treatments.

Surgery

In general, surgery for lumbar disease is most successful when the major component is lower extremity pain, weakness or paresthesias that fails to respond to non-surgical treatments. Surgery for back pain is much less predictable, but in select individuals (e.g., isthmic spondylolisthesis) may be quite successful. Surgical consultation should be obtained any time there is a significant neurologic deficit such as the loss of bladder or bowel control or a loss of motor function. Referral is also appropriate for severe radicular pain and less severe pain that does not subside over a six to 12 week period.

CARE OF THE PATIENT AFTER LUMBAR SURGERY

As with any surgery, inflammation of the wound or drainage will prompt the surgeon to evaluate for possible wound infection. Other worrisome signs and symptoms are fevers, chills, and increasing pain. Persistent or recurrent leg pain or increasing neurologic deficit warrants further investigation.

Lumbar Discectomy

In appropriately selected individuals, lumbar discectomy is an extremely successful procedure, producing dramatic relief of symptoms. With severe root irritation, the patient may still have twinges of the leg pain. In addition, the lumbar area will be stiff and sore, with the pain resolving rapidly over the first few weeks. The stiffness will persist for several months. Walking is encouraged as a form of exercise. Stamina will gradually improve. By six weeks, stretching and back strengthening exercises are added. For laborers, it is particularly important to regain trunk strength prior to resuming employment to decrease the risk of re-injury. Some surgeons will utilize a work hardening program to this end. After three to six months, the uncomplicated lumbar discectomy patient may resume activity without restriction.

Lumbar Decompression With and Without Fusion

Many of the same principles used in the discectomy patient apply in this situation. However, the surgery is generally much more extensive. There is more muscle stripping and, if a fusion has been performed with the patient's own bone, the pelvic area is also uncomfortable from muscle stripping and bone removal.   Some surgeons will use some form of orthosis in these individuals. Walking is an important exercise early in the course. When there is fusion, some surgeons will delay stretching exercises for eight to 12 weeks to allow the fusion to mature. For heavy laborers, the return to work should be delayed until four to six months after surgery.

Trauma

Injuries severe enough to require surgery will usually be stabilized with some form of internal fixation. This hastens the ability of the surgeon to mobilize the patient. Most spine surgeons will use some form of orthosis for three to six months, as fusion is a part of the surgical procedure. Depending on the extent and severity of the injury, including neurologic injury, the surgeon will modify the rehabilitation plan as needed.

Failed Back

Even with strict indications, the spine surgeon will have patients who continue to have lumbar or lower extremity symptoms assuming that the pathology was addressed at the time of the original procedure, conservative modalities were employed, and narcotics were avoided. The cause of this pain may be quite elusive. One subset will include chronic inflammation of the nerve roots and meninges. This condition, arachnoiditis, produces a characteristic appearance on myelography, computerized tomography, and magnetic resonance imaging. Typically, the individual will describe the pain as worse at night, having a burning character, and often in a non-dermatomal distribution. The prognosis for arachnoiditis is guarded.   It may respond to an integrated pain management program but it is likely to remain chronic.

Unless there is demonstrable pathology that can be addressed surgically, these patients are not helped by surgery and are best served by a chronic pain management program. Surgery may be indicated in well motivated individuals when there is persistent neural compression by recurrent or retained disc fragments or bony compression. Other indications include iatrogenic instability and non-union of attempted fusion.

BIBLIOGRAPHY

Frymoyer J.W.: Medical Progress. Back Pain and Sciatica. N. Engl. J. Med., 1988: 318:291-300.

Frymoyer J.W. (Ed): The Adult Spine: Principles and Practice. New York: Raven Press, 1991.

Hoppenfeld S.: Orthopaedic Neurology. Philadelphia: J.B. Lippincott, 1977.

Macnab I.: Backache. Baltimore: Williams and Wilkins, 1977.

Rothman R.H. and Simenone F.A. (Eds): The Spine, Second Edition. Philadelphia: W.B. Saunders, 1982.

5

THE HIP

By Matthew J. Kraay, M.D.
and Randall E. Marcus, M.D.

Orthopaedic complaints involving the hip area are often seen in adults and these problems can significantly affect activity, function, and quality of life. The magnitude of these disorders are readily apparent to most primary care physicians, especially those who care for significant numbers of elderly patients.

Recent estimates indicate that more than 275,000 hip fractures occur annually in the United States, 95% of which occur in patients over 50 years of age. The estimated health-care cost of all hip fractures in the United States approximated $7.2 billion in 1984, and this figure continues to increase as the geriatric portion of our population also increases in size.

Arthritis, whether primary or secondary, develops in many adults, not infrequently during the more active years. Based on estimates from the 1980s, over 100,000 total hip replacements are performed yearly in treatment of hip disease. Total hip arthroplasty can provide pain relief and restore function to many severely affected patients. Early diagnosis and appropriate medical management of many of these problems can often prevent or delay progression of these disorders.

Although primary bone tumors are generally uncommon in the middle-aged and elderly adult population, metastatic involvement of bone is common and frequently involves the hip. Treating these often complex problems frequently requires the cooperative efforts of both medical and orthopaedic specialists.

The primary care physician will frequently care for patients with a variety of problems involving the hip. Early recognition, accurate diagnosis, and institution of appropriate care can result in resolution of many of these conditions and delay progression of others. Of equal importance is the need for appropriate referral of certain problems to the orthopaedic surgeon for more urgent treatment or surgery. This chapter will first review the historic, physical, radiographic, and laboratory evaluation of disorders of the hip in general, and then more thoroughly discuss several of the more common and worrisome disorders affecting the hip that may confront the primary care physician.

HISTORY

Certain aspects of the history can provide insight into the etiology of hip complaints. As with any medical problem, accurate diagnosis and appropriate treatment starts with a thorough history.

Orthopaedic problems involving the hip most frequently present with pain as the chief complaint. Critical to identification of the problem that the patient presents with is the accurate localization of pain around the hip joint itself. Although this is frequently suggestive of the etiology of the pain, confirmation often depends on additional information obtained on physical examination and confirmed by radiographic, laboratory, or other evaluation.

Pain from articular hip joint pathology (e.g., arthritis) is typically localized in the groin, whereas pain from a trochanteric bursitis is typically localized to the lateral side of the hip over the greater trochanter. Disorders of the sacroiliac joint usually present with "hip pain" localized over that joint itself. Frequently, patients will complain of "hip pain" localized to the buttocks or along the course of the sciatic nerve posterior to the hip joint. In these patients, further characterization of the pain and physical findings often identifies a lumbar spine disorder as the etiology of this referred type of "hip pain." Similarly, pain truly originating from the hip joint can be referred to the anterior thigh or knee.

Further characterization of pain with regard to quality, severity, relieving or aggravating factors, and temporal relationship to an initiating or recurring event can be helpful in identifying the underlying etiology. Arthritic pain typically is worse with weight-bearing and relieved somewhat by rest. Progression of arthrosis resulting in marked loss of the joint space, regardless of the underlying cause, is frequently associated with development of night pain. Patients with loosening of total hip replacement components will often complain of pain with initial weight-bearing on the extremity that resolves with continued activity. "Hip pain" associated with lumbar spine disorders can usually be identified when the typical findings of neurogenic claudication or radiculopathy are present (see chapter 4). Acute septic arthritis is typically associated with acute onset of severe pain localized to the hip joint and markedly aggravated with any movement of the hip.

The patient with a hip problem should be questioned regarding a history of remote as well as recent trauma. Young patients with a previous history of significant injury to the hip (e.g., dislocation or fracture) may develop late avascular necrosis of the femoral head or secondary degenerative arthritis of the hip. Nondisplaced or even displaced fractures of the hip frequently occur as a result of seemingly minor trauma in the elderly patient with osteoporosis. Stress fractures of the femoral neck and pubic rami can occur in the active young patient or in the severely osteoporotic, sedentary patient.

The patient should be thoroughly questioned regarding presence of any associated constitutional symptoms. Presence of fever or chills, or history of recent febrile illness may suggest an infectious etiology. Malaise, fatigue, or weight loss may be associated with neoplastic disease or chronic inflammatory diseases such as rheumatoid arthritis or its variants.

The nature of any previous surgery or procedures on the hip should be established if possible. Frequently, adults with secondary degenerative arthritis will have a history of childhood treatment of congenital hip dysplasia, Legg-Calve'-Perthes disease, slipped capital femoral epiphysis, septic arthritis, or other pediatric hip disorders. The primary care physician must be aware of problems related to prior surgical treatment of hip disorders that affect the adult population, including the possibility of secondary infection, loosening, or failure of a total hip prosthesis or other hip implant.

Assessment of the functional limitations imposed by disorders of the hip are less helpful in establishing a diagnosis but are important determinants of the quality of life experienced by the patient. The patient's ability to walk and sit for a reasonable amount of time, use assistive devices for ambulation, and perform one's own activities of daily living are important considerations in therapeutic decision making.

A thorough review of the patient's general medical history can also provide considerable insight into the etiology of many hip disorders. A history of excessive ethanol use or use of steroid medication justifies concern about complications related to associated osteopenia or avascular necrosis. The effect of other medications on bone mineral metabolism can clearly contribute to the development of hip pathology. Antibiotic treatment can sometimes modulate the acute symptoms of septic arthritis, making both diagnosis and recovery of the infective organism difficult. Many other systemic diseases can have primary or secondary manifestations related to the hip.

PHYSICAL EXAMINATION

A thorough physical examination can provide considerable additional information about hip pathology. Assessment of gait is an important aspect of this examination, which can reveal much about the functional limitations imposed by hip joint disease. While observing the patient walking on a level surface, the duration of time in stance phase, stride length and velocity, posture, deformity, and compensatory mechanisms can be assessed.

One of the most commonly seen abnormalities in a patient with hip pathology is an antalgic limp. This is characterized by shortened duration of stance phase on the involved extremity in response to pain with weight-bearing on that extremity.

An abductor limp can often be observed in patients with hip disease. This limp is secondary to muscular weakness and atrophy from long-standing hip dysfunction, altered hip biomechanics, or neurologic deficit. Normally, during midstance phase of gait, the strong hip abductors cause the pelvis to rotate upwards, shifting the body's center of gravity and trunk laterally over the weight-bearing extremity. In patients with abductor weakness, a positive Trendelenburg sign may be observed when the pelvis does not rotate upwards normally in a single leg stance (see Fig. 5-1). Hip abductor weakness manifests as an abductor limp or gluteus medius lurch, whereby the trunk and center of gravity is thrown to the ipsilateral side during stance phase in order to compensate for the inadequate function of the hip abductors (see Fig. 5-2). Patients with painful hips may demonstrate a compensatory abductor lurch since this mechanism decreases the joint reaction force and pain in the hip.

Patients with hip extensor weakness or limited hip extension due to arthritis and deformity may compensate by exaggeration of their normal lumbar lordosis or forceful extension of the trunk with walking, referred to as an extensor or gluteus maximus limp or lurch (see Fig. 5-3).

Further inspection should identify the presence of any noticeable swelling, deformity, abnormal posturing, erythema, or other discoloration in the region of the hip. The hip may be slightly flexed and externally rotated in the case of acute septic arthritis, in order to minimize intracapsular pressure within the hip joint. Fractures about the hip are frequently associated with deformity, usually consisting of shortening and external rotation of the extremity. Estimation of leg length equality can be done by a variety of techniques, perhaps the simplest of which consists of measuring from the anterior superior iliac spine to the ipsilateral medial malleolus with the patient supine, and comparing this with the opposite extremity (See Fig. 5-4).

The hip joint itself is located deep to a substantial investment of musculature and soft tissue, which makes palpation of the joint difficult. Nevertheless, palpation of the surrounding bony landmarks and soft tissues can assist in evaluation of disorders in this region. Tenderness over the pubic rami, greater trochanter, and ischial tuberosity may result from tendinitis, or strain at the site of muscular attachment of the adductor, abductor, and hamstring muscle groups, respectively. Localized bony pathology to these areas, whether it be trauma, tumor, or infection, may often be associated with localized tenderness or

Figure 5-1. The Trendelenburg sign is seen in the figure on the right. With weakness of the abductor musculature, a sag of the pelvis in single-leg stance is demonstrated.

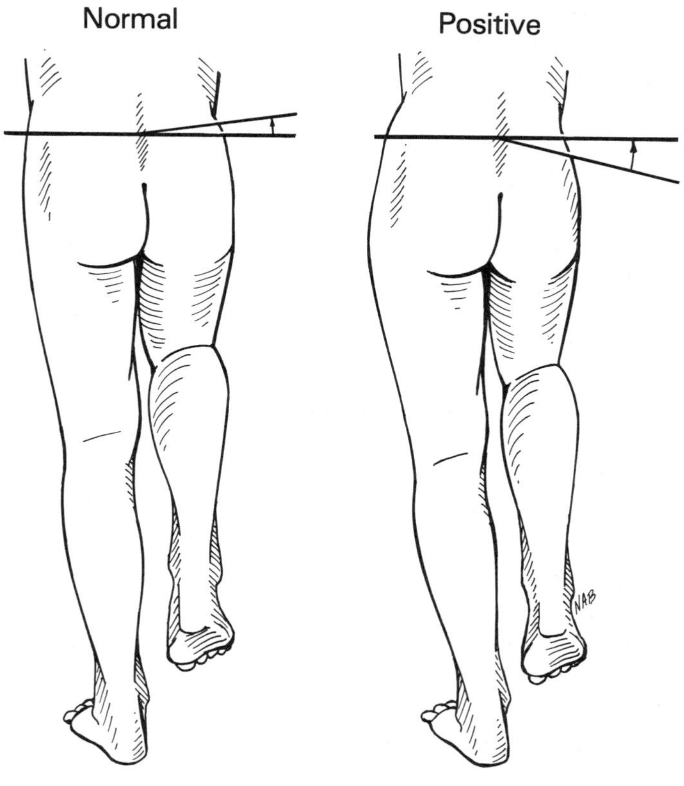

Figure 5-2. The abductor limp is seen with hip abductor weakness. The trunk and center of gravity is thrown to the ipsilateral side during stance phase in order to compensate for inadequate function of the hip abductor musculature.

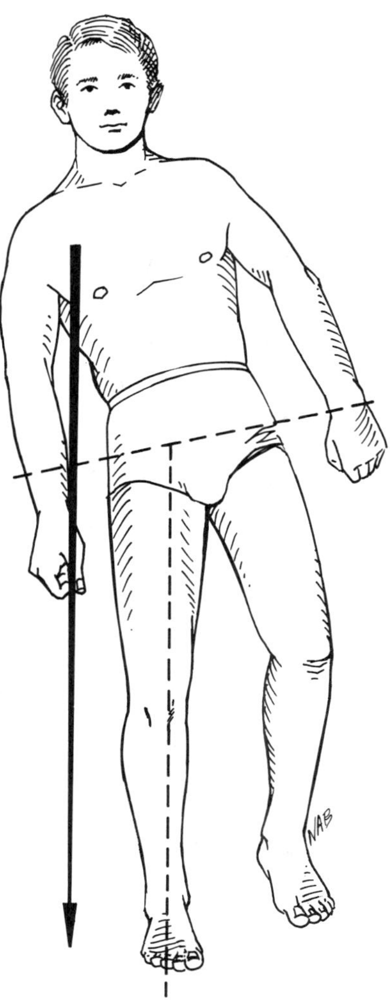

Figure 5-3.   The extensor limp is seen with hip extensor weakness or limited hip extension due to arthritis. Forceful extension of the trunk with walking is demonstrated.

EXTENSOR LIMP

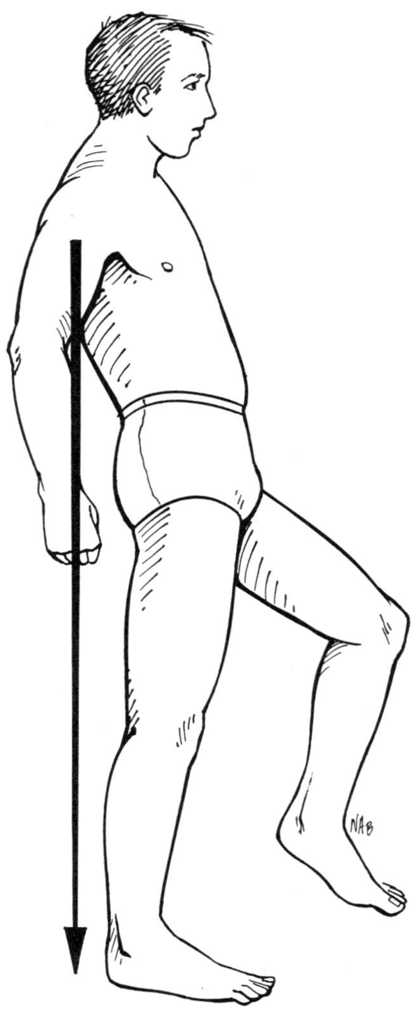

Figure 5-4. Limb length measurement for estimation of leg length.

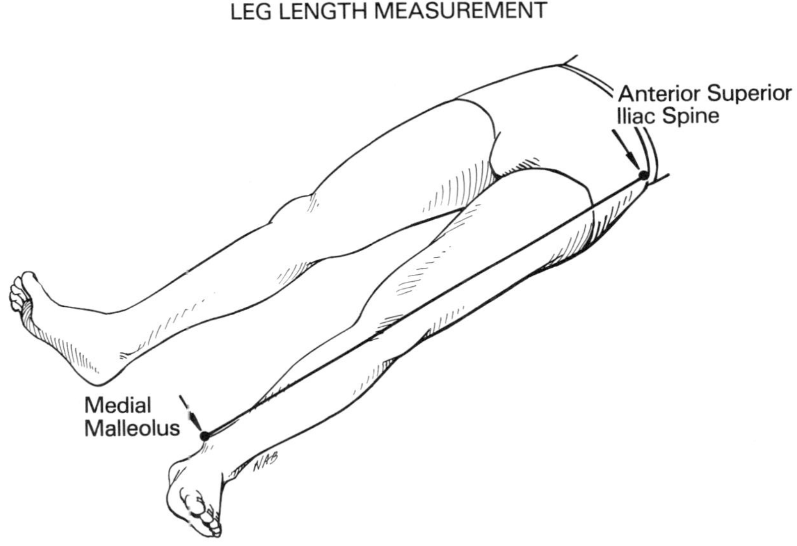

palpable swelling. Inflammation overlying the bony prominence of the greater trochanter or, rarely, the ischial tuberosity can result in a bursitis, presenting as an area of localized tenderness.

The sciatic nerve can often be palpated in a soft tissue depression midway between the greater trochanter and the ischial tuberosity when the hip is flexed (see Fig. 5-5). Irritation of the nerve in the area of the hip, or especially from nerve root compression in the lumbar spine, can result in tenderness on palpation of this area. Palpation of the area of the sacroiliac joints and along the lumbar spine can frequently identify areas of "hip pain" that do not originate from the hip joint itself.

Assessment of range of motion of the hip is an important part of the examination of the hip. Patients with significant hip pathology, such as septic arthritis, fracture of the proximal femur, or advanced arthritis of the joint will often have marked pain with even the slightest motion of

Figure 5-5. The sciatic nerve can often be easily palpated below the sciatic notch when in the lateral position with the hip flexed.

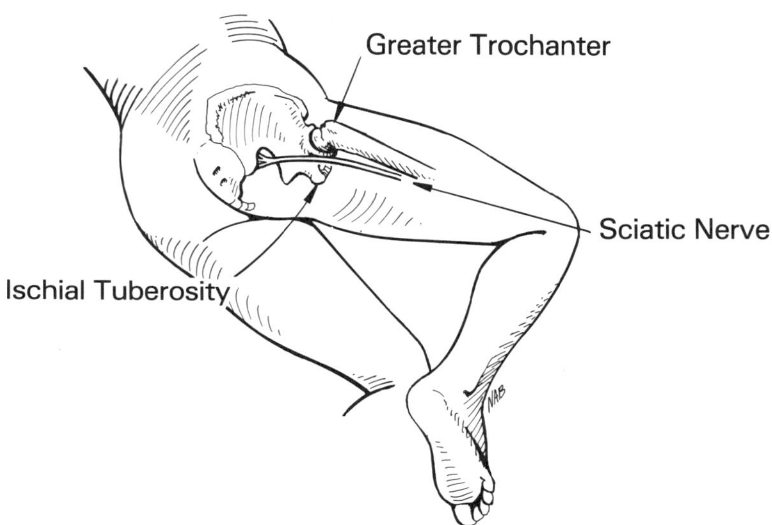

the hip. With the patient supine, initial gentle internal and external rotation of the extremity, the "roll test," will identify those patients who can be subjected to more vigorous range of motion evaluation.

When evaluating range of motion of the hip, attention should be directed towards stabilization of the pelvis to eliminate motion between the pelvis and the spine that may be otherwise perceived to originate at the hip joint. With the patient supine on the examination table, flexion and presence of any flexion contracture of the hip can be assessed. The examiner's hand should be placed under the patient's lumbar spine and the hip flexed upwards until the lumbar lordosis flattens. At this point, the pelvis is stabilized, and the extremity being examined can then be further flexed to its maximum, normally approaching 120 to 135 degrees. With the pelvis stabilized by flexion of the contralateral hip in this manner, the extremity can then be extended and presence of any flexion contracture or limitation of extension back to neutral can be determined (see Fig. 5-6).

Full extension of the hip is best assessed with the patient lying prone on the examination table with the knees slightly flexed to relax the hamstring muscles. With one arm stabilizing the patient's pelvis, the other hand can then raise the thigh and the maximum of extension, normally 20 to 30 degrees, can be determined.

The range of abduction (normally 45 to 50 degrees) and adduction (normally 20 to 30 degrees) can also be determined with the patient in the supine position. The examiner should stabilize the trunk by placing the forearm across the pelvis at the level of the anterior superior iliac spine, using the hand to hold on to the contralateral hemipelvis at the same level (see Figs. 5-7A,B). With the examiner's opposite hand on the ankle, the extremity can be abducted and then adducted across the midline over the contralateral extremity. The end point of motion occurs when the pelvis begins to move with abduction or adduction of the limb.

Figure 5-6. Hip extension is examined in the supine position. The lumbar spine is flattened and the pelvis is stabilized by flexion of the contralateral hip. A flexion contracture is seen in the patient's right hip.

HIP EXTENSION

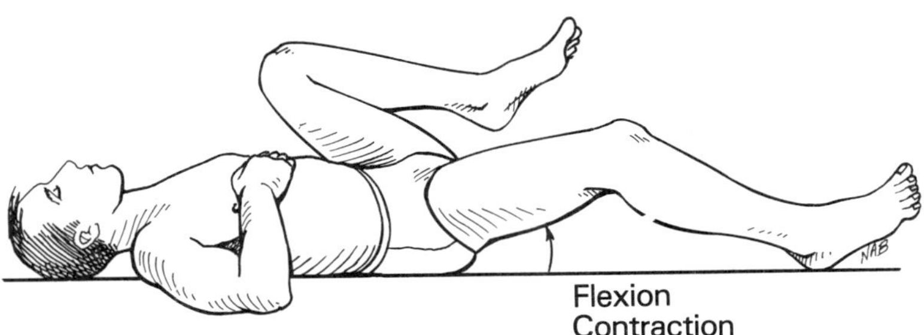

Figure 5-7. Examination of hip abduction and adduction.

(A) Demonstration of normal left hip abduction of 45 to 50 degrees. Note the trunk is stabilized by the examiner's forearm lying across the pelvis at the level of the anterior superior iliac spines.

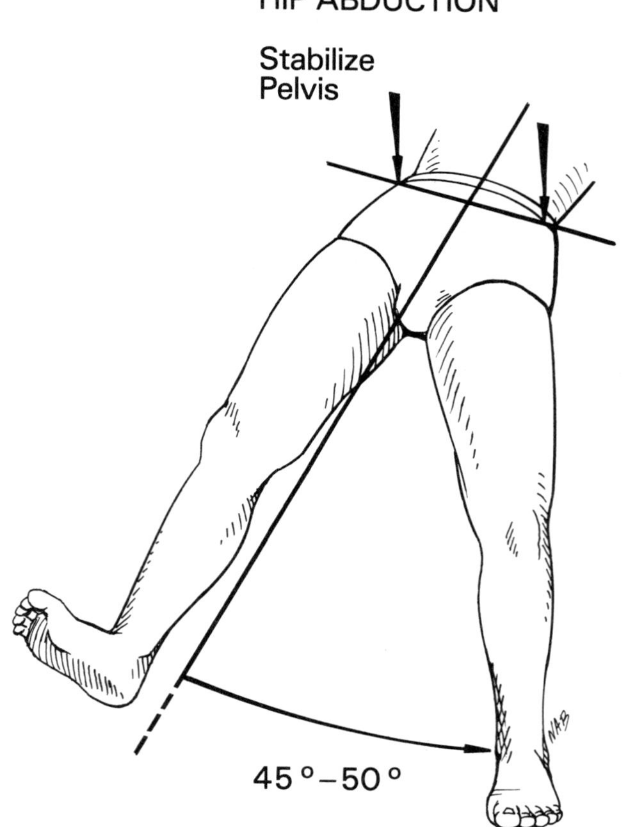

(B) Demonstration of normal left hip adduction of 20 to 30 degrees. Again, the pelvis should be stabilized with the examiner's arm.

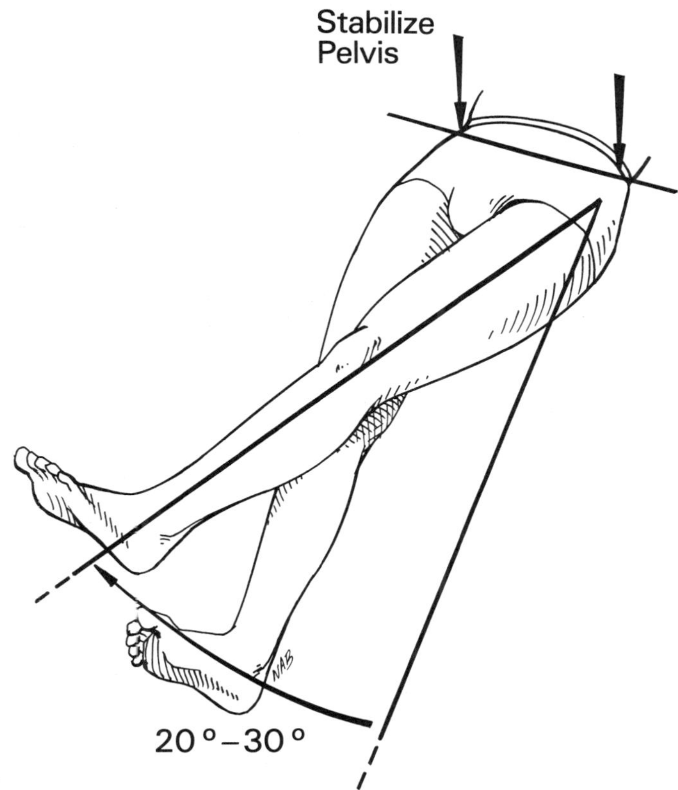

Internal and external rotation of the hip can be determined in either the flexed or extended position. The angular result can differ in certain pathologic conditions, depending on the position in which the measurement was obtained, and thus this should be recorded. Range of motion in extension is perhaps a more accurate assessment of functional limitation since the hip is normally in this position with ambulation. With the patient either supine, with knees flexed and hanging over the edge of the table, or lying prone with knees flexed, the extremity can be internally and externally rotated while the thigh is stabilized with the opposite hand and range of motion determined (see Fig. 5-8). Range of motion in flexion can similarly be determined with the patient either sitting or supine, with both the hips and knees flexed to 90 degrees. The normal limits of internal and external rotation vary from individual to individual but are approximately 35 and 45 degrees, respectively.

Active range of motion is probably best determined at the time of motor strength evaluation. Both active range of motion and strength of the hip flexor, extensor, abductor, adductor, and internal and external rotator groups can be assessed, following the guidelines for the neurologic examination of the lower extremity (see chapter 4).

RADIOGRAPHIC EVALUATION

Plain radiography, including an anterior-posterior view of the pelvis, and anterior-posterior and lateral views of the involved hip, serves as a good screening examination for most hip problems and is mandatory in cases of suspected hip trauma. Consideration should be directed towards assessment of general and local bone quality, femoral head sphericity, acetabular dysplasia, deformity of the proximal femur, presence of joint space narrowing, degenerative changes including osteophytes, and the presence of a fracture or other bone or soft tissue abnormality (e.g., tumor).

Standard or computer tomography is often useful in diagnosis and defining the pathologic anatomy of certain hip disorders. Not infrequently, nondisplaced fractures of the femoral neck can be visualized only with tomography when plain radiographs fail to reveal a fracture

Figure 5-8. Hip rotation in the sitting position. The thigh should be stabilized by the examiner's hand; the knee should be flexed and hang over the table.

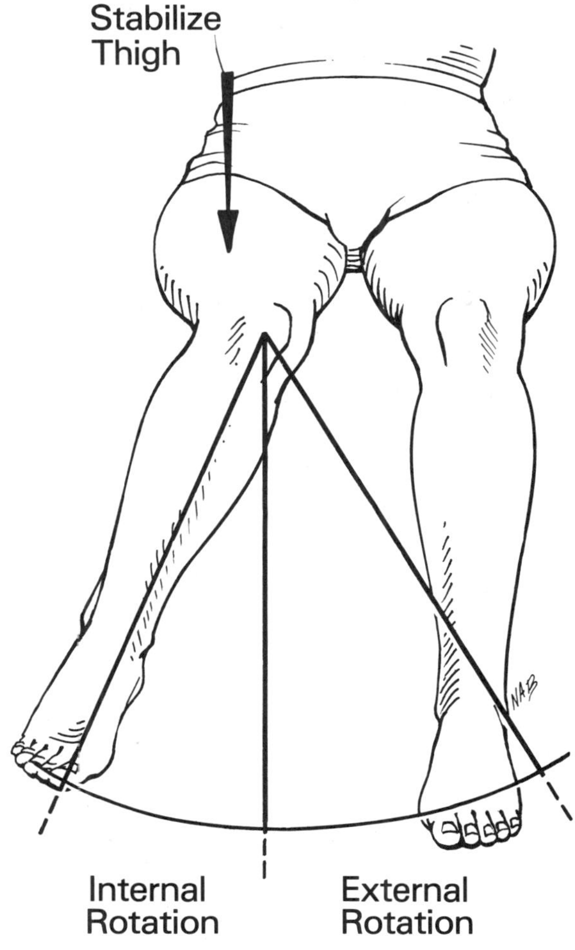

line. Obviously, the extent of tumorous masses or areas of subchondral collapse in cases of osteonecrosis can be more accurately defined with computed tomography than with plain radiographic techniques.

Radionuclide imaging techniques are valuable diagnostic tools in a variety of hip disorders. Technetium bone scanning can be useful in the evaluation of avascular necrosis, infection, implant loosening, and neoplastic conditions affecting the hip. Stress fractures, nondisplaced fractures of the femoral neck, and avascular necrosis secondary to previous trauma can also be evaluated with this technique. Gallium or indium scanning techniques are especially useful in evaluation of infection in the hip.

Magnetic resonance imaging has been very useful for evaluation and staging of both bone and soft tissue tumors. Soft tissue, intra-articular and epiphyseal extension, as well as marrow involvement, is detected most reliably with this technique when compared with the other commonly used imaging techniques. Magnetic resonance imaging is also the best modality in the diagnosis and staging of avascular necrosis.

Arthrography, which includes aspiration and synovial fluid culture, is an important diagnostic technique in cases of suspected infection. This technique is also essential in the evaluation of cases of suspected prosthetic loosening or infection.

SPECIFIC HIP DISORDERS

Fractures

Fractures of the hip can occur as a result of seemingly minor trauma in the elderly patient with osteopenia. Because of the tenuous vascular supply of the femoral head, it is important to distinguish between intracapsular femoral neck fractures and peritrochanteric fractures when considering treatment. In general, displaced fractures of the proximal femur will present with a history of trauma, pain in the area of the hip, and resultant inability to bear weight on the affected limb. Physical findings often include local swelling, tenderness and ecchymosis, a positive "roll test," and shortening and external rotation of the injured extremity.

The potential risk of avascular necrosis of the femoral head with displaced femoral neck fractures frequently warrants urgent orthopaedic intervention, especially in active, younger patients. Delay in treatment aimed at reestablishing vascularity to the femoral head, by open reduction and internal fixation of the fracture, has been associated with less favorable results. Elderly patients frequently have significant medical problems that affect operative mortality and should be expediently stabilized prior to surgery. In the older, less active patients with poor bone quality, excision of the displaced femoral head, which frequently develops late avascular necrosis, and hemiarthroplasty may be the most appropriate method of treatment. In certain instances, otherwise medically fit patients with premorbid arthritis of the hip joint who sustain fractures of the hip may be candidates for total hip arthroplasty (see chapter 10).

The primary care physician should also be aware of the not uncommon presentation of the impacted, non-displaced femoral neck fracture. This often occult injury can be associated with little more than mild hip pain and discomfort with full weight-bearing on the involved extremity. Plain radiographs frequently fail to demonstrate the fracture line and a high index of suspicion is necessary to make the diagnosis. Tomograms or a technetium bone scan done at 48 to 72 hours post-injury are valuable techniques for confirming the diagnosis. When properly identified, this fracture can be easily treated with multiple pin fixation. Failure to recognize this occult injury, however, can result in displacement of the fracture with a higher risk of avascular necrosis and a more lengthy and complicated surgical procedure.

Peritrochanteric fractures of the hip are associated with an insignificant incidence of avascular necrosis. As a result, these injuries require less emergent treatment than the femoral neck fractures. Stabilization with the current sliding hip screw devices, typically used to treat these fractures, allows for early mobilization of the patient with all of its resultant benefits. Problems with penetration of the screw into the hip joint by cutting out through osteopenic bone in the femoral head and development of localized bursitis over the prominent screw and side plate just below the greater trochanter can occur.

Stress fractures of the femoral neck and pubic rami occur in two distinctly different groups of patients: the active young patient and the elderly sedentary patient with osteoporosis. In the former, recurrent pain on exertion warrants evaluation for a possible stress fracture. Plain radiographs can fail to reveal the fracture in many instances; however, technetium bone scan reliably identifies the stress fracture in most patients.

Infection

Acute septic arthritis involving the hip is an orthopaedic emergency. Adults who develop joint sepsis frequently have an underlying medical condition that predisposes them to the development of septic arthritis. Predisposing factors include sources of extra-articular infection (e.g., urinary tract infection, pneumonia), chronic illness (e.g., diabetes mellitus, alcoholism), immunosuppressed states (e.g., malignancy or steroid or immunosuppressive therapy), or underlying joint pathology.

Patients with septic arthritis of the hip typically present with acute onset of swelling, tenderness, warmth, and irritability of the involved joint. The hip may be held in a flexed, externally rotated position to minimize pressure within the joint capsule. Fever is present in the majority of patients and blood cultures are positive in approximately 50% (see chapter 10).

Prolonged exposure of the articular cartilage to the proteolytic enzymes produced by the inflammatory response has a deleterious effect on cartilage matrix integrity and chondrocyte viability. While treatment of septic arthritis involving other more accessible joints is somewhat controversial, most will agree that adequate decompression of the septic hip is probably only achieved with surgical arthrotomy. The diagnosis is usually confirmed by aspiration and synovial fluid analysis which demonstrates a total leukocyte count of greater than 50,000 cells/mm and a differential count of greater than 80% polymorphonuclear leukocytes. Results can sometimes be equivocal since only 70% of patients with culture positive septic arthritis will have synovial fluid total leukocyte counts of greater than 50,000/mm.

Staphylococcus species are the most common agent causing septic arthritis; however, streptococcus species and gram negative organisms are also frequent pathogens. In younger, sexually active adults, gonococcal infections with the clinical presentation consisting of migratory polyarthritis, tenosynovitis, and typical cutaneous manifestations is not uncommon. Fortunately, involvement of the hip is not common, and the infection usually responds dramatically to appropriate antibiotic treatment.

Chronic low grade infections in and around the hip can be difficult to diagnose. Infrequently, low grade infections can present as a relatively rapid, progressive arthrosis of the hip. Often these infections occur around orthopaedic implants or prostheses, resulting in pain, bone destruction, and loosening of the device. Technetium, gallium, and indium imaging techniques have been helpful in establishing the diagnosis in these situations. Chronic infection often persists unless the implant is removed, the wound debrided, and the patient treated with an extended course of appropriate antibiotics. Treatment with oral antibiotics before establishment of the diagnosis is generally inadequate and hinders recovery of the infective organism and jeopardizes further treatment.

Because of problems with bone loss and difficulty in eradicating established infections around prosthetic implants, prevention and prompt recognition of periprosthetic infections is critical. Late prosthetic infections typically develop as a result of hematogenous seeding from a remote source of infection (e.g., urinary tract infection or febrile bacterial illness) or from a transient bacteremia at the time of dental, surgical, or other invasive manipulation (e.g., colonoscopy, esophagogastroduodenoscopy).

The primary care physician will frequently be performing diagnostic manipulative procedures on the gastrointestinal and genitourinary tracts in patients with implanted orthopaedic devices. In these circumstances, prophylactic antibiotic coverage is recommended for patients with orthopaedic implants, similar to the American Heart Association guidelines for patients with prosthetic heart valves. Early recognition and referral for aggressive treatment of acute periprosthetic infections may be associated with improved results, often not requiring removal of the implant to obtain resolution of the infection.

Arthritis

Arthritic involvement of the hip joint occurs frequently in the adult population and significantly affects the patient's quality of life. Destruction of the joint space can result from many diseases, including primary osteoarthritis, rheumatoid arthritis or its variants, post-traumatic arthritis, osteonecrosis, or secondary osteoarthritis in association with systemic disease (e.g., hemophilia, sickle cell hemoglobinopathy), congenital hip dysplasia, or remote sepsis. Symptoms include pain (generally perceived in the area of the groin and anterior thigh), stiffness, shortening or restriction of range of motion, and deformity associated with a variable degree of functional limitation. Pain may lessen somewhat with activity in early rheumatoid involvement; however, pain typically increases with activity and weight-bearing in osteoarthritis. Progression of arthrosis to the point of complete loss of the joint space, regardless of etiology, is often associated with development of night pain, rest pain, and significant functional limitation.

In general, treatment for most of these disorders is medical and aimed at slowing progression of the underlying disease and relief of pain. Nonsteroidal anti-inflammatory drugs have become the mainstay of management for the pain and inflammation associated with these disorders. Treatment of rheumatoid arthritis and its variants with steroids and other immunosuppressives can greatly slow the progression of joint destruction and deformity. Simple measures such as weight-loss, maintenance of general physical fitness, and activity modification, including use of a cane in the contralateral hand, can often help the patient's symptoms.

There are several instances in which early surgery may significantly delay progression of joint destruction. Young patients with early secondary osteoarthritis from underlying congenital acetabular dysplasia or deformity of the proximal femur are examples of this situation. In these patients, osteotomy of the pelvis or proximal femur may correct the anatomic abnormality responsible for development of the arthritis, and improve the hip biomechanics.

Patients with early stages of osteonecrosis or avascular necrosis of the femoral head may also benefit from early surgical management. In these patients, diagnosis requires a high index of suspicion, since early stages of the disease present with either absent or subtle radiographic findings. Radionuclide and magnetic resonance imaging techniques have been useful in establishing the diagnosis in these patients (see Fig. 5-9). Patients with a history of ethanol abuse, steroid treatment, previous trauma (especially dislocation of the hip or femoral neck fracture), contralateral hip osteonecrosis, and the collagen vascular diseases, as well as sickle cell and thalassemia diseases, are at risk for development of avascular necrosis. In nearly 25% of affected patients, however, the etiology remains idiopathic. In appropriately selected patients, surgery directed at removing the necrotic bone and reestablishing vascularity to the femoral head can prevent progression of the disease process.

Neoplasm

While primary malignancies of bone are uncommon in the adult, metastatic lesions of bone may occur in up to 60% of patients with cancer. The proximal femur and pelvis, including the acetabulum, are common sites for metastases to bone. More than 80% of all metastases to bone originate from primary malignancies of the breast, lung, prostate, thyroid, and kidney. Not infrequently, the primary site may be unknown and the metastasis may be the first lesion detected. The rate of metastasis to bone may be as high as 84% with cancer of the breast and prostate, 50% with thyroid cancer, and approximately 40% with lung and renal cancer. The orthopaedic surgeon is frequently requested to biopsy these lesions in order to establish a diagnosis and assist with further treatment.

Due to the high biomechanical stresses on the proximal femur, symptoms from pathologic fractures or impending fractures associated with metastatic lesions in the proximal femur are common. Frequently, these patients will require combined surgical and medical management. Surgical mortality, complication rate, and rehabilitation are improved if impending pathologic fractures are treated prophylactically. Depending on the location and character of the lesion, treatment can consist of

Figure 5-9. Avascular necrosis of the hip.

(A) X-ray of a patient whose right hip shows increased sclerosis and slight collapse of the superior articular surface of the hip.

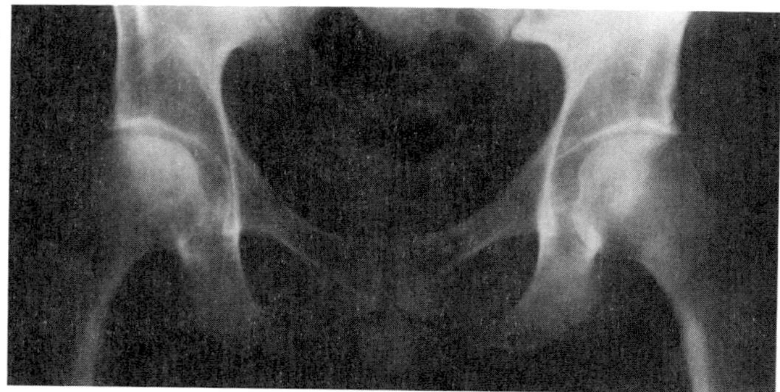

(B) The MRI examination of the same patient's hips showing approximately 50% involvement of the avascular necrosis in the right hip. The left hip in this patient was normal.

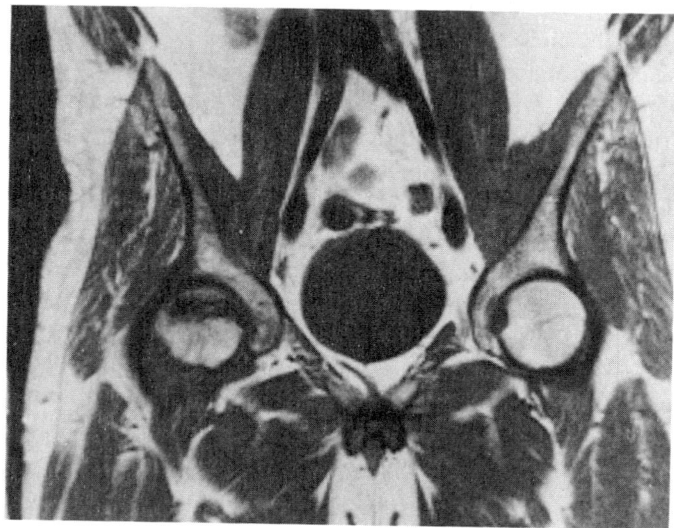

internal fixation and stabilization of the fracture or prosthetic replacement. Involvement of the chondral or subchondral surface of the acetabulum or femoral head with tumor generally necessitates total hip prosthetic replacement. Indications for prophylactic stabilization of metastatic lesions include lesions greater than 2.5 cm in diameter, involvement of more than 50% of the cortex of a long bone, pathologic avulsion of the lesser trochanter, and persistent pain despite irradiation. Patients with pathologic fractures will generally benefit from fracture treatment with regards to pain relief, mobility, and other quality of life concerns, irrespective of life expectancy. Rarely, soft tissue sarcomas or other lesions (e.g., pigmented villonodular synovitis) will present as a mass or painful lesion located in the area of the hip (see chapter 9).

Bursitis

As many as 15 separate bursae have been described about the hip. Distinct inflammatory syndromes are associated with three: the trochanteric, iliopsoas, and ischial bursae. Trochanteric bursitis is a relatively common disorder, presenting typically with gradual onset of pain over the lateral aspect of the greater trochanter and the proximal thigh. Symptoms are usually exacerbated by walking, stair climbing, and direct pressure from lying on the involved side. Diagnosis is usually confirmed by identification of point tenderness over the area of the greater trochanter. Abduction of the hip against resistance may also exacerbate pain. Inflammation around the site of muscular attachment of the gluteus medius and maximus, near the greater trochanter, may be responsible for or contribute to symptoms in some cases. Bursal or tendinous calcification may be seen radiographically in the area of the greater trochanter. Degenerative arthritis of the lumbar spine and hip, leg discrepancy, and repetitive trauma (e.g., running) may contribute to development of trochanteric bursitis. Injection of the involved area with local anesthetic and corticosteroid can be both diagnostic and therapeutic. Other measures, including nonsteroidal anti-inflammatory medications, local application of heat, and ultrasound, can be of benefit. Surgery is rarely indicated for treatment of trochanteric bursitis.

Enlargement or inflammation of the iliopsoas bursa (iliopectineal bursa) is a rare cause of pain or a mass around the hip. Because of its location, tenderness or swelling is located anterior to the hip joint and just lateral to the femoral vessels. Patients with iliopsoas bursitis may hold the hip in a flexed, externally rotated position, and limp to avoid hyperextension of the hip. Trauma or underlying osteoarthritis, rheumatoid arthritis, or other inflammatory condition of the hip may be associated with development of iliopsoas bursitis. Diagnosis is established by demonstration of the bursa by arthrography. Treatment consists of corticosteroid injection and other conservative measures. Surgical excision is rarely indicated and usually reserved for cases of recurrence.

Ischial bursitis, or "weaver's bottom," is also an unusual cause of pain around the hip. In most instances, a history of trauma or prolonged sitting on hard surfaces is present. Pain and point tenderness are usually well localized to the area of the ischial tuberosity. Local injection of corticosteroid and use of a cushion provide relief of symptoms.

Meralgia Paresthetica

Meralgia paresthetica results from entrapment and compression of the lateral femoral cutaneous nerve (L2-L3) at the level of the inguinal ligament, just medial to the anterior superior iliac spine. Symptoms consist of a characteristic burning pain with associated hypesthesia and occasional numbness over the proximal anterolateral thigh. Because the nerve is entirely sensory, neurologic deficit involves only this modality. Frequently, symptoms are exacerbated by extension or abduction of the extremity and prolonged standing or walking. Pain may be elicited by compression over the area of nerve entrapment. Associated conditions include diabetes, pregnancy, obesity, and local extrinsic compression (e.g., corset, belt, or tight pants). Treatment includes local corticosteroid injection, weight loss, and removal of any external compression over the area.

Bibliography

Berrettoni B.A. and Carter J.A.: Mechanisms of Cancer Metastasis to Bone. <u>J. Bone and Joint Surg.</u>, 1986; 68A:308-312.

Bywaters E.L: The Bursae of the Body. <u>Ann. Rheum. Dis.</u>, 1965; 24:215-218.

Cummings S.R., Rubin S.M., and Black D.: The Future of Hip Fractures in the United States. <u>Clin. Orthop.</u>, 1990; 252:163-166.

Goldenberg D.L. and Reed J.I.: Bacterial Arthritis. <u>N. Engl. J. Med.</u>, 1985; 312:764-771.

Green N.E.: <u>Disseminated Gonococcal Infections and Gonococcal Arthritis</u>. A.A.O.S. Instructional Course Lectures Number XXXII. St. Louis, MO: C.V. Mosby, 1983.

Harrington K.D.: Impending Pathologic Fractures from Metastatic Malignancy: Evaluation and Management. In Anderson L.D. (ed): A.A.O.S. Instructional Course Lectures. Volume XXXV. St. Louis, MO: C.V. Mosby, 1986.

Hoppenfeld S.: <u>Physical Examination of the Spine and Extremities</u>. Norwalk, CT: Appleton-Century-Crofts, 1976.

Kenzora J.E., McCarthy R.E., Lowell J.D., and Sledge C.B.: Hip Fracture Mortality-Relation to Age, Treatment, Preoperative Illness, Time of Surgery, and Complications. <u>Clin. Orthop.</u>, 1984; 186:45-55.

Krey P.R. and Bailen D.A.: Synovial Fluid Leukocytosis - A Study of Extremes. <u>Am. J. Med.</u>, 1979; 67:436.

Simon M.A. and Karluk M.B.: Skeletal Metastases of Unknown Origin. <u>Clin. Orthop.</u>, 1982; 166:96-103.

Swiontkowski M.F., Winquist R.A., and Hansen S.T.: Fractures of the Femoral Neck in Patients Between the Ages of Twelve and Forty-nine Years. <u>J. Bone and Joint Surg.</u>, 1984; 66A:837-846.

Thrall J.H. and Ellis B.I.: Skeletal Metastases. <u>Radiol. Clin. North Am.</u>, 1987; 25:1155-1170.

White B.L., Fisher W.D., and Laurin C.A.: Rate of Mortality for Elderly Patients after Fracture of the Hip in the 1980's. <u>J. Bone and Joint Surg.</u>, 1987; 69A:1335-1340.

Wilson P.D. and Gordon S.L. (ed): NIH Concensus Development Conference - Total Hip Joint Replacement. <u>J. Arthroplasty</u>, 1983; 1:189-234.

6

THE KNEE

By Donald B. Goodfellow, M.D.

The knee is the largest and most complex joint in the human body; consequently, the investigations of injury and disease processes affecting the knees pose subtle complexities to even the most experienced examiner.

While a detailed discussion of the anatomy of the knee is outside the focus of this text, there are a number of anatomic factors that help to explain the vulnerability of this joint to both disease and injury processes (see Fig. 6-1). Possessing the largest surface area of articular cartilage, as well as synovium, the knee joint is quite susceptible to diseases primarily affecting these structures. Many factors are responsible for making the knee the most vulnerable of the weightbearing joints to either repetitive or incidental trauma. The complicated internal structure of ligaments, meniscal cartilage and the differential radiuses of the medial and lateral femoral condyles lead to a complex array of motions involving rocking, rotation, and gliding, making the concept of the knee as a simple hinge overly simplistic. Situated between the largest (femur and tibia) and strongest (quadriceps, hamstrings and gastrosoleus) lever systems in the body, the skeletal architecture provides very little intrinsic restraint, causing the knee to rely almost exclusively on its sophisticated arrangement of ligaments to provide stability against intrinsic and extrinsic forces. It is protected by relatively thin layers of soft tissue, exposing it to direct trauma as well. The more familiar the examiner becomes with the structure and function of the knee, the more precise and accurate he will be with his evaluation.

Figure 6-1. Anterior view of the right knee.

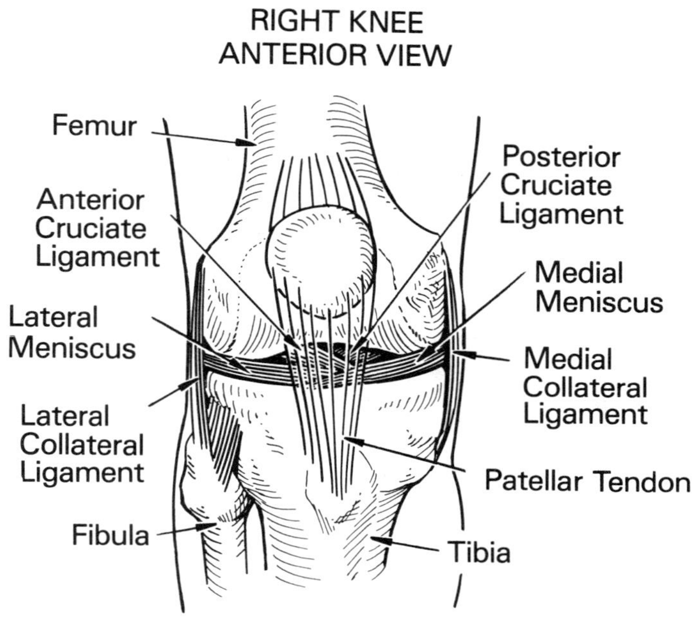

HISTORY

Without a thorough history, the evaluation of the knee has no beginning and could conceivably seem endless; its importance is paramount. The trick is to be thorough yet efficient, obtaining the most information in the least amount of time by artfully limiting extraneous information, but gleaning even the most minute of important details. In obtaining the history of a disease process, a different line of questioning is generally required, as opposed to that of an injury. A more thorough evaluation of past medical and family history, as well as a detailed review of systems in association with other disease processes and other joint involvement, becomes quite important. One must remember, however, that it is almost human nature to try to assign the onset of an affliction to even the most minor of traumas. It is the purview of the examiner to obtain enough information to assign an appropriate amount of significance to such an event.

In contrast, obtaining information regarding the mechanism of how an injury occurs is critical. The direction and magnitude of the force applied, the weightbearing status of the limb at the time of the injury, whether this occurred with or without contact, and other associated injuries are of major importance. In the case of recurring injuries, the activities with which these episodes occur and certainly any past surgical history further helps to delineate the pathology.

Armed only with the age and sex of the patient, the seasoned examiner can make some assumptions that would limit the probability of problems. For instance, the young adolescent male presenting with knee problems is most commonly affected by either Osgood-Schlatter's disease or, less likely, a discoid meniscus or osteochondritis dissecans, whereas the young adult female is most likely to present with patellofemoral problems. However, one cannot be overly prejudicial in this regard as further information is obtained. Specific questions regarding which knee, whether other joints are involved, and whether they occurred in an acute or chronic situation by sudden or insidious onset should be obtained straightaway.

The patient will generally present with one of three complaints: pain, loss of function, or swelling. Rarely a patient will be seen whose only complaint is that of crepitus or noise within the joint.

When pain is a presenting complaint, it should be kept in mind that there are only a few sources of pain within the joint. The primary source of pain is the synovial membrane. This can be an intrinsic problem, such as the hypertrophic tissue characteristic of rheumatoid arthritis or, secondary to that caused by injuries or those that stimulate the synovium, such as infection or pseudogout. The other major source of pain is any kind of tension situation within the synovial cavity or other soft tissue, which causes stimulation of nerve endings. Examples of this are a hemarthrosis which causes tension within the joint, or a partial rupture of the medial collateral ligament, which is often much more painful than a complete rupture.

The nature and site of the pain must be determined. Was its onset insidious or acute; related to activity or occurring at rest; is it intermittent or constant; does it occur at any particular time during the day? Affirmative answers to these questions can lead to a specific diagnosis, which should be correlated with the physical examination and ancillary studies. It is well-known, for example, that an intense aching pain that occurs primarily at night may be related to an osteoid osteoma. The patient's perception of the site of pain is also of diagnostic importance. A generalized discomfort is more likely to be caused by a disease process, whereas localized pain is more likely due to an injury. Once again, a correlation with the physical examination is important. This is particularly true when the patient relates the pain as being in the anterior distal thigh, as this presentation often masquerades for problems related primarily to hip pathology.

Loss of function can present as either stiffness, insecurity, or limitation of motion. Stiffness is defined as a resistance to motion. It can occur because of swelling within the joint itself or within the soft tissue surrounding the joint. One must keep in mind that there is a normal physiologic variation of stiffness that occurs primarily at the beginning and towards the end of the day. The degree and duration are of importance. Classically, in patients with rheumatoid arthritis, it can take as long as two to three hours in the morning to begin to lose the feeling of stiffness in early affected joints. When involving the joint itself, it is commonly felt that this is due to a breakdown in the lubrication system, due to aging or damage to the articular cartilage. It can also occur in edematous tissues such as diseased synovium, or injured muscle-tendon units.

Insecurity can be manifested in terms of giving way, locking, or shifting. Giving way can be a manifestation of muscle weakness, or more commonly the interposition of a small fragment of meniscal or articular cartilage between the joint surfaces while they are under stress. True locking, on the other hand, occurs when a larger fragment meniscus such as a bucket-handle tear, or a large osteochondritis dissecans fragment, becomes truly wedged in the joint, acting as a painful block, usually to extension. This term needs to be delineated from the more common sensation of catching or stiffness. Catching can generally occur when opposing surfaces of articular cartilage under stress are irregular, such as occurs in chondromalacia. Stiffness, on the other hand, is something that does not usually abruptly change, as does true locking. Shifting is a manifestation of subluxation of either the patella or the knee joint itself. It occurs as a sudden aberrant motion within the joint. It suggests significant ligamentous or patellar instability. The patient will frequently state that they felt the knee or kneecap "go out of place."

Limitation of motion is not a common chief complaint. However, it can occur in conjunction with complaints of locking or swelling. The gradual loss of motion that occurs with aging is often unrecognized by the patient due to its insidious nature. Range of motion from 10 degrees to 90 degrees allows the majority of activities of daily living to be performed with minimal disability.

Although usually associated with pain, sometimes the presence of swelling alone will constitute the primary complaint of the patient. The swelling can be generalized or local, involve the joint cavity, or surrounding soft tissues. It can occur suddenly after an injury, usually within the first two to six hours, indicating a hemarthrosis, or can occur on a more insidious basis, indicating a synovial effusion within the joint. Localized swelling can be due to direct trauma, such as a hematoma, overuse syndrome, such as tendinitis or bursitis, or as the result of a tumor or infection. Specific swelling in the back of the knee usually constitutes a Baker's cyst, which was first described as a tuberculous infection of the semimembranosus, gastroc-soleus bursa. This will be described in more detail under the specific problems at the end of the chapter.

Crepitus alone is a rare presenting complaint. In most circumstances, it is related to patellofemoral problems, but in certain circumstances can represent a physiologic process, similar to that of cracking your knuckles. On rare occasions, a snapping can occur as an irritation, particularly of the iliotibial band. Hearing or sensing a pop which occurs at the time of an injury makes one suspicious of a ligamentous injury.

Once again, the importance of history is to help direct the physical examination, which must then correlate with the known information. It can help to limit the probabilities, but does not limit the possibilities.

PHYSICAL EXAMINATION

Just as the history should not be a tedious endeavor, the physical examination should also be an efficient investigation. Armed with the knowledge of the history, one should have a general understanding of what to expect on the physical examination, but certainly should not be surprised by the unexpected. A complete examination of the knee is often not necessary, provided the physical examination confirms a specific diagnosis suspected following the history. If, however, one is unable to do this on a brief, but thorough, evaluation, then further investigations and testing may be necessary. As in all circumstances, the knee joint cannot be isolated in the examination. The associated joints, nerves, muscles, connective tissues, etc. must all be evaluated as well. The examination should progress through a series of observations, palpations, and manipulations. In most circumstances, particularly those involving an injury,you are generally fortunate enough to be able to evaluate an uninjured or uninvolved knee first to obtain knowledge of the individual's physiologic variations.

Observations

Observations should begin with an assessment of the overall alignment of the lower extremity, as it compares to the unaffected or uninvolved side. This must be observed in relationship to the hip, foot, and ankle (see Fig. 6-2). Any hyperextension or flexion deformity should also be noted, along with any rotational abnormalities, such as intoeing, outtoeing, or "squinting" of the patella (see Fig. 6-3). Similarly, the alignment of the patella in relationship to the joint line (i.e., either patella alta or patella infera) should be noted, as well as the attachment site of the patellar tendon (i.e., the tibial tubercle) in relationship to the overall alignment of the leg.

Gait

Normally, the knee comes to full extension only at heel strike. During stance phase, slight flexion occurs and the quadriceps must contract at this point to prevent giving way. At toe off, the knee flexes to about 40 degrees and continues to flex through midswing to approximately 65 degrees. The quadriceps then contracts to begin acceleration of the leg, with the knee returning to full extension once again at heel strike. The hamstrings must contract just prior to heel strike to decelerate the leg and prevent hyperextension of the knee at heel strike. The stride length of each leg should be equal and the patient should spend approximately equal time on each leg during the stance phase.

Figure 6-2. Lower extremity deformities.

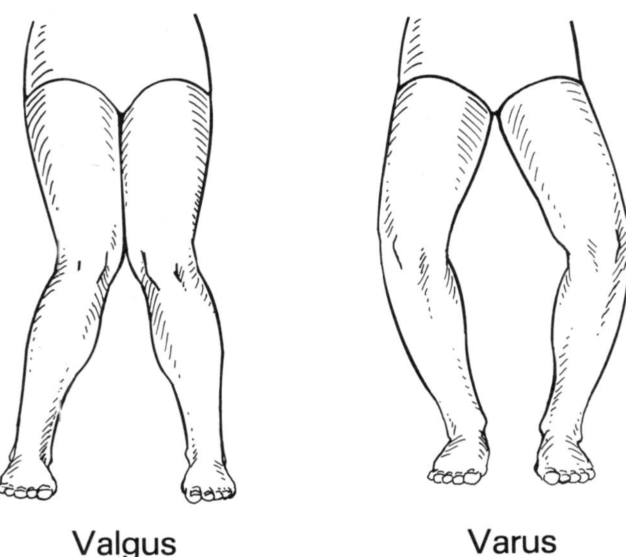

Figure 6-3. Extensor malalignment. Pronation, external tibial torsion, abnormal Q-angle, and femoral anteversion are shown.

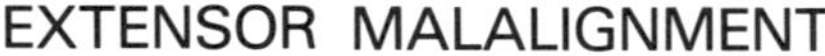

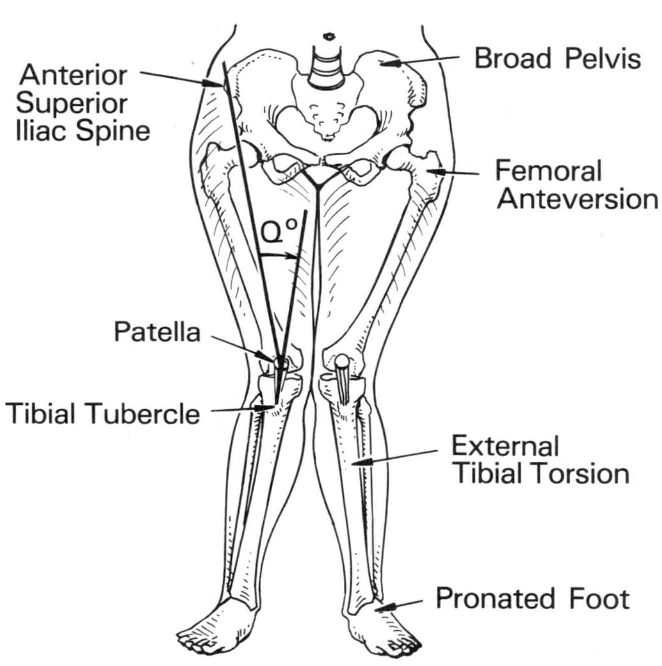

Abnormalities in gait pattern can occur for a number of different reasons. Weak quadriceps can manifest as a hard heel strike with excessive hip extension and rotation to force the knee into a hyperextended position to prevent buckling. Alternatively, the patient may use his hand to force the thigh into an extended position to stabilize the knee, or walk with an extreme back knee gait to keep the knee in full extension. Weak hamstrings do not decelerate the knee properly and result in a hyperextension at heel strike. Ligamentous instability can result in either a varus or valgus thrust, or an insecurity due to buckling or shifting within the joint. Pain within the knee joint usually presents itself as an antalgic gait, which means that the patient spends less time in stance phase on that leg compared to the opposite. This also usually manifests itself as a shortened stride on the unaffected side.

Functional tests such as squatting, duck walking, hopping, stair climbing, running in place, and observation during sporting activities are usually not required to establish specific diagnoses, and are usually left for assessments regarding return to activity following treatment.

Continued observation should now be focused on the knee itself, assessing any generalized or localized swelling, the presence of ecchymosis, erythema, abrasions, or other skin manifestations of injury or disease. Any obvious muscular atrophy or defects within the muscles should be noted as well.

Range of Motion

Both active and passive range of motions of the knee should be noted. The anatomically neutral position of the knee occurs when the femur and tibia are in a straight, fully extended position. Positive degrees of motion are measured for flexion and negative degrees of motion are used to describe hyperextension of the knee (see Figure 6-4). Normal values would be 140 degrees of flexion and as much as 5 degrees to 10 degrees of hyperextension. However, there can be a significant amount of normal variation and it is, therefore, important to compare the involved and uninvolved sides. If there is significant bilateral hyperextension, the patient should also be checked for generalized ligamentous laxity. It is generally best to check active extension with the patient in a sitting position, and any difference between the active and passive extension should be noted as an extension lag.

A decrease or absence of active extension is seen in partial and complete rupture of the quadriceps mechanism. In the supine position, while supporting both heels, any tendency to hyperextension on the involved side should be considered as a posterior sag, and is often indicative of posterior cruciate ligament injuries. While in the supine position with the hip flexed to 90 degrees, the knee should be extended to examine the flexibility of the hamstrings. Normally, one would expect to achieve full extension of the knee and often in very lax individuals such as dancers or gymnasts, further flexion of the hip is obtainable even with the knee in full extension. In the prone position with only the trunk and thighs supported and the rest of the lower extremity hanging over the end of the bed, one can check for subtle loss of extension by a difference in heel height between the two extremities. In this position, one can also check for quadriceps contraction by passively flexing the knee as far as possible, keeping the hip in full extension.

There are a number of causes for a decrease in range of motion. The most common is that of swelling within the joint, either by an effusion or a hemarthrosis. A mechanical block such as a bucket-handle tear of the meniscus or loose body in the joint can adversely affect the range of motion. A subtle loss due to the advancement of osteoarthritic spurs can occur with primarily a loss of full extension and subtle degrees of loss of flexion. As the osteoarthritis advances, range of motion can continue to deteriorate. Soft tissue swelling or pain such as occurs in

Figure 6-4. Measurement of knee range of motion. Any hyperextension is measured in negative degrees. Normal range is -5 degrees to 140 degrees but should always be compared with the opposite extremity.

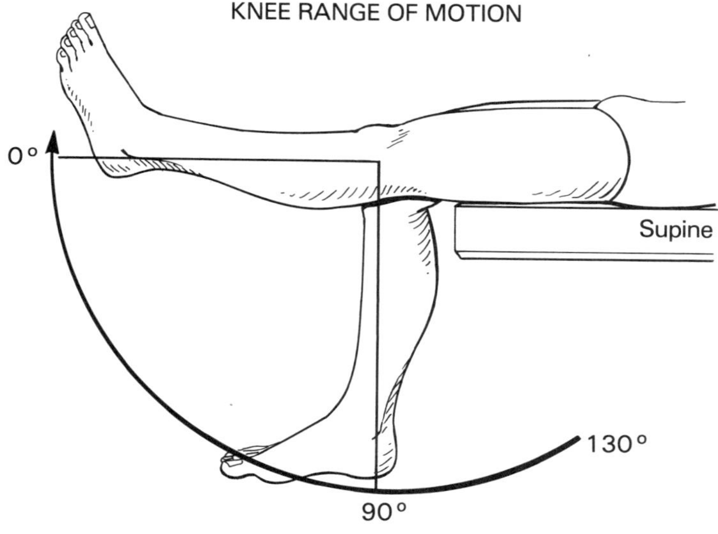

rheumatoid arthritis or damaged ligaments will also produce muscle spasm, limiting the range of motion. The synovitis associated with either infective or crystalline diseases will often produce a restriction of motion, which is out of proportion to what one would expect from simply the swelling alone. Obviously, fractures and significant ligamentous disruptions may allow abnormally increased range of motions often in abnormal directions.

Although the vast majority of motion occurs with extension and flexion, the knee does possess the ability to rotate both internally and externally. Ten degrees of rotation in either direction is generally felt to represent a normal range and abnormal increases will generally represent severe ligamentous damage.

Palpation

A general assessment of the temperature of the knee, both in the generalized and localized fashion, should be compared to the uninvolved knee. Although this has little diagnostic significance by itself, it may allow the examiner the opportunity to localize specific areas of damage.

Effusion

In the presence of a large effusion, the generalized swelling is usually obvious. The classic sign of a ballottable patella is almost certainly present but often superfluous. However, in the assessment of small effusion, the test using a ballottable patella is often inaccurate and misleading. In an attempt to force the fluid out of the suprapatellar pouch, the patella is often forced in a distal direction, entrapping the anterior fat pad and giving the erroneous impression of a ballottable patella. A more accurate assessment can be obtained by placing one hand over the suprapatellar pouch, gently forcing the fluid into the peripatellar areas distally. With the opposite hand placed with the fingers and thumb on opposite sides of the patella, and alternatively tapping and squeezing, a fluid wave is created and can be palpated as a thrill or rebound phenomenon by the opposite digits (see Figure 6-5).

Figure 6-5. Testing for a small knee effusion. Placing one hand over the suprapatellar pouch, without forcing the patella distally, excess fluid is forced into the peripatellar areas. With the opposite hand alternately tapping, or squeezing produces a fluid wave or thrill.

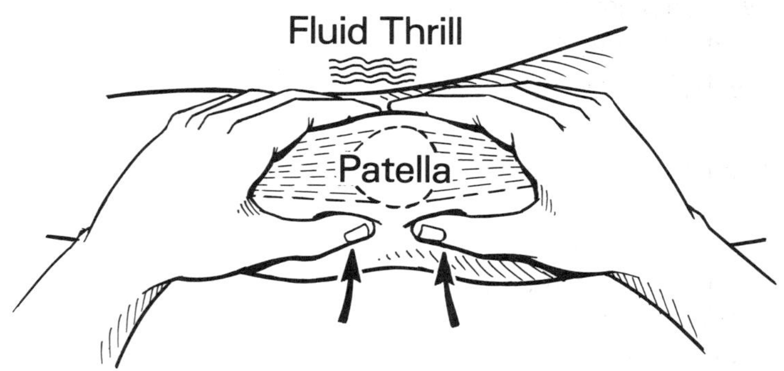

Although it is often difficult to distinguish synovial thickening from a small or moderate effusion, a sensation of bogginess or lumpiness within the joint is more indicative of synovial thickening, as opposed to a smooth appearance seen with an effusion.

Crepitus

Crepitus can be either felt or heard. It is most common to find this over the patellofemoral joint as a representation of articular cartilage degeneration. Occasionally, a thickened synovial plica can create a similar sensation. The presence of crepitus in the patellofemoral joint is not always of significance, unless it is accompanied by other painful palpations. It should be noted that approximately 50% of patients over the age of 50 years will have asymptomatic patellofemoral crepitus. Crepitus along the joint lines again can represent either localized synovial thickening, unstable meniscal fragments, or degenerative articular cartilage.

Tenderness

Generalized tenderness is commonly associated with disease processes, whereas localized tenderness signals the site of damage. This is where a precise knowledge of the surface anatomy of the knee is of utmost importance in distinguishing different diagnoses. A difference as small as 1 centimeter can mean the difference between a correct and incorrect diagnosis. For example, pain along the medial joint line just posterior to the medial collateral ligament is most commonly associated with a tear of the posterior horn of the medial meniscus. However, just anterior and superior to this area is the attachment point for the medial collateral ligament, commonly the site of injury to the medial collateral ligament. Palpation of the knee in all four quadrants should be routinely carried out.

Anterior Quadrant Palpation

An assessment of the tone and bulk of the quadriceps, along with any palpable defects as seen in a quadriceps rupture, should be noted. In particular, assessment of the vastus medialis is important when assessing the function of the patellofemoral joint. While palpation of the inferior surfaces of the patella can be carried out with alternately medial and lateral subluxations, intervening synovial tissue can make the interpretation of the findings somewhat dubious. However, the finding of tenderness at either the proximal or distal pole of the patella is suggestive of quadriceps or patellar tendinitis respectively. The presence of tenderness at the tibial tubercle (the distal insertion of the patellar tendon) in an adolescent is indicative of Osgood-Schlatter's disease. In the adult, it is most commonly associated with a sequela of Osgood-Schlatter's disease, which is an ununited loose ossicle. Thickening or swelling within the prepatellar bursa is indicative of prepatellar bursitis commonly seen in patients who spend a significant amount of time "walking" on their knees (roofers and other construction workers). Tenderness to palpation on either side of the patellar tendon in the area of the fat pad is indicative of an impingement of the fat pad, most frequently seen in adolescent females. Palpating along the medial border of the patella, over the medial femoral condyle, one will often find a small band of tissue representing the medial plica. If this is painful and simulates the symptoms of the patient, this is consistent with a medial plica syndrome.

Medial Quadrant Palpation

Palpation of the medial meniscus attachment and its adjacent synovium is performed along the medial joint line. Tears of the posteromedial portion of the medial meniscus are the most frequently found at surgery consistent with the most common finding of tenderness at the posteromedial corner of the knee joint. Palpation along the midtibial region medially represents the broad insertion of the medial collateral ligament distally. The femoral epicondyle represents its proximal insertion site. Local tenderness is indicative of damage to the structure, and it should also be palpated during the ligamentous exam to determine any laxities within the ligament itself. Just medial to the tibial tubercle and along the proximal flare of the medial tibial condyle is the insertion of the pes anserinus. There is a large underlying bursa in this area, which is commonly involved in overuse syndromes seen in runners and swimmers, particularly those that perform breast stroke. This represents the insertion of the sartorius, gracilis, and semitendinosus tendons.

Lateral Quadrant Palpation

The lateral joint line also represents the attachment of the lateral meniscus, and tenderness here is most commonly found in the middle region of the lateral joint. Assessment of the lateral collateral ligament with its attachment at the fibular head and lateral epicondyle of the femur can be best performed with the knee in a figure-of-four position (with the ipsilateral ankle crossed over the contralateral thigh) where the ligament can be palpated as a tight cord approximately the size of a pencil. Attaching just posterior on the fibular head and extending proximally, the bicipital tendon can also be palpated for both thickening and tenderness, indicative of a tendinitis. The iliotibial band should be assessed for tenderness, both as it crosses the lateral epicondyle of the femur and at its insertion point on Gerdy's tubercle of the tibia. Snapping or tenderness that occurs at the lateral epicondyle is generally accompanied by a tight iliotibial band, causing an overuse friction syndrome. Gentle tapping over the area of the common peroneal nerve as it wraps around the fibula, approximately 3 to 4 cm distal to the proximal tip, should be assessed for any positive Tinel's signs indicative of nerve damage. Although an uncommon site of injury, the proximal tibiofibular joint should also be assessed for stability and pain, particularly in patients with intermittent peroneal nerve paresthesias.

Posterior Quadrant Palpation

The posterior fossa is a diamond-shaped structure, bounded by the hamstring tendons proximally and the two heads of the gastrocnemius distally. Within it runs the posterior tibial nerve, and popliteal artery and vein. Assessment of the popliteal pulse is best done with the knee in 90 degrees of flexion and with the hamstrings an calf muscles relaxed. Both heads of the gastrocnemius muscle should be palpated for tears and defects. The medial head just proximal to its insertion into the tendon is a common site for injury, particularly in runners and tennis players. A cystic swelling within the fossa, commonly known as a Baker's cyst, can act as a reservoir for joint fluid. Approximately 50% of Baker's cysts readily communicate with the joint. The cyst is an enlargement of the normal gastroc-semimembranosus bursa, which can be present and asymptomatic in adolescents or indicative of recurrent effusions in adults.

Manipulation

Ligamentous Examination

Assessing the knee for ligamentous instability can be challenging for even the most experienced examiner, particularly if complex injuries are involved. No amount of reading can substitute for the careful observation of an experienced examiner and the repetitive performance of these manipulations under a critical eye. In the acute situation where pain and spasm are present, the examination can be most difficult. However, by placing the patient in a relaxed position and with a gentle careful examination, a diagnosis can most often be made.

In situations such as team physician's face, where the mechanism of injury is observed and the patient can be evaluated immediately before pain and secondary muscle spasm occurs, the assessment of the ligaments is much easier. It should also be remembered, however, that during exercise the ligaments of the knee undergo a normal increase in physiologic laxity and, once again, evaluation of the uninjured opposite leg is extremely important. Re-evaluation of the patient on several occasions is also helpful in determining the extent of damage.

The prerequisite of having the patient in a relaxed position cannot be overemphasized. It is also quite helpful to evaluate the uninjured knee first, so that the patient has an understanding of what manipulations are going to be performed. It is often best to save any painful manipulations to the very end of the examination, since they will often elicit involuntary guarding of the knee.

Collateral Ligaments

With the patient lying in the supine position on the table and the examiner facing the patient from the side, the ankle is secured in the ipsilateral axilla of the examiner. To test for medial collateral ligament function, the fingers of the ipsilateral hand are placed along the medial joint line of the knee. The thenar eminence of the opposite hand is then placed against the fibula head. A valgus force is applied by pushing medially against the knee from the lateral side as a lateral force is produced on the ankle. The degree of opening produced by this maneuver should be noted with the knee near full extension, as well as flexed at approximately 30 degrees (see Fig. 6-6). Any perceived difference between the uninjured and injured knee suggest injury to the medial collateral ligament. In addition, if this instability is perceived with the knee near full extension, damage to one or both of the cruciate ligaments should also be suspected.

To test for injury to the lateral collateral ligament, the positions of the hands should be reversed with the ipsilateral hand of the examiner placed along the medial flare of the tibia and the opposite hand placed

Figure 6-6. Assessment of collateral ligament stability. Applying a valgus stress to the knee, the degree of opening on the medial side can be measured. To assess lateral stability, a varus stress is applied while palpating lateral opening.

KNEE EXAMINATION
MEDIAL COLLATERAL LIGAMENT

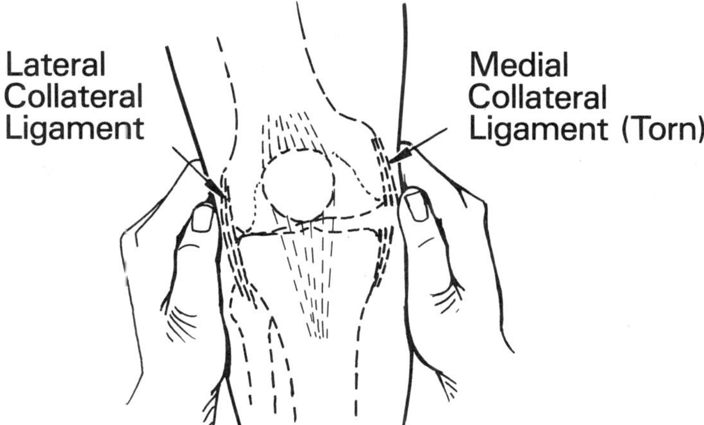

along the lateral joint line, palpating the area of the lateral collateral ligament. This time a varus stress is produced by pushing laterally against the knee from medially with a medial force against the ankle. Once again, the amount of gapping that occurs on the lateral joint line should be noted and compared with the opposite knee.

Cruciate Ligaments

The intracapsular ligaments of the knee are the primary restraints to anterior and posterior subluxation of the tibia on the femur. They are often the most difficult to assess but are also the most crucial in determining the treatment of isolated or combined injuries to ligaments of the knee.

There are any number of tests that have been described to determine the integrity of the anterior cruciate ligament, most of which, including the anterior drawer sign, are difficult, if not impossible, to perform in the face of an acute injury with a hemarthrosis. The Lachman test is by far the most specific and sensitive test for the integrity of the anterior cruciate ligament (see Fig. 6-7). By placing the palm of the hand underneath the calf of the leg, the knee is flexed to approximately 20 degrees to 30 degrees.   Care must be taken to avoid any excessive external rotation of the leg. The leg should be in as much rotation as the opposite leg in a relaxed position. The index finger and thumb of the opposite hand are then placed over the anterior joint line and an anteriorly directed force is applied to the calf. Any motion that can be perceived between the femur and tibia indicates a positive examination and, in almost all circumstances, represents damage to the anterior cruciate ligament.

Figure 6-7. The Lachman test. With the knee flexed to 30 degrees, anterior force is applied to the proximal tibia. Any perceived motion between the tibia and femur is a positive test.

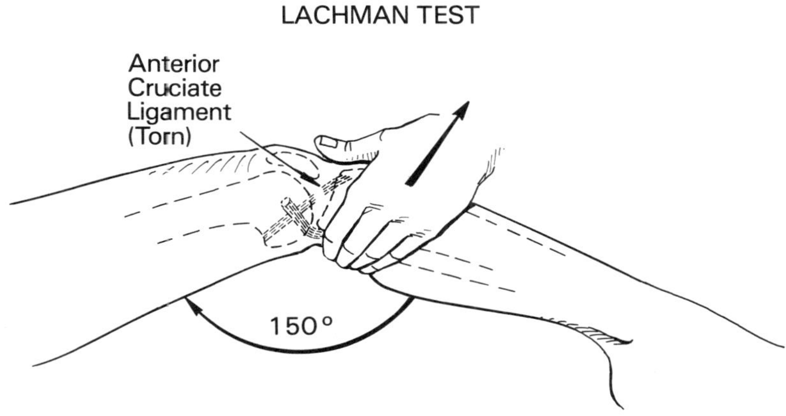

A number of other tests, including the Slocum, pivot shift, jerk, and flexion rotation drawer tests, are almost impossible to perform in an acute situation without adequate anesthesia and are extremely examiner-dependent and are, therefore, not very reliable tests. They are best performed either under anesthesia, or in a chronic situation by an extremely experienced examiner.

To examine the posterior cruciate ligament's integrity, first observe any tendency towards excessive hyperextension or varus of the involved knee compared with the opposite knee, while simultaneously lifting both heels off the bed with the knees in full extension and the patient in a supine position. Next, have the patient flex both knees to 90 degrees and, from the side, observe any tendency towards a posterior sag or loss of the normal contour of the anterior tibia in relation to the opposite knee (see Fig. 6-8). In particular, look for a loss of the prominence of the tibial tubercle in comparison with the opposite knee. While the patient remains in this position, the examiner should stabilize the foot by gently sitting on it. The examiner's hands are then wrapped around the knee

Figure 6-8. Posterior drawer test. With the knee flexed to 90 degrees, the amount of posterior displacement of the proximal tibia in relation to the femoral condyles is measured. This should be compared with the opposite knee.

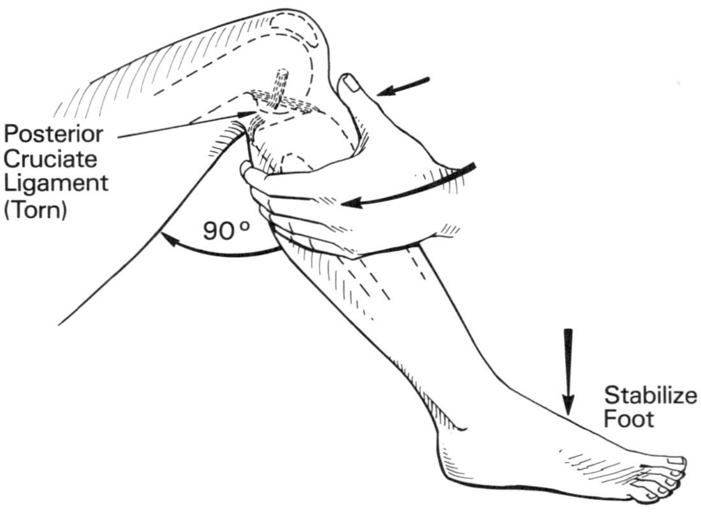

with the thumbs placed over the anterior joint line, both medially and laterally, while the fingers palpate the tendons of the hamstrings and biceps to insure their relaxation. The examiner should first note the position of the anterior surfaces of both the medial and lateral tibial plateaus in relationship to the femoral condyles. In a normal situation, there will be a one-centimeter drop-off on both the medial and lateral sides with the tibia, being more prominent. A straight posterior force is then applied to the tibia and a discrete endpoint should be obtained in a normal situation. In an abnormal situation, the tibia will move posteriorly, and the degree of posterior displacement should be noted in relationship to the femoral condyles. If there is no discrete endpoint, this should also be noted. Similarly, an anterior displaced force on the back of the tibia can be performed, while again noting the degree of displacement in relationship to the femoral condyles. This represents the posterior and anterior drawer test. The posterior drawer is quite accurate for diagnosing damage to the posterior cruciate ligament; however, the anterior drawer test can be quite inaccurate in an acute situation due to muscle spasm. Additionally, any tendency to internal or external rotation of the tibia while performing these tests should be noted. Any differential between the amount of dropback on the medial or lateral side of the joint can indicate damage to the structures supporting the posteromedial and lateral corners of the joint (i.e., the arcuate ligament complex laterally and the posterior oblique and semimembranosus medially).

Once again, it is extremely important to compare the uninvolved with the involved side for all tests of ligamentous instability. Any perceived difference in any of the examinations of the knee indicate significant damage to the primary restraint against that motion. That is to say, that a "mildly positive" Lachman test indicates damage to the anterior cruciate ligament while a grossly positive Lachman test indicates not only damage to the anterior cruciate ligament, but most likely damage to some of the secondary restraints to anterior instability as well.

Meniscal Signs

A number of rotational tests have been described in an effort to help diagnose derangements of the medial and lateral meniscal cartilages. The intent of all these tests is to trap an abnormally mobile or torn meniscal fragment between the femoral and tibial condyles, producing either pain as the fragment is being entrapped or a small pop along the appropriate joint line as the fragment is released from its entrapment. The two most common tests are the McMurray's test and the Apley compression and distraction test. McMurray's test (see Fig. 6-9) was originally described in an effort to diagnose tears of the posterior horns of either the medial or lateral meniscus. To perform this test, the patient is asked to lie in a supine position on the examining table. The examiner cups the heel in the palm of one hand, while placing the fingers and thumb along the joint lines of the knee. The knee is then flexed to beyond 90 degrees,

Figure 6-9. The McMurray's test for meniscal tears. By alternately rotating the flexed knee internally and externally, an abnormally mobile meniscal fragment can be trapped between the femoral and tibial condyles. Producing either pain or pop is a positive test.

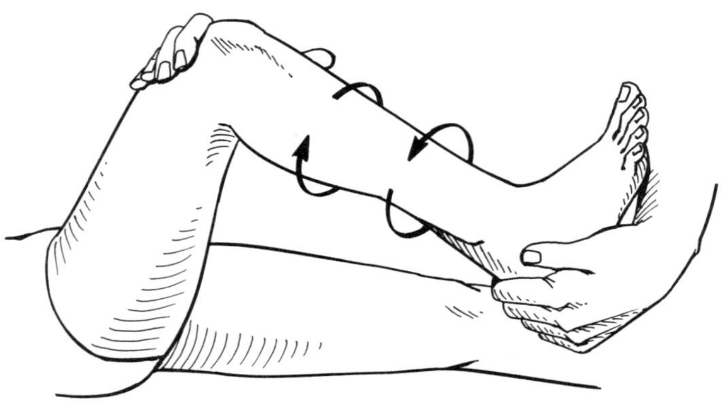

and the foot is taken from a position of abduction and external rotation to one of adduction and internal rotation. A pop or click felt along the medial or lateral joint line indicates possible damage to the posterior horn of the respective meniscus. A less reliable sign of this test is pain perceived by the patient on either the medial or lateral side. Once again, it is important to perform this on the uninvolved knee, as occasionally a click can be felt on the lateral side of the knee in a normal individual.

The Apley's test (see Fig. 6-10) is a modification of the McMurray's test, designed to distinguish a ligamentous injury to the knee from a meniscal injury. The patient is placed in the prone position with the hip extended and the knee flexed again beyond 90 degrees. The compression portion of the test is performed by placing downward pressure on the foot and internally and externally rotating the knee, again attempting to either elicit a clicking or pain along the joint line. The test is then performed while traction is applied to the foot, while stabilizing the thigh and again internally and externally rotating the foot, trying to elicit discomfort. Lesions of the meniscus should be suspected if there is pain with the compression test but not with the distraction test. In contrast,

Figure 6-10. Apley test. Compression traps the abnormal meniscal fragment resulting in pain. Distraction places tension on stretched ligaments resulting in pain.

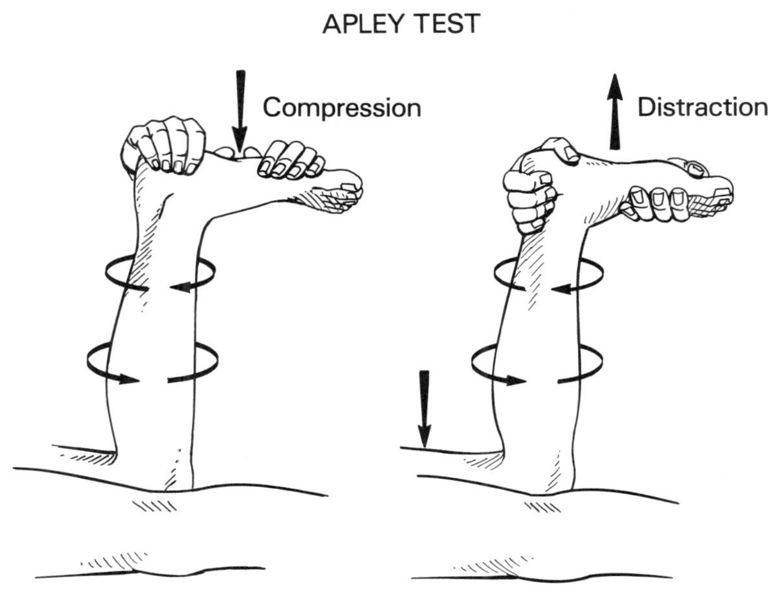

ligamentous injuries should be painful when this test is performed with the joint in distraction. However, if there is significant synovitis or patellofemoral pain, the results of this test are nullified. Similarly, all of the rotational tests will produce pain in patients with significant medial or lateral collateral ligament injuries. Functional tests for meniscal problems such as squatting or duck walking have been used in the past but are usually quite painful and difficult for many patients to perform. In addition, it is felt that these may cause some significant injuries as well and are usually not recommended at this time.

Extensor Mechanism

The examination of the extensor mechanism begins with the

evaluation of the alignment and gait of the patient, as previously noted. A more specific evaluation is often necessary, since it is one of the more common presenting complaints of all patients but particularly adolescent and young adult females. Observation of the patellar tracking is best done with the patient in the sitting position, with the legs draped over the side of the examining table. The examiner should first take note of the starting position of the patella, and whether this represents an abnormally high (alta) or low (baja) patella in relationship to the tibia. By then placing the index finger and thumb gently alongside the patella, the patient should be asked to extend the knee from a flexed position to a fully extended position. The course the patella takes through the trochlear groove should, therefore, be observed. In abnormal tracking, an abrupt shift to the lateral side of the knee just prior to full extension will often occur. Any crepitus perceived in this area should also be noted at this time. The patient should then be placed in the supine position on the examining table, and the alignment of the knee cap in relationship to the long axis of the femur and its insertion onto the tibia should be measured. This measurement is the Q-angle (see Fig. 6-3). The central point of the patella is the common point between the insertion of the patellar tendon on the tibial tubercle and the anterior superior iliac spine. A Q-angle of up to 14 degrees is generally considered normal but once again should be compared with the uninvolved side if possible.

Direct palpation of the medial and lateral facets of the patella with the appropriate attempt at displacement should be performed as well and any elicited pain noted. Unfortunately, since synovium is interposed, the specificity of this portion of the examination is quite suspect. Similarly, by placing direct pressure on the patella with the knee in full extension, entrapment of the synovium in the suprapatellar pouch can also elicit pain, which makes this test somewhat unreliable. The most reliable test for retropatellar pain is performed with the knee in 20 degrees to 30 degrees of flexion in order to place the patella directly within the trochlear groove. This can be done by either placing a pillow underneath the knee or having the patient simply cross one leg over the other. Compression is then applied, first to the medial and then to the lateral side in an attempt to elicit pain. With the knee in this position, the amount of displacement in both a medial and lateral direction should also be observed. The degree to which this occurs is usually measured in relationship to the medial or lateral extent of the femoral trochlea. Apprehension perceived by the patient, particularly with lateral displacement, with the feeling of the knee about to "go out" is usually diagnostic of patellar subluxation or dislocation (see Fig. 6-11).

Neurovascular Examination

Muscle Testing

The primary extensor of the knee is the quadriceps, which is innervated by the femoral nerve with primarily L3 and L4 root innervation. With the patient in a sitting position, and the leg draped over the table, the patient should be asked to extend the knee actively. One hand should then be used to palpate the tone and bulk of the muscle, as the other hand is used to provide a downward displacement force as the patient resists this maneuver.

The primary flexor of the knee is the hamstrings, which include the semimembranosus, semitendinosus, and biceps femoris. They are all innervated by the tibial portion of the sciatic nerve. However, the semimembranosus and semitendinosus receive the majority of their innervation from L5, whereas the biceps femoris receives most of its innervation from S1. With the patient in the supine position, the patient is asked to actively flex the knee. Again, while both stabilizing and palpating the posterior thigh with one hand, the other hand is used to provide an extension force, which should be resisted by the patient, and the degree of strength noted. Once again, both legs should be evaluated for comparison.

The patellar tendon reflex is felt to represent an L4 reflex. Pulses should be tested in the femoral, popliteal, dorsalis pedis, and posterior tibial areas as well, particularly in older individuals where major surgery is contemplated.

At this point a regional or general examination should be performed, as indicated by findings on both the history and physical examination or if a specific diagnosis has not been obtained at this point.

Figure 6-11. In patients with symptomatic patellar subluxation and dislocation, lateral displacement of the patella will produce significant apprehension with the feeling the knee is about to "go out".

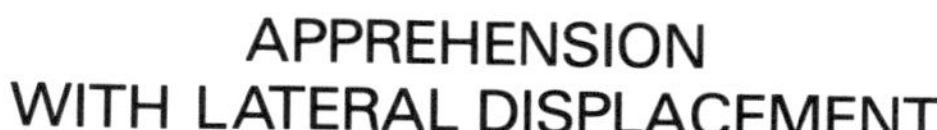

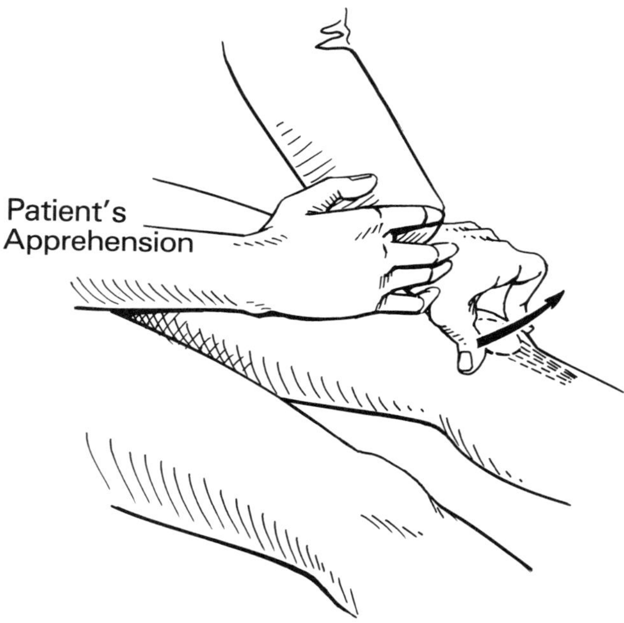

ANCILLARY INVESTIGATIONS

Radiologic Evaluation

All patients being evaluated for knee pain should have standard radiographs. At the bare minimum, an anterior-posterior standing radiograph with comparison to the opposite knee, along with a lateral taken with the knee in partial flexion, should be obtained. On the anterior-posterior film, a sufficient enough length of the femur and tibia should be obtained in order to make a measurement of the degree of varus or valgus. In addition to any defects, fractures, etc., a comparison of the medial and lateral joint spaces should also be performed. On the lateral, a measurement of the ratio between the length of the patella and the length of the patellar tendon, as measured from the distal pole of the patella to the tibial tubercle, should be obtained. The normal ratio is felt to be 1 to 1.2, with a higher ratio indicating patella alta and a lower ratio indicating patella baja. To evaluate further the patellofemoral joint, a skyline or Merchant view should be obtained. There are a variety of techniques to obtain these films with each one having its own criteria for abnormality. It is important, therefore, to know which technique is being applied when reviewing the radiographs. In situations where arthritis is suspected, particularly in osteoarthritis, a posterior-anterior flexed-knee view should also be obtained. The patient's knee needs to be in about 45 degrees of flexion while standing. This has been shown in a number of instances to demonstrate more precisely the degree to which the articular surface has been damaged and can be substituted for the normal tunnel view when looking for osteonecrosis or osteochondritis dissecans.

In trauma situations, either oblique films, looking for compression fractures not seen on the plain anterior-posterior radiograph, may also be needed. Stress views for ligamentous instability or for epiphyseal fractures should be performed only by experienced examiners and usually require a sufficient degree of anesthesia to prevent any muscle guarding. In instances of fractures of tibial plateau, tomograms are very helpful in determining the degree of depression and the number of fracture fragments present. In all cases where a diminished pulse is obtained in a trauma situation, or where a knee dislocation is suspected, an arteriogram needs to be considered.

Arthrograms, which were once the hallmark for diagnoses of torn medial and lateral menisci, are slowly being replaced by magnetic resonance imaging (MRI) or diagnostic arthroscopy.

The use of computed tomography scans to evaluate bony trauma can also be helpful and are more recently being used to evaluate subtle patellofemoral malalignment problems in some centers. Certainly, their use in determining the staging and extent of tumors remains extremely important.

Nuclear scans, particularly technetium bone scans, are often used in evaluating problems about the knee. In suspected osteonecrosis where the plain film x-rays are normal, a technetium bone scan can be extremely helpful in making the diagnosis. Once again, in staging of tumors, this remains a hallmark looking for skip lesions and metastatic disease. More recently, scans have been used in helping to make a diagnosis of reflex sympathetic dystrophy about the knee. The use of technetium in diagnosing acute and chronic osteomyelitis is also well-known. Frequently using gallium scans to look for indolent infections can also be of some benefit.

Magnetic resonance imaging is gaining increasing importance in diagnosis of traumatic lesions about the knee and, in particular, ligamentous and meniscal pathology. Presently, it is still a poor test for the evaluation of the articular cartilage but is felt to be more reliable than an arthrogram in diagnosing meniscal pathology. In most circumstances, it is also quite sensitive in the evaluation of the integrity of the anterior and posterior cruciate ligaments. It, too, can be used to evaluate osteonecrosis, tumors, or infection. Similarly to the computed tomography, MRI has been used in an attempt to evaluate subtle problems of patellofemoral tracking. Although cost still remains a problem, its noninvasiveness has a significant appeal. There is a long learning curve involved in evaluating the information obtained by MRI, but it will continue to increase in importance in the evaluation of problems about the knee.

Laboratory Tests

Of all the laboratory tests that can be performed, arthrocentesis in the evaluation of the synovial fluid is probably the most fruitful. There are a number of techniques described to perform this. I have found the following to be the most successful and the least painful to the patient. The patient is placed in the supine position with a small roll under the knee if there is a tense effusion or in relaxed, extended position otherwise. Sterile technique is an absolute necessity in this circumstance in order to prevent any introduction of infection into the joint, and to insure an uncontaminated culture. The superior lateral aspect of the suprapatellar pouch is then sterilely prepared, and local anesthesia is instilled into the skin, subcutaneous tissue, and the capsule of the joint. A second syringe with a larger bore needle is then inserted as the fluid is milked into the patellar pouch by placing gentle compression across the front of the patella and patellar tendon. As much of the fluid as possible is aspirated and, depending on the circumstances, should be evaluated for cell count with differential, culture and sensitivity, crystal evaluation and, in the case of a hemarthrosis, the observation for fat or bony spicules within the fluid.

At this point, by leaving the needle in place and removing the syringe and sending the fluid for the appropriate tests, one of several medications can then be injected into the joint, if indicated. A local anesthetic can be injected in the case of trauma to allow for a better evaluation of ligamentous stability and to provide a degree of pain relief. In some circumstances, cortisone can be injected, along with a mixture of local anesthesia. The needle is then withdrawn and compression applied until bleeding has stopped. A simple bedside evaluation of the synovial fluid can be performed. Obviously, fluid for culture should be sent immediately or appropriately stored. The fluid can then be placed in appropriate laboratory tubes, and a simple test for the amount of turbidity within the fluid can be performed: Newspaper print should be clearly visible through the fluid if it is normal. Any degree of turbidity is considered abnormal and usually represents an elevated white blood cell count.

Additionally, blood tests as indicated by the history and physical examination can then be performed, including rheumatoid factor, complement levels, antinuclear antibody, etc. A simple screen test for rheumatologic or infectious processes is an erythrocyte sedimentation rate, which is also often used as a measure of activity of the disease process.

Arthroscopy

The role of arthroscopy as a diagnostic tool is now subjugated to the more primary role of assisting in surgical procedures within the joints. Furthermore, with the increasing sophistication of magnetic resonance imaging, the role of arthroscopy in simple diagnosis continues to lessen as well. It should never be used as a substitute for a thorough clinical examination. However, in situations where all other noninvasive or minimally invasive tests have failed to disclose a diagnosis, arthroscopy still plays a role. It certainly allows for selective synovial biopsies and, in experienced hands, accounts for a 98% or 99% accuracy rate in making the appropriate diagnosis. In the case of trauma, in particular ligamentous disruption within the joint, it still has an appropriate role in determining the entire extent of damage and associated injuries. Even in those circumstances where it is being used as a surgical tool, it is also used to confirm the diagnosis at the time of the definitive treatment.

Isokinetic Testing

Isokinetic testing was originally designed to be used as a rehabilitation tool and to follow a patient's progress through the rehabilitation process. It is a very precise way of defining the degree of weakness within the major muscle groups in and about the knee. In some circumstances, it also can be used to distinguish a malingerer from someone who has true disability. The torque curves generated by repetitive cycles of hamstring and quadriceps functioning cannot be precisely reproduced by the malingerer but in someone with true pain very symmetric and consistent cycles will be observed.

SPECIFIC PROBLEMS

Trauma

The single most important point to remember in trauma is that a hemarthrosis indicates a significant and disabling injury until otherwise proven. Up to 80% of hemarthroses represent a tear of the anterior cruciate ligament. Patellar dislocations account for the next 15% with osteochondral fractures accounting for the majority of the rest. In less than 1% an isolated meniscal lesion is responsible for a hemarthrosis.

However, the absence of a hemarthrosis or an effusion does not rule out a significant injury to the knee. In significant ligamentous and capsular disruption, synovial fluid cannot be contained within the joint cavity. In those circumstances, however, there usually is significant soft tissue swelling. Even though an effusion cannot be elicited, a careful evaluation for both the possibility of compartment syndromes as well as direct vascular compromise should be repeatedly performed. Once again, in those circumstances where a dislocation of the knee is suspected, an arteriogram should almost always be performed.

Ligamentous injuries of the knee are often overlooked in cases of multiple trauma, particularly those resulting in hip dislocations or ipsilateral fractures of the femur and tibia. Frequent re-evaluations should be performed in the first few days after multiple injury, with particular note of any effusions or swelling about the knee.

It was once felt that significant ligamentous injuries did not occur in children with open epiphyses without the avulsion of bone. While it is true that epiphyseal fractures and avulsion fractures are more common, an increasing number of children have been found to have intersubstance ligamentous damage, primarily because of our more sophisticated evaluation techniques, including arthroscopy.

Minor fractures about the knee, particularly when they are associated with hemarthrosis, should alert the evaluator to a significant ligamentous injury. The Segond fracture, or lateral capsular sign, is very commonly associated with anterior cruciate disruption. A patellar dislocation can often result in a small fracture of the lateral femoral condyle or the medial facet of the patella. Fat seen on an aspirative hemarthrosis of the knee should alert one to an intra-articular fracture, even though it cannot be seen on plain film x-rays. Further investigation with either tomograms or CT scans may be necessary to delineate the fracture.

Bursitis

A bursa is a synovial sac found between skin and tendon, tendon and bone, or individual tendons that helps to reduce the friction as these structures move against one another. In the knee there are multiple bursae (see Fig. 6-12), but the three most commonly involved with injury or disease processes are the prepatellar, pes anserinus, and popliteal. Injury to the bursa can occur either as a repetitive process or overuse syndrome or direct trauma. Infection is usually caused by a direct inoculation, although the site may be nearly invisible.

The prepatellar bursa lies anterior to the patella and is a common site for both repetitive and direct trauma. Individuals that work on their knees, such as roofers, carpet layers, or cement masons are commonly aggravated by prepatellar bursitis pain. In addition, since they are very susceptible to minor puncture type injuries in the area, they often have an infective bursitis as well. With the advent of outdoor carpeting in the form of Astroturf, we have seen many more traumatic prepatellar bursitis in football players and soccer players due to direct trauma as they fall.

The pes anserinus bursa, which lies between the tendons of the pes anserinus and the tibial plateau, is most commonly involved with repetitive trauma. Runners with rotational malalignments or a tendency towards pronation are commonly afflicted. Similarly, swimmers who frequently perform the breast stroke have a high incidence of pes anserinus bursitis.

The popliteal or Baker's cyst is the most frequently palpated bursa about the knee. It is the bursa between the semimembranosus and medial head of the gastrocnemius, and approximately 50% of these communicate with the knee joint. These can be congenital and often are found in asymptomatic adolescents. In patients with recurrent effusions, the cysts can increase or decrease in size depending on the state of the effusion within the knee. In those patients, controlling the source of the effusion will usually control the amount of swelling within the bursa. In circumstances where the synovium itself is primarily involved, such as rheumatoid arthritis, the cyst can increase in size dramatically. An abrupt rupture of the cyst can occur, simulating either a deep-vein thrombophlebitis or a cellulitis of the posterior calf area. If aspiration of this cyst fails to reveal any fluid, one has to be particularly concerned that a soft-tissue neoplasm, such as synovial cell sarcoma may be the cause.

Figure 6-12. Knee bursae, lateral view.

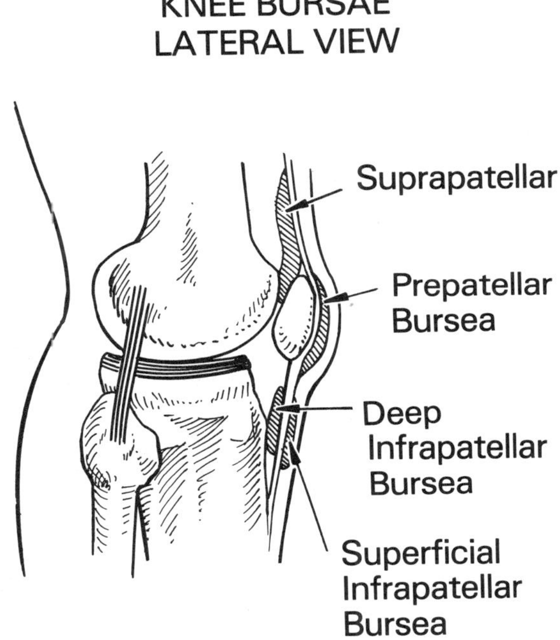

Swelling within the bursa can occur either because of recurrent trauma or direct trauma. Obviously, infective agents can also cause significant swelling. Occasionally, particularly in the prepatellar bursa, a chemical synovitis either from calcium or uric acid crystals can produce a severe bursitis, often indistinguishable from an infection.

If the diagnosis is in doubt, then aspiration of the bursa under sterile technique with appropriate laboratory evaluation should be performed. Relative rest, avoiding any of the inciting problems, along with ice application, and use of nonsteroidal anti-inflammatory agents should be performed in those circumstances where trauma is involved. Obviously, infection should be treated with appropriate antibiotics. Occasionally, after aspiration of the bursa and in circumstances where infection has been ruled out, cortisone injection can provide rapid relief. Corrective orthotics and modification of either running or swimming techniques can provide lasting relief once the initial problem is brought under adequate control. If repeated problems arise, consultation with an appropriate sports medicine or orthopaedic specialist should be obtained. Rarely, surgery is indicated to excise the bursa. Also, in circumstances where either repeated infections or recalcitrant infections are encountered, surgical drainage of the bursa may need to be considered.

Tendinitis

Tendinitis or, more precisely, tendinosus with peritendinitis can involve any of the tendinous structures about the knee. It is generally caused by overuse, resulting in the fatigue failure of collagen fibrils within the tendon. Repeated injury causes degeneration with neurovascular granulation tissue and its self-perpetuating inflammatory response within the peritenon. At first, the complaint is usually stiffness or pain following a period of rest after exercise. If the condition continues without treatment, patients will begin to have problems during the warm-up period and continue on following the exercise. Without treatments, symptoms will progress to pain throughout the entire exercise process and again after periods of rest and, finally, to pain even with activities of daily living or at rest. The farther the patient has progressed along this spectrum, the longer it will take for healing to occur.

The most common site for injury is at the junction of the tendon to the bone. This represents an area of stress concentration where the collagen fibrils are more susceptible to injury. The diagnosis is specific to the site of pain. For example, patellar tendinitis cannot occur without pain directly to palpation of the patellar tendon. Commonly, thickening within the tendon synovial sheath will also be elicited, and a loss of flexibility is commonly encountered. Weakness can also be a primary or secondary problem.

Treatment for tendinitis is relative rest, limiting the patient's activities to the point where pain is not perceived. This can be anything from the cessation of the inciting activity all the way to the point of cast immobilization and ambulatory aids. Ice and other physical therapy modalities such as ultrasound can be used to decrease inflammation and swelling. Flexibility and strengthening of the involved muscle should be done on a gradually increasing basis, beginning with isometric contractions, followed by isokinetic, isotonic, both eccentric and concentric, contractions. Nonsteroidal anti-inflammatory agents can be used also to help alleviate both pain and swelling, but steroid injections in and around tendons present a significant risk for rupture and should not be performed in most circumstances. Any mechanical problems that can be adjusted with orthotics should also be performed, and resumption of vigorous activity should wait until the patient becomes asymptomatic. A gradual resumption of the activities should take place in terms of both duration and demand upon the involved structure.

In recalcitrant cases, surgery is sometimes indicated. The technique is generally to fenestrate the tendon in line with its fibers, excising the abnormal granulation and degenerated mucinous tissue to encourage revascularization and stimulate a healing process.

Since greater than 95% of these injuries occur because of errors in training, most of these could be prevented by a sensible regimen of exercise and gradual increase in activity level. Certainly, in people who have had previous problems, this needs to be encouraged.

Infection

Intra-articular infection of the knee is not an uncommon diagnosis and must be considered in all cases of patients who present with an effusion. The mechanism by which the infection occurs can be by direct inoculation, hematogenous spread from an antecedent infection elsewhere, or direct spread by osteomyelitis. In children, it is most commonly associated with osteomyelitis. In children presenting with fever, inability to bear weight on the leg, and distal anterior thigh pain, do not forget to assess the hip joint in your evaluation, as hip pathology can often present with anterior thigh symptoms.

Depending on the infective agent, the patient can present with either insidious or acute onset of pain. Temperature elevation is common but not always present, and initial x-rays are usually negative, even in the cases of osteomyelitis. The diagnosis is made by arthrocentesis with fluid being analyzed by gram stain, cell count with differential, and culture and sensitivity. In those cases where osteomyelitis is suspected, a bone scan or MRI may be helpful in the diagnosis. The sedimentation rate is almost always elevated and can be a useful tool in evaluating the progress of the treatment.

Appropriate antibiotic coverage should begin immediately. The age of the patient and the suspected organism should lead to an initial broad coverage, which can then be narrowed as the culture and sensitivity reports become available. There remains controversy as to whether surgical drainage is always necessary or whether repeated aspiration is sufficient for treatment. Certainly, in those instances where loculated fluid is suspected, or where the patient has had a slow response to antibiotic coverage, drainage should be considered. Whether this is done arthroscopically or by direct arthrotomy depends on the experience of the surgeon and to some extent on the pathology encountered. In those cases where surgery is indicated in treatment of osteomyelitis, and there has been direct inoculation of the knee joint, drainage of the knee should also be performed.

In the differential diagnosis, do not overlook the possibility of a chemical synovitis produced by either pseudogout or gout itself, and the fluid should be evaluated for crystals unless the diagnosis is obvious by other means. In rare cases, an acute flare of rheumatoid type disease can be very difficult to distinguish from infection. However, cell counts above the level of 50,000 to 60,000 are quite suggestive of infection, particularly with a predominance of polymorphonuclear leukocytes.

Meniscal Injuries

Patients with meniscal injuries have different presentations at differing ages. This is an exceedingly rare injury in preadolescence, and most patients of this age presenting with symptoms such as popping, locking, or swelling suggestive of meniscal pathology are found to have a discoid lateral meniscus. In the adolescent or young adult, the patient is most likely to remember a twisting or squatting injury, resulting initially in mild to moderate pain, usually not enough to prevent further participation immediately. Within six to eight hours, they will develop a fairly significant effusion, with associated stiffness. The pain will become more localized to the joint line area. With avoidance of rotational movements upon the knee, the symptoms can be minimized; however, popping and recurrent sharp pain, associated occasionally with giving way, occur with pivoting activities. Acute locking, associated with bucket handle tears of the meniscus, are more likely to occur in this age group, although it is still an uncommon finding. Almost all of these patients will present with an effusion, joint line tenderness, and a positive McMurray's test. Patients who present with a lack of full extension are likely to have a displaced bucket handle tear of the meniscus. However, a displaced osteochondritis dissecans fragment must be considered, but can usually be diagnosed on plain radiographs.

Middle-aged men and women will often present with either no history of trauma at all, or recollection of a very minor twisting. Most commonly, they complain of an aching discomfort on the medial aspect of the knee at night. Many will report an inability to sleep in the lateral position with both knees touching. Swelling and stiffness are intermittent and associated with exercise. At first, the symptoms can be relieved simply by rest and avoidance of athletic activities, but generally there is an increasing frequency of recurrence. Pain is localized to the posteromedial joint line, and an effusion is commonly present. McMurray's test frequently produces pain, but infrequently produces a popping sensation. Radiographs may show mild or moderate narrowing of the medial joint line. It should be noted that women presenting with these complaints are more likely to have patellofemoral arthrosis than a torn medial meniscus.

Older individuals presenting with joint line tenderness and recurrent swelling are often found to have tears of the meniscus in association with osteoarthritis. In those individuals with an insidious onset, the symptoms are more likely to be related to osteoarthritis. However, a number of these patients will have had a relatively minor fall or twist when the symptoms were acutely exacerbated. These patients are much more likely to obtain better results with meniscal surgery.

The symptoms associated with tears of the meniscus are caused by tension on the unstable portion of the meniscus, as it is entrapped between the two articular surfaces, causing a localized synovitis. This synovitis in turn produces a localized tenderness along the joint line and the recurrent effusions. The McMurray's test is designed to reproduce this tension by entrapping the fragment between the articular surfaces, and therefore reproduce the pain.

The meniscal pathology is suspected by both history and physical examination. The diagnoses can be confirmed by one of three ways. The arthrogram, which was once the standard, is losing some of its popularity and is being replaced, primarily by the use of magnetic resonance imaging. The accuracy of arthrography is related to the experience of the radiologist, who usually is about 90% accurate with medial pathology and about 70% accurate with lateral pathology. Magnetic resonance imaging, which is less invasive but more expensive, is also examiner-dependent, but in some series has shown an accuracy of 95% with medial pathology and 85% with lateral pathology. Arthroscopy, which is the most expensive and invasive, is also the most accurate, with a 95% to 99% accuracy rate with both medial and lateral pathology. Deciding whether to proceed directly with arthroscopy or to perform either arthrography or MRI is based on the suspicions of the operating surgeon. In those individuals with classic history and physical findings, imaging studies can often be superfluous. In those individuals, particularly middle-aged women, where the diagnosis is often obscured or complicated by the coexisting patellofemoral problems, further imaging studies can help to delineate the exact pathology.

The trend in recent times, and particularly since the advent of arthroscopic surgery, has been to preserve meniscal tissue. Therefore, in the rare circumstance where the meniscal tear is within the vascular zone of the meniscus, i.e., the outer 15% to 20%, meniscal repair should be performed preferentially. However, 95% of the tears occur in areas that are not amenable to repair, and these require surgical excision. Only the mobile fragment and any tissue necessary to preserve a uniform contour of the meniscus should be removed. Rarely is total meniscectomy required.

Ligamentous Injuries

Collateral Ligaments

The collateral ligaments are most commonly injured when direct medial or laterally directed forces are applied with minimal rotation. In those cases where there is direct contact, the contralateral side of the knee will suffer the ligamentous injury. The degree of disability is proportional to the extent of the tear and is generally classified into three levels of severity. Any laxity found while stressing the ligament represents a severe injury to that ligament. The extent of swelling is also dependent on the severity of the injury. When a rapid effusion develops, a significant injury to a cruciate ligament must be considered. However, a mild effusion occurring over the next 10 to 12 hours after injury can occur in isolated cases. It is sometimes difficult to distinguish less severe forms of ligamentous injury from a torn meniscus. In those circumstances, there will be no increased laxity. The tenderness can be along the collateral ligament, which obviously crosses the joint line. Also, a significant effusion is more commonly associated with meniscal pathology. The Apley's test, although described to help differentiate between the two injuries, is often of little help. The McMurray's test, although often painful, should not produce a click or a pop in the presence of ligamentous injury. The treatment of injuries to the collateral ligament is dependent upon the integrity of the cruciate ligaments. Therefore, the status of these ligaments must be established beyond doubt. In order to rule out damage to the cruciate ligaments, a negative Lachman test must be present, and there should be no increased laxity on a posterior drawer. When in doubt, an examination under local or general anesthesia or arthroscopy or other imaging techniques should be done to establish the status of the intra-articular ligaments. In those cases of isolated injury to the collateral ligaments, nonsurgical measures are indicated, with a protected range of motion and progressive rehabilitation exercise to regain strength and mobility within the extremity. In combined injuries, surgery is often indicated.

Cruciate Ligaments

Injuries to the anterior cruciate ligament occur far more commonly than injuries to the posterior cruciate ligament. Understanding the mechanism of injury is helpful in establishing the diagnosis of an anterior cruciate ligament injury. Generally, these occur as a deceleration, rotation injury on a fixed foot, with a valgus stress. They can also occur with hyperextension or severe varus and valgus stress. About 75% of the patients will either perceive or hear a pop within the knee at the time of the injury. The initial pain is quite intense, and the patient is rarely able to continue with the activity. The knee will often feel unstable, particularly with any kind of rotational movements, and the patient may report feeling the knee shift in and out of place at the time of the injury. A rapid effusion usually develops within six hours and is often quite large. Initially, there is significant disability, with inability to even walk without support.

The diagnosis of torn anterior cruciate ligament should be suspected in all cases of acute hemarthrosis. The Lachman test is the most sensitive finding on physical examination. Radiographs are most commonly normal; however, occasionally, there will be a Segond fracture or lateral capsular avulsion fracture seen. Occasionally, a tibial eminence fracture will be present, particularly in an adolescent.

In the chronic anterior cruciate deficient knee, the patient usually reports repeated effusions after episodes of giving way or shifting, especially with pivoting maneuvers. The Lachman test will be positive, and pivot shift or other evaluations for rotational instability will be positive in these circumstances, or will produce significant apprehension on the patient's part.

The treatment of a torn anterior cruciate ligament is dependent on the extent of associated pathology, as well as the future demands of the patient. 45% of patients with acute tears of the anterior cruciate ligament will have associated tears of either the medial or lateral menisci. Greater than 60% of those patients with chronic insufficiency of the anterior cruciate ligament will have meniscal pathology. Conservative management for the low-risk individual may consist of treating the associated injuries of meniscal pathology arthroscopically and initiating a rehabilitation program to reestablish normal strength in the quadriceps and hamstrings, followed by the use of a brace for athletic activities. In the higher-demand individuals, reconstruction of the anterior cruciate ligament should be considered.

The diagnosis of posterior cruciate ligament is made more difficult by a number of factors. First, they occur far less frequently than their anterior counterparts. Second, they are often associated with significant multiple trauma. Third, their physical findings are often far more subtle than those found in the anterior cruciate injury. The most common mechanism of injury is that of hitting the tibia against the dashboard of a car and can be associated with ipsilateral femur fractures or hip dislocations. A high degree of suspicion and repeated physical examinations, particularly in those patients who develop any effusion in the knee, are necessary to establish the diagnosis. A more subtle presentation is that of falling on the knee. If the foot is in dorsiflexion during the fall, the majority of the force will be directed towards the patella. However, if the foot is plantarflexed, the force is directly posterior at the tibial tubercle and can often injure the posterior cruciate ligament. Also, patients who abruptly hyperflex their knee, particularly with any degree of rotation, can suffer an isolated injury to the posterior cruciate ligament as well. The majority of patients present with much less of an effusion, due to the extra-synovial location of this intracapsular ligament. Although some present with subtle findings of a posterior sag, the posterior drawer test is still the most sensitive on examination. Once again, even a subtle difference between the injured and uninjured leg indicates a significant injury to the posterior cruciate ligament. Radiographs should be obtained to look for an avulsion fracture of the posterior tibia. Magnetic resonance imaging studies can be helpful in the difficult or multiple-trauma patients, and arthroscopy can certainly be diagnostic, as well as helpful in finding associated injuries.

The treatment of the posterior cruciate ligament remains controversial among orthopaedic experts. In most circumstances where the ligament is an isolated injury, it can be initially treated conservatively, although there is increasing concern of late degenerative changes, particularly on the medial compartment of the knee. In those cases where conservative management is chosen, careful repeated evaluations to determine if there is any evidence of increasing arthritic changes must be maintained. In those cases of associated injuries or where conservative measures have failed, surgical reconstruction can be effective and should be considered. Injuries with a displaced avulsion fracture of the tibia are usually best treated by surgical repair.

In those instances where there is a combination of ligamentous injuries, particularly when both the anterior and posterior cruciate ligaments are torn, arteriogram must be considered. These combined ligamentous injuries are usually best treated by surgical repair and reconstruction.

Anterior Knee Pain

This is the most common presenting complaint of adolescent and young adult males and females. It represents a myriad of diseases and injuries associated with the extensor mechanism of the knee. In young adolescent males, it is the most common presenting complaint for Osgood-Schlatter's disease. In women, from early adolescence to middle age, it is the most commonly presented complaint in the knee, and it is most commonly associated with patellofemoral malalignment.

Anterior knee pain is frequently seen when there has been an abrupt change in the activity level of the involved patient. This is commonly seen at transition periods, such as the change from junior high school to high school or from high school to college athletics. In addition, it is associated with certain athletic activities in particularly, such as basketball, rowing, and the breaststroke in swimming. It is also the most common presenting complaint for runners of all distances.

The diagnosis of Osgood-Schlatter's disease is usually quite easily made on physical examination, with the finding of severe pain at the tibial tubercle and pain with resistance to extension of the knee. Radiographs will often show fragmentation of the tibial tubercle as well. The treatment for Osgood-Schlatter's disease is usually to advise activity modification in relationship to symptoms. Ice following exercise and a general stretching program are also advised. When the pain is severe enough to cause a limp or the need for pain medication, cessation of the inciting activity should occur until such time as the symptoms resolve. The disease is usually self-limited to a period of four to six months and is associated with the adolescent growth spurt. In rare recalcitrant cases, immobilization is sometimes necessary for treatment. Although surgery is rarely indicated, an occasional patient will develop an ununited ossicle at the tibial tubercle, which can cause enough symptoms to require surgical excision.

It is questionable whether the diagnosis of chondromalacia of the patella can ever be made on clinical evaluation or can only be made from a pathologic specimen. Regardless of whether it is called chondromalacia, patellofemoral stress syndrome, patella malalignment, or lateral compression syndrome of the patella, it is the most common diagnoses of the knee in the adolescent and young adult female. This often represents the pain associated with an overuse syndrome related to excessive demands on the patellofemoral joint. At the knee, a great many biomechanical forces are changing during the adolescent growth spurt. With increased lever arms of both the femur and tibia during rapid growth in the associated leg, and muscle strength and flexibility increasing, forces are brought to bear on the patellofemoral joint during even normal daily activities. Coupled with increasing demands of athletics and perhaps some subtle malalignments of the patellofemoral joints themselves, one is likely to get anterior knee pain.

The patient most commonly presents with a dull ache, which occurs following running, jumping, or climbing activities. It can also be associated with sitting for long periods of time, particularly in a confined situation, like the backseat of a car or a movie theater. It rarely causes night pain, and there are often times when the patient is totally asymptomatic. It is rarely, if ever, associated with swelling, and if associated with giving way or shifting, the diagnosis of patella subluxation or dislocation should be considered instead.

On physical examination, anterior knee pain is commonly associated with malalignment syndromes of the lower extremity (see Fig. 6-3). Pronation of the foot and ankle, external tibial rotation, valgus alignment of the knee, and femoral anteversion are common findings. If the Q-angle of the knee is greater than 14, one should suspect the diagnosis of patella subluxation or dislocation. The vastus medialis is often either atrophic or dysplastic. An effusion or swelling is rare early in the disease process. Crepitus is also extremely rare but can be found in the older adult. Peripatellar tenderness is common, and patella compression generally produces pain reminiscent of the symptoms. If patella tracking is significantly abnormal, or if apprehension is present on patella manipulation, then the diagnosis of subluxation or dislocation should be entertained again. Joint line pain is sometimes found, particularly along the medial side of the knee, but McMurray's test and ligamentous stability should be normal. It is not uncommon to find an associated loss of flexibility in the hamstrings, quadriceps, and iliotibial band in these patients.

The hallmark of treatment of this problem is physical therapy. Certainly, any orthotic devices to help correct pronation should be used, particularly in athletes. Flexibility should be restored by gentle stretching exercise programs, and restoration of the normal quadriceps strength should be performed as well. Full-arc quadriceps exercise programs, however, should be avoided, because they tend to increase the demand on the patellofemoral joint and are usually counterproductive. Straight-leg raising exercises, terminal knee extensions, and multi-angle isometrics should be used. In greater than 90% of the cases, this approach alone can be successful in returning these young patients to their previous level of activity. When this approach fails, the consideration of this being more of a malalignment problem, with either subluxation or dislocation, must be entertained. In the majority of these cases, surgery is necessary to realign the normal patellofemoral mechanics.

If subluxation and/or dislocation have occurred, referral to an orthopaedist is necessary to determine whether surgery is indicated. The surgery generally is some form of realignment procedure, which may be as minor as a lateral release or as extensive as femoral and tibial osteotomies.

Osteoarthritis

Osteoarthritis of the knee can either be primary or secondary. Primary osteoarthritis is a multi-factorial disease that probably has some genetic basis, as well as some factors related to both alignment and activity. Secondary osteoarthritis can occur as a result of damage caused by disease or trauma. It is therefore necessary, in obtaining the history, to review the family history as well as the past medical and surgical history related to the involved knee.

In general, primary osteoarthritis presents as an insidious onset of pain associated with an increased stiffness and occasional swelling. The stiffness generally lasts less than half an hour in the morning and is associated with a change in position, such as standing after a period of sitting. It is generally bilateral and relatively symmetric. On physical examination, the patient will often have an antalgic gait for the first several steps, which will then smooth out. There are often subtle malalignments, with either mild varus or valgus. The knee itself will sometimes feel mildly warm. Early on in the disease, there is rarely a large effusion and, if one is present, one should also suspect the diagnosis of a degenerative medial meniscus tear. The joint-line will primarily be tender and associated osteophytes are common. Mild crepitus can occur early, with more moderate or marked crepitus appearing at late stages of the disease. A subtle loss of motion is commonly present, with 5 degrees to 10 degrees of a flexion contracture and a loss of 20 degrees to 30 degrees of flexion. If there has been an acute exacerbation of an underlying discomfort, one should also consider the diagnosis of a torn meniscus.

Radiographs will generally show a narrowing of the involved joint compartments with marginal osteophytes. In the evaluation of the radiographs, however, one should remember that the disease can be present for a considerable period of time before radiographs will demonstrate significant findings. The flexed knee posterior-anterior study will often be more dramatic in the appearance of the joint space narrowing than the standard standing film. Radiographs taken in the supine position can be misleading with regard to joint space narrowing.

The findings of secondary arthritis are quite similar to those of primary arthritis; however, the history of a previous meniscectomy, septic arthritis, or disease such as gout, are usually obvious. With a history of previous fracture or other severe injury, the radiographs may show associated changes.

Initial treatment of osteoarthritis is directed primarily towards decreasing the load demands of the knee, as well as decreasing associated symptoms, particularly swelling and stiffness. The use of orthotics can be helpful in correcting minor malalignments, as well as providing an increased absorbing force within the shoe to counteract the loss of ability of the articular cartilage of the knee to absorb shock. Modification of activity should also be discussed, although ultimately the final decision about decreasing activity levels rests with the patient. Nonsteroidal anti-inflammatory agents are obvious mainstays in the medical treatment of this process, along with the use of ice after exercise and, occasionally, moist heat, particularly at night. Maintenance of general flexibility and strengthening around the legs can also be helpful, although obtaining these without placing undue stress on the knees is paramount. As the disease progresses over time, occasional steroid injections can be used to buy an additional amount of time, prior to consideration of any surgical management. Recently, intra-articular lavage has gained some degree of popularity, although its long-term benefits have yet to be established. The use of arthroscopic debridement has been shown to be most effective in patients who have had an acute exacerbation of their problem related to an injury, or where a mechanical problem develops, such as a loose body or a meniscal flap. In the younger patient, where a varus or valgus alignment is present without evidence of mechanical instability, osteotomies to realign the knee can be quite effective in gaining symptomatic relief for as long as seven to 10 years. Ultimately, when other modes of treatment have been exhausted, the use of a total knee or hemi-knee arthroplasty may be indicated. In cases where severe bone loss or histories of repeated infections in the knees have been present, fusion of the knee joint should be considered.

Osteonecrosis

Osteonecrosis generally presents as the acute onset of severe pain, usually in women over 50 years old, although occasionally men can be affected as well. It is rarely associated with the systemic steroids and alcoholism and so forth that is commonly seen in avascular necrosis of the hip. The patient will generally relate the symptoms to some trivial trauma but will undoubtedly remember the precise moment of onset. The pain is localized to the involved femoral condyle, and the effusion, when present, can be either small or large. The pain seems to be out of proportion to the findings on physical examination.

Initial radiographs can be negative; however, the technetium bone scan becomes positive very early on and is quite diagnostic. More recently, magnetic resonance imaging has been shown to be very effective in determining the precise location and size of the defect.

Treatment is determined by the size and location of the defect. In circumstances, where the lesion is small and collapse is mild, treatment with non-weight-bearing and appropriate pain and nonsteroidal anti-inflammatory medications can be successful. However, the majority of osteonecrosis cases require surgery. Arthroscopic debridements, with osteotomies to realign the joint, or total knee replacements may be considered, depending again on the size and location, degree of compression, and age of the patient.

Special Considerations of Patients with Total Knee Replacements

Patients with total knee replacements are particularly susceptible to two problems. One is loosening of the prosthesis and the other is infection. In the present state of technology, the expected duration of a total knee replacement is between 12 and 15 years. Normally, following the surgery, the patient will complain of intermittent stiffness and lameness for approximately six to eight months. Depending on the prosthetic design, the patient should be able to regain a range of motion from approximately 0 degrees to 120 degrees of flexion. The alignment of the knee should not change over time, and an effusion should not be present on a recurrent basis. The prosthetic device does make considerable noise with clicks and pops, but these should be consistent with each particular motion. Any patient presenting with persistent pain or swelling should be evaluated for both aseptic or septic loosening of the prosthesis. Early on in the loosening process, the patient will sometimes complain of pain when first standing that goes away after several steps.

In the advent of loosening, comparing radiographs with the original postoperative films will show increased lucency around the prosthetic device or the cement-bone interface. If an effusion is present, it should be aspirated using the sterile technique and sent for culture as well as cell count.

If an infection is caught early, occasionally the prosthetic device can be saved with aggressive debridement and intravenous antibiotics. However, in the majority of cases, the prosthesis requires removal. If the infection can be brought under control, a replacement prosthetic device can be inserted at a later date. In the cases of aseptic loosening, revision can be done at the time of prosthetic removal.

Because infection is such a devastating problem in patients with total knee replacements, antibiotic prophylaxis is considered necessary for gastrointestinal, genitourinary, and dental manipulations. The appropriate antibiotic can be chosen, based on the patient's allergic history and the normal flora found in the appropriate area.

Bibliography

DeHaven K.:   Diagnosis of Acute Knee Injuries with Hemarthrosis. Am. J. Sports Med., 1980; 8:9-14.

Henry J.H. (ed): Patellofemoral Problems. Clinics in Sports Medicine., 1989; vol. 8, no. 2.

Hunter L.Y. and Funk F.J., Jr (ed): Rehabilitation of the Injured Knee. St. Louis:C.V. Mosby Co., 1984.

Noyes F., Grood E., Butler D., et al.:   Clinical Laxity Tests and Functional Stability of the Knee: Biomechanical Concepts. Clin. Orthop., 1980; 146:84-89.

Renström P. and Johnson R.J.:   Anatomy and Biomechanics of the Menisci. Clinics in Sports Medicine., 1990; 9 (3): 523-538.

7

THE FOOT AND ANKLE

by Randall E. Marcus, M.D.

It is estimated that one-third of the musculoskeletal complaints seen in primary care involve the foot and ankle. This region of the body receives tremendous stress and strain in normal weight-bearing activities, and problems related to injury as well as degenerative conditions will be seen by the physician on a daily basis.

This chapter begins with a brief review of the anatomy and biomechanics of the foot and ankle. Specific examination of the region with recommendations for initial testing will be outlined. Common problems resulting in complaints of foot and ankle pain and deformity are presented. Each condition is discussed with its presentation and pertinent findings on examination. Recommendations for treatment by the primary care physician and indications for referral to a specialist are provided.

ANATOMY AND BIOMECHANICS

The ankle is a hinged joint in which the talus fits into a mortise formed by the distal tibia (medial malleolus) and the distal fibula (lateral malleolus). The posterior aspect of the mortise or socket is composed of the distal posterior tibia (posterior malleolus) and by the transverse talofibular ligament. The lower portion of the tibia and fibula are held together by the interosseous ligament, as well as, the anterior and posterior inferior tibiofibular ligaments (see Fig. 7-1).

The capsule of the ankle joint is composed of various ligaments, the most important of which are the medial and lateral collateral ligaments. The medial collateral ligament or deltoid ligament is attached above the medial malleolus and distally radiates anteriorly to the navicular and neck of the talus. Three ligaments compose the lateral collateral ligament and stabilize the lateral side of the joint. The anterior talofibular ligament runs forward from the lateral malleolus to the neck of the talus, the posterior talofibular ligament runs backward from the lateral malleolus to the talus, and the calcaneofibular ligament passes downward from the tip of the lateral malleolus to the lateral surface of the calcaneus. When the foot is plantarflexed, the anterior talofibular ligament lies in a vertical direction and is, therefore, the ligament most likely to be injured in ankle sprains.

The movements of the ankle joint are dorsiflexion and plantarflexion. If the intermalleolar interval is narrowed by injury or arthritis, the talus cannot engage in the mortise and range of motion, particularly dorsiflexion, is restricted.

The talus forms a gliding synovial joint with the calcaneus and articulates with it through facets on the middle and upper surface of the calcaneus. The two bones are held firmly together by the interosseous ligament. Inversion and eversion movements are possible at the talocalcaneal articulation. The distal end of the talus forms a rounded head that articulates in the socket in the navicular. The calcaneocuboid joint lies lateral to, but in the same transverse plane as, the talonavicular joint. These joints, although separate from each other, are described as the transverse tarsal joint. The remaining tarsal bones are the three cuneiforms which lie medial to the cuboid and distal to the navicular (see Fig. 7-2).

At all the tarsal joints, the principal movement is gliding in an upward and downward direction to produce plantarflexion and dorsiflexion of the distal part of the foot. The talonavicular and the calcaneocuboid joints also have a side-to-side gliding that contributes to inversion and eversion motion. However, this latter movement takes place chiefly at the talocalcaneal (subtalar) joint. In stabilizing the hindfoot, it is usually necessary to arthrodese the talocalcaneal, the talonavicular, and the calcaneocuboid joints. This surgical procedure is known as a triple arthrodesis.

Figure 7-1. Lateral view of the ankle illustrating the lateral collateral ligament complex.

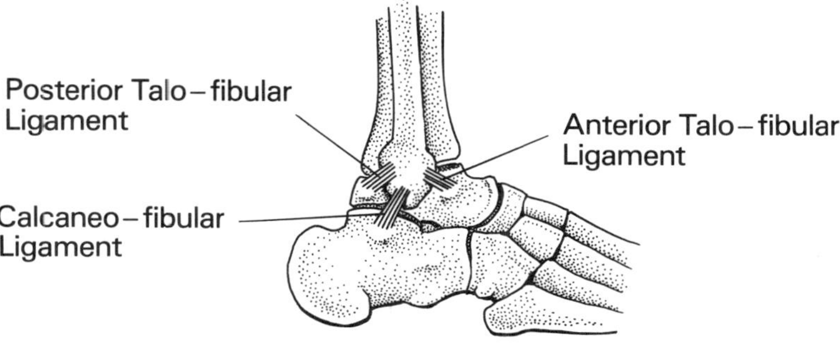

Figure 7-2. Dorsal anterior view of the foot and ankle.

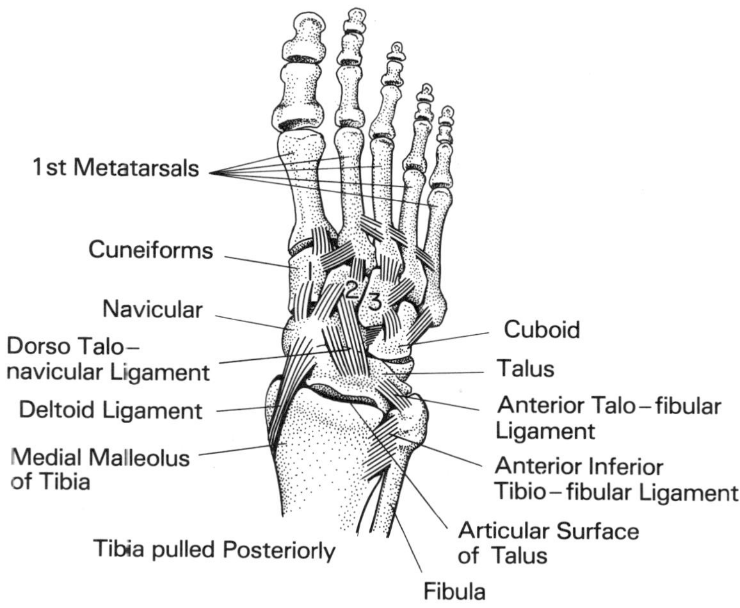

There are five metatarsals that articulate with the tarsal bones. The first is the stoutest and strongest; the second is longest and projects fore and aft of the metatarsals on either side of it; and the fifth has a pointed projecting base. The contiguous sides of the bases of the lateral four metatarsals have articular facets. The interlocking of the various metatarsal bones at Lisfranc's joint results in a very stable configuration. The peroneus brevis tendon has a strong insertion at the base of the fifth metatarsal. This is a common site for avulsion fractures resulting from inversion injuries of the foot.

The foot is described as having two longitudinal arches. It is designed for walking and should be regarded as a spring rather than a rigid arch. The three medial digits, their metatarsals and cuneiforms, and the navicular and talus are collectively known as the medial longitudinal arch of the foot. The lateral longitudinal arch consists of the lateral two digits, their metatarsals, the cuboid, and the calcaneus. The foot is arched not only longitudinally but also transversely, the dorsum being convex both anteroposteriorly and from side to side; the plantar aspect is concave in both directions.

The metatarsophalangeal articulation is a condyloid joint. It is enclosed in a capsule that is strengthened by thickenings medially and laterally, by strong rounded collateral ligaments and, on the plantar aspect, by the thick, dense, fibrous structure, and the plantar ligament which is fused with the deep layer of the flexor tendon sheath. The plantar ligament of the first metatarsophalangeal joint is replaced by the sesamoid bones in the tendon of the flexor hallucis brevis muscle. These sesamoid bones can be a source of pain under the first metatarsophalangeal joint when they are contused, fractured, or otherwise inflamed.

The first toe consists of two phalanges and the lateral four toes have three articulated phalanges, each with medial and lateral collateral ligaments and a thickened plantar ligament along its plantar surface. Imbalances in the extrinsic and intrinsic musculature surrounding these toe joints can result in contractures of the ligaments and deformity of the toes.

EXAMINATION OF THE FOOT AND ANKLE

An adequate history is critical for proper diagnosis of foot and ankle problems. Specific questions regarding the patient's past medical history, including factors such as cigarette smoking and diabetes, are of particular importance in the foot and ankle. Both of these factors contribute to possible neurovascular problems in the lower extremities.

Physical examination is divided into observation and inspection, palpation, and manipulation. The foot should be observed in weight-bearing and non-weight-bearing stances.

Deformities such as pes planus (flatfoot), consisting of depression or complete loss of the longitudinal arch, can readily be detected. The most common cause of pes planus is the hypermobile flatfoot, which is usually inherited and manifests in childhood. The common complaints are pain and fatigue with weight-bearing activities. In most cases, conservative treatment, consisting of a longitudinal arch support and Oxford-type shoe with a counter that is firm enough to grasp the heel is successful in treating this problem. Only rare cases require surgical intervention. The rigid flatfoot, a less common etiology of pes planus, is characterized with abnormalities of the tarsal bones usually due to bridging between the talus and the os calcis or between the navicular and os calcis. This foot is characterized as being quite rigid in the hindfoot area, often with spasm of the peroneal musculature. Surgical intervention is often required in the treatment of this condition and the patient should be referred to a specialist (refer to chapter 8).

The cavus foot is a deformity characterized by an excessively high longitudinal plantar arch and is often associated with neurological disease such as Friedreich's ataxia or Charcot-Marie-Tooth neuropathy. Presence of a cavus foot should alert the examiner to a further generalized neurologic evaluation of the patient. Referral of these patients to a specialist, is recommended (refer to chapter 8).

The patient's gait should be evaluated for abnormalities such as a limp or excessive pronation (an eversion of the foot) or supination (inversion of the foot). These problems can often be corrected with proper orthotics. Observing the patient's gait is important not only in treating foot and ankle problems but also in other associated abnormalities of the lower extremities. Patients who have excessive pronation often will present with medial knee pain exacerbated with walking or running. These patients can often be treated with orthotics consisting of a medial arch support. A limp can often be associated with pathologic conditions of the hip such as when the patient throws himself laterally over the painful side while walking (abductor lurch).

Careful palpation of the foot and ankle will often point out the anatomic structure in which the abnormality is located. Particular attention should be paid to palpation of the pulses at the posterior tibial and dorsal pedal region. Proximal vascular abnormalities will occasionally be diagnosed.

Neurologic examination of the foot and ankle consisting of sensory, motor, and reflex examination is an important part of the physical examination. In addition to recognizing local neurologic problems, systemic problems such as diabetic peripheral neuropathy with loss of proprioception and vibratory sense can be diagnosed.

Manipulation of the foot and ankle, consisting of performing range of motion examination to the ankle (dorsiflexion and plantarflexion), subtalar (inversion and eversion), and midtarsal joints (side-to-side gliding and plantarflexion and dorsiflexion)should be performed. The flexibility and range of motion of the metatarsophalangeal joints should also be noted. Stiffness of the first metatarsophalangeal joint is commonly found in hallux rigidus, an arthritic degeneration of the first metatarsophalangeal joint.

SPECIAL TESTS

Radiologic evaluation of the ankle consists of an anterior-posterior, lateral, and mortise views. The mortise view is an anterior-posterior view taken with the ankle rotated internally so as to attain a true frontal view of the mortise. Standing anterior-posterior, lateral, and oblique views of the foot are indicated when one suspects a bony problem in this area.

A technetium bone scan limited to the foot and ankle is often used in determining the etiology of more obscure problems such as stress fractures that ordinarily are not seen on early radiographs.

Tomograms and computerized axial tomograms (CAT scans) are particularly helpful in detecting congenitally fused bones such as in the rigid flatfoot. Magnetic resonance imaging (MRI) is useful in evaluating the foot and ankle, especially in the presence of occult fractures, as well as in suspected avascular necrosis of tarsal bones.

Electromyogram and nerve conduction studies are occasionally used in the evaluation of foot and ankle problems, particularly in nerve compression disorders such as tarsal tunnel syndrome. This is a compression of the posterior tibial nerve that can produce burning pain about the medial ankle and dorsum of the foot. Finally, vascular studies, particularly non-invasive Doppler studies, are of great help in evaluating circulatory problems in the foot and ankle. A foot and ankle problem often cannot be adequately treated surgically until the vascular problem is corrected.

ANKLE PAIN

Sprain

Ankle ligament injuries or sprains can be divided into first, second, and third degree injuries. A first degree sprain is a stretch injury to the ligament characterized by minimal swelling, rare ecchymosis, and full ligamentous stability. A second degree injury is a partial tear of the ligament and is usually associated with ecchymosis and moderate pain, but full stability, on examination. Specifically, the ligament is at least partially intact and comes to a firm endpoint on examination. A third degree sprain is a complete tear of the ligament characterized by marked ecchymosis, swelling and pain. On examination, there is no firm endpoint to stress of the ligament. Most sprains are either first or second degree injuries and occur to the lateral collateral ligamentous complex of the ankle. Radiologic evaluation of the ankle is recommended to confirm the diagnosis and exclude a fracture. For first and second degree sprains, elevation and ice pack application for 48 hours is recommended. An Aircast™ (see Fig. 7-3) is an excellent way to treat these injuries. If there is a moderate amount of pain and swelling, the patient is placed on crutches and should be non-weight-bearing on the injured foot for the first two weeks. The cast is worn over a sock and inside a shoe. Progressive weight-bearing ambulation is utilized after the initial two-week period. Continued use of the air cast for all weight-bearing activities in the first six weeks of treatment or until the ankle examination returns to normal is recommended. For third degree injuries, referral to an orthopaedic specialist is indicated, and treatment usually involves either casting or surgical intervention for repair or reconstruction of the ligament.

Fracture

Ankle fracture is also a commonly seen injury. This is diagnosed with point tenderness over the area of pain and is associated with moderate ecchymosis and swelling. Radiologic confirmation of diagnosis is necessary.

Nondisplaced fractures about the malleolus are often treated with either an Aircast™ or a short leg fiberglass cast. Sometimes a relatively benign-appearing, minimally displaced lateral malleolar fracture can be associated with complete disruption of the syndesmotic ligaments, and surgical intervention is indicated. It is important when obtaining radiologic views of the ankle to obtain a good view of the mortise in the anterior-posterior plane. There should be approximately equal distance between the tibia, fibula, and talus medially, dorsally and laterally on this view. If there is spread in any one of these planes, a serious ligamentous injury may be associated with the fracture, and referral to an orthopaedic specialist is indicated for treatment (See Fig. 7-4).

Tendon Injury

The three most common tendon injuries in the ankle are to the Achilles tendon, peroneal tendons, and posterior tibialis tendon.

Figure 7-3. The Aircast™ is an excellent ankle orthosis used to treat ankle sprains.

(A) Demonstration of the product's ability to resist inversion and eversion.

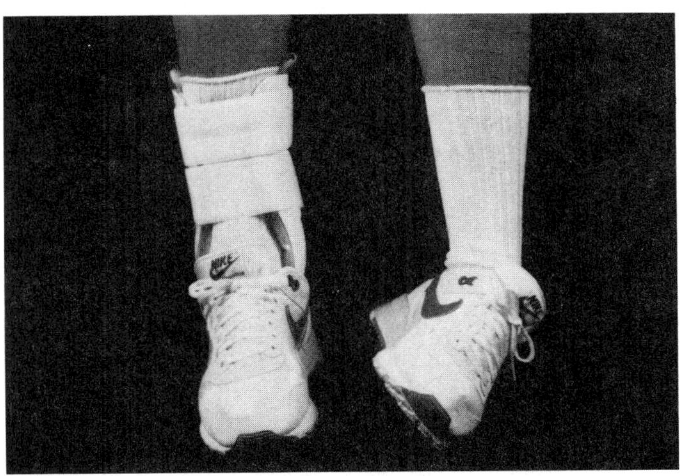

(B) Demonstration of the ambulatory nature of this type of functional management (Aircast™ Inc., Summit, New Jersey).

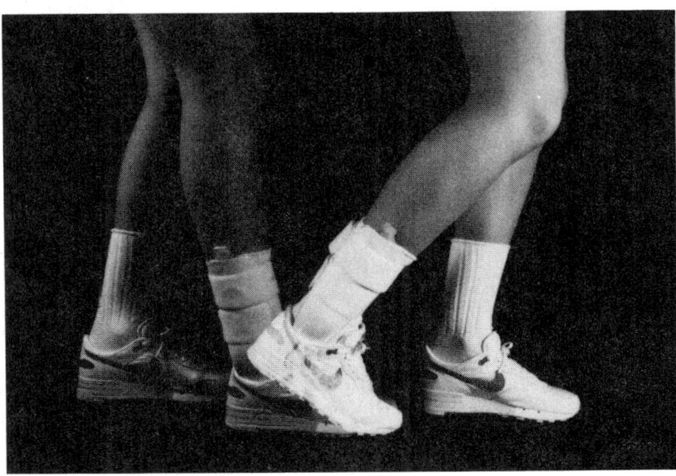

Figure 7-4. The mortise type anterior view of the ankle joint demonstrating a significant lateral shift of the talus. Note the increased space between medial malleoulus, which has a nondisplaced fracture, and the talus and fibula. This patient had a significant disruption of the syndesmosis ligaments between the tibia and fibula, necessitating surgical intervention.

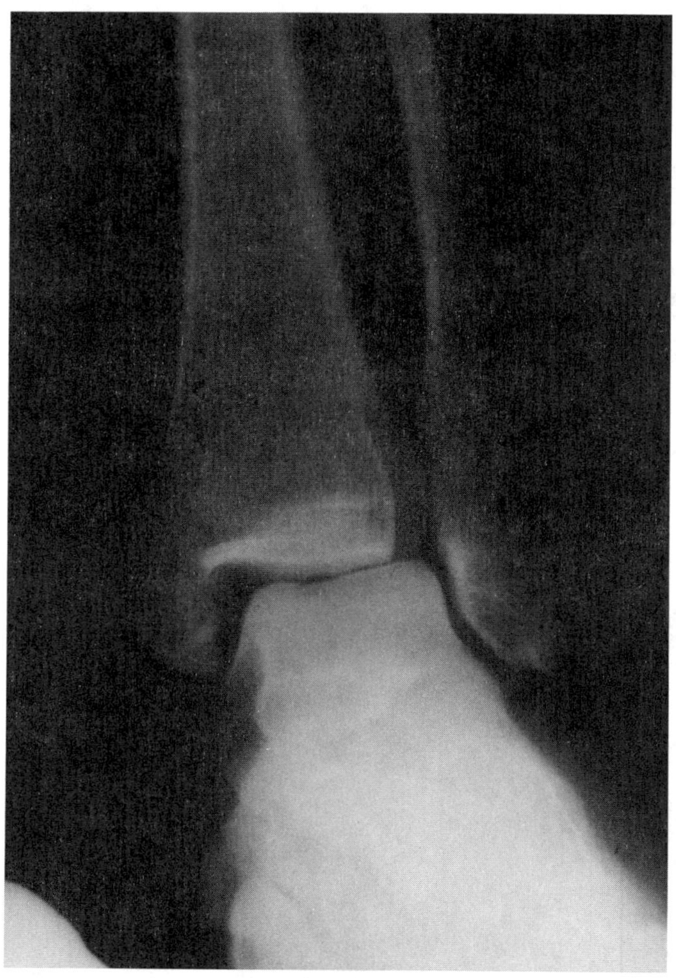

Achilles Tendon

Achilles tendon tendinitis is a common problem in joggers and participants in aerobics classes. Typically, examination reveals tenderness about the Achilles tendon with exacerbation of the pain on dorsiflexion of the ankle. There may be some swelling about the Achilles tendon area and increased skin temperature. Occasional nodules may be felt in the tendon itself. It is obviously important to determine whether the Achilles tendon is intact. It should be palpated throughout its length. The Thomas test is performed to confirm the integrity of the tendon. The patient is placed in the prone position, the knee is flexed to 90 degrees, and the gastroc-soleus muscle in the posterior calf is squeezed by the examiner. If the test is positive for Achilles tendon rupture, no motion is seen at the ankle. If the Achilles tendon is intact and the Thomas test is negative for rupture, the ankle plantar flexes when the muscle of the gastrosoleus is squeezed.

Treatment of Achilles tendinitis is with nonsteroidal anti-inflammatory medications, rest, and a higher heel in the patient's shoes. Women should use a one to two inch heel and men should use a one inch heel lift in their shoes on a temporary basis. Running or jumping type activities should be stopped on a temporary basis. Once the injury has healed, stretching exercises to the ankle, particularly in dorsiflexion, are recommended.

Rupture of the Achilles tendon is a serious injury and should be referred to an orthopaedic specialist. Most ruptures in active individuals are treated with surgical repair of the Achilles tendon; however, casting can also be utilized. There is evidence that surgical repair is associated with a decreased incidence of re-rupture of the tendon.

Peroneal Tendon

Peroneal tendinitis commonly presents as pain about the lateral aspect of the foot and ankle posterior to the lateral malleolus. It often can be seen in patients who perform running or jumping activities. Typically, pain is noted along the path of the peroneus brevis tendon, which runs along the posterolateral aspect of the foot and ankle and inserts about the prominence on the base of the fifth metatarsal. Resisted eversion of the foot exacerbates the pain. Subluxation of the peroneal tendons at the lateral malleolus is also a cause of lateral foot and ankle pain. With eversion and inversion of the ankle against resistance, subluxation of the tendons can be seen behind the lateral malleolus. This problem often necessitates surgical intervention and should be referred to a specialist. Tendinitis of the peroneal tendons can be treated with rest and nonsteroidal anti-inflammatory medication.

Posterior Tibial Tendon

Rupture of the posterior tibialis tendon is a difficult and often missed diagnosis. Typically, the patient presents with transient pain about the medial ankle and lateral foot pain. This injury typically occurs in the middle-aged patient who has had longstanding pes planus alignment of the foot.

On physical examination, the patient classically has an asymmetrically increased pes planus deformity of the ipsilateral foot with asymmetrically increased pronation on gait evaluation (see Fig. 7-5). Further evaluation reveals absence of function of the posterior tibialis tendon. The tendon is examined by holding the foot in an everted and equinus position and asking the patient to invert against resistance. This test should be performed on both the injured and normal extremity in order to evaluate the function of the tendon. Radiologic evaluation usually reveals the sagging of the talonavicular or cuneonavicular joint in the lateral x-ray film.

Unless there has been a laceration to the area, the loss of tibialis posterior tendon function is almost always due to attrition from degeneration of the tendon. This problem should be referred to a specialist for treatment, which involves orthotics and/or surgical intervention with tendon transfers or triple arthrodesis.

Arthritis

Arthritic changes in the ankle due to either rheumatoid or osteoarthritic disease is another cause of ankle pain. Typically, the

Figure 7-5. The posterior view of a patient with a ruptured posterior tibialis tendon of the right ankle. Note the asymmetrically increased pes planus and pronated deformity of the right foot and ankle compared with the left.

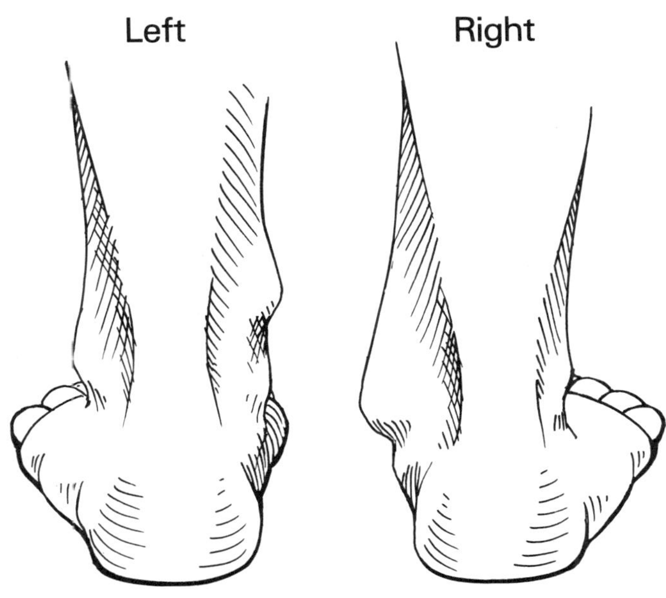

patient presents with pain on weight-bearing activities. Examination reveals swelling, stiffness and crepitus with range of motion of the ankle. Radiologic evaluation shows loss of the joint space at the tibial-talar articulation.

Treatment with nonsteroidal anti-inflammatory medications, as well as intra-articular steroid injections, is helpful in both diagnosis and pain relief. If this treatment fails, referral to an orthopaedic specialist for ankle fusion is indicated. Ankle fusion has been shown to produce excellent results with minimal changes in the patient's gait. In rare circumstances, ankle joint replacement is indicated, but long-term results have not been as good.

FOOT PAIN

The foot can be divided into the hindfoot which includes the calcaneus and talus and their articulations, the midfoot which involves mid-tarsal joints and their articulations, and the forefoot.

The Hindfoot

One of the most common problems seen in the hindfoot is heel pain. Typically, the patient complains of pain located in the plantar aspect of their heel, which is worse when they begin weight-bearing in the morning and often subsides after standing and walking activities have begun. Usually, no history of injury is noted; however, this is a common complaint in runners and aerobic dancing participants. The problem is also commonly seen in patients who participate in sports on hard surfaces, such as squash and racquet ball.

The condition is caused from inflammation of the plantar fascia at the attachment of the plantar aponeurosis on the calcaneus. Oftentimes a spur will develop along the plantar aspect of the calcaneus at the plantar fascia origin. This condition is called a plantar fasciitis.

Physical examination reveals point tenderness at the heel pad, particularly at the medial heel area. The plantar aponeurosis can be palpated from the great toe to the medial process of the tuberosity of the calcaneus. This tissue is often tender to palpation, particularly with the first toe held in extension.

Radiologic evaluation often reveals a spur at the medial tuberosity of the calcaneus. It is generally thought that the spur is the result of traction and inflammation of the periosteum.

Treatment involves the use of a custom-molded orthotic with medial arch support and stress relief at the heel. The orthotic should be worn in a rubber-soled shoe and should be utilized at all times for weight-bearing activities. It should be stressed to the patient that walking barefoot or without the orthotic should be avoided. Nonsteroidal anti-inflammatory medications can also be utilized in addition to the orthotic in the treatment of this condition. On rare occasions during an acute flare-up, corticosteroid injection into the plantar fascia origin at the calcaneus can be utilized. Multiple injections should be avoided because of the possibility of necrosis of the heel pad. Almost all patients note gradual relief of symptoms using these modalities. Surgical intervention is rarely indicated in the treatment of plantar fasciitis.

Arthritis of the subtalar joint with progressive valgus of the hindfoot is seen in conditions such as rheumatoid arthritis or osteoarthritis. The condition presents as pain in the hindfoot with increasing pes planus alignment of the foot and pronation. There is often pain and crepitus with range of motion of the subtalar joint. Radiologic evaluation reveals sclerosis and narrowing of the subtalar joint. Treatment includes nonsteroidal anti-inflammatory medications as well as intra-articular steroid injection. Orthotics with extra-depth shoes are often helpful. If conservative care fails, the patient should be referred for surgical intervention which includes triple arthrodesis.

Fractures of the hindfoot, particularly the calcaneus, often result in disruption and post-traumatic arthritis of the subtalar joint. When conservative care fails, subtalar or triple arthrodesis is often indicated.

The Midfoot

Midfoot problems are relatively rare. Occasional fractures of the midfoot, especially stress fractures, can be seen in runners. In many cases, plain radiographs are difficult to interpret and will not reveal occult injuries. A bone scan is recommended in this situation and occasional use of magnetic resonance imaging (MRI) is recommended. Treatment of stress fractures is symptomatic. A change in weight-bearing activities and the use of a rubber-soled shoe will usually give satisfactory results. Occasional use of a short leg walking cast is helpful. Patients with multiple or recurrent stress fractures should be referred for metabolic and osteoporosis evaluation. The diabetic patient with peripheral neuropathy is prone to neuropathic fractures of the midfoot. These often present as painless swelling or crepitus located in the foot. Careful radiologic evaluation is indicated in any patient with neurologic abnormality and painless swelling of the foot. Neuropathic fractures or dislocation should be referred to a specialist for treatment, which includes brace support or surgical intervention.

The Forefoot

One of the most common causes of forefoot pain is metatarsalgia. The patient complains of pain with weight-bearing activities located along with metatarsal heads, most commonly the second or third. The pain is often accompanied by a callosity along the plantar aspect of the symptomatic metatarsal head. Tenderness is directly under the metatarsal head and not in the web space between the toes.

A custom-molded soft orthotic with a metatarsal pad and stress relief at the symptomatic metatarsal head is quite helpful in alleviating this problem. The use of a shoe with a wide toe box, which allows the transverse metatarsal arch to spread properly with weight-bearing activities, is also important. Surgical intervention is rarely indicated for this problem (see Fig. 7-6).

Hallux valgus and bunions are common complaints related to the first ray. Typically, this complaint is seen in women who have worn pointed-toed, high heeled shoes on a regular basis. The pain is located over the first metatarsal head medially and is accompanied by thickening of the skin and callosity along the distal metatarsal head. A prominent medial eminence or spur along the distal medial metatarsal head is seen. The first toe gradually becomes deformed with lateral deviation and pronation. In many cases, a medial deviation of the first metatarsal (metatarsus primus varus) is also observed (see Fig. 7-7).

Figure 7-6. A typical custom-molded soft orthotic with a metatarsal pad, used in the treatment of metatarsalgia.

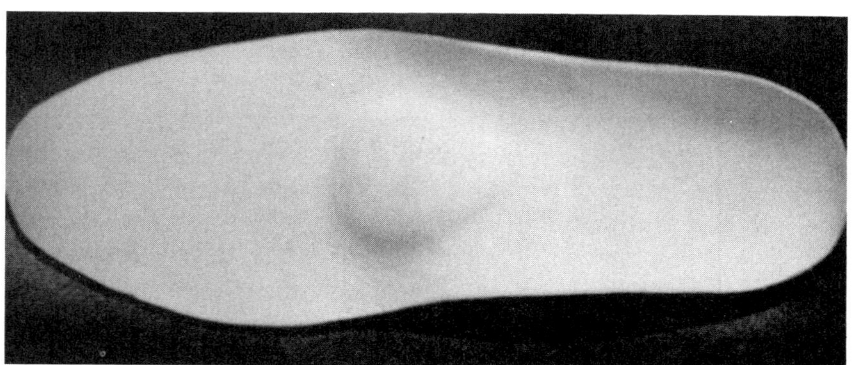

Figure 7-7. The dorsal view of the forefoot demonstrating a 35 degree hallux valgus with lateral-valgus deviation of the great toe. A prominent medial eminence is seen along the medial aspect of the first metatarsal head (bunion). The angle of deviation between the first and second metatarsal measures 15 degrees, consistent with metatarsus primus varus.

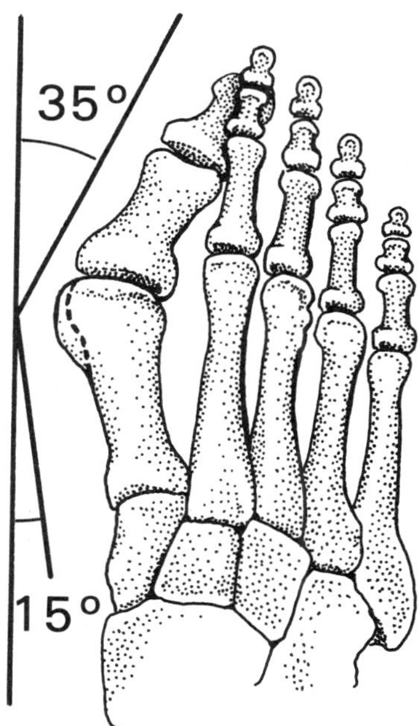

Conservative care for this problem consists of changing the patient's footwear. Oftentimes tracing the patient's foot in a weight-bearing position and overlying a tracing of the patient's shoe is helpful in convincing the patient to wear a shoe with a wider toe box. Stretching exercises are occasionally helpful and relieving the patient's shoe over the medial eminence is also useful. Early recognition of the problem before it becomes painful is essential in preventing further deformity and the need for surgical intervention in these patients.

Surgery is indicated when the deformity and prominence at the metatarsal head becomes painful. Surgical techniques for correction of the problem involve osteotomy of the metatarsal, bunionectomy and removal of the medial eminence, in addition to correction of the alignment of the first toe. If the patient persists in wearing improper shoes, recurrence of the deformity and symptoms can be seen.

Hallux rigidus or degenerative arthritis of the first metatarsophalangeal joint is another complaint related to the first ray of the forefoot. The patient often presents with pain at the first metatarsophalangeal joint on weight-bearing. Examination reveals tender spurs along the dorsum and medial aspect of the joint. Range of motion at the joint is markedly restricted particularly in dorsiflexion. Pain and crepitus are associated with motion in the joint.

Treatment for hallux rigidus involves use of nonsteroidal anti-inflammatory medications as well as intra-articular steroid injections. Use of a metatarsal pad can also be helpful in this condition.

Surgical intervention is indicated with failure of conservative care and involves debridement of the joint and/or fusion. Arthroplasty of the joint is rarely indicated and provides only temporary relief.

Gout often presents as severe pain in the first metatarsophalangeal joint. Typically, the patient has no history of injury and notes the acute onset of pain, swelling and erythema about the joint. Definitive diagnosis can be made by aspiration of the joint and identification of urate crystals under polarized microscopy. Treatment with nonsteroidal anti-inflammatory medication or colchicine is usually curative for the attack. A careful medical history to elicit any causes of the acute gouty attack is helpful. A serum uric acid level is also recommended in these patients. Medical treatment of the uric acid metabolic problem is controversial and usually reserved for patients with recurrent attacks.

The bunionette or tailor's bunion is an enlargement on the lateral distal aspect of the fifth metatarsal. This can often become painful with rubbing on the lateral aspect of the shoe. Examination reveals a tenderness about the prominence of the lateral aspect of the fifth metatarsal head. Radiologic evaluation will often show a spur about the lateral metatarsal head or an enlargement of the head itself.

Adjustments to the patient's shoe or a wider toe box shoe will often alleviate the symptoms. If this fails, referral for surgical intervention with removal of the spur or prominence is indicated.

Pain between the metatarsal heads, particularly in the second or third web space, is often associated with an interdigital plantar neuroma

(Morton's neuroma). Classically the patient presents with pain on weight-bearing in the third web space of the foot. Less commonly, the pain is located in the second web space. The pain is often exacerbated by walking or running and relieved by rest. The pain may be intermittent and is particularly problematic with the use of a pointed-toed or high heeled shoe. The pain, often described as burning, tends to be localized in the plantar aspect of the web space with occasional radiation and numbness in the adjoining toes (see Fig. 7-8).

Findings on physical examination are point tenderness in the web space, which is exacerbated with transverse compression of the metatarsal heads on either side of the affected web space.

Treatment with a metatarsal pad and a wider toe box in the shoe is often successful. Use of nonsteroidal anti-inflammatory medications and occasional use of local infiltration with steroid is also helpful. If the patient does not respond to conservative treatment, surgical excision of the neuroma is indicated.

Fractures of the shafts of the metatarsals are another cause of forefoot pain. Stress fractures or "march" fractures are fatigue-type fractures along the shaft of the metatarsals. The most common location is the second or third metatarsals. The patient presents with pain in the

Figure 7-8. Dorsal view of forefoot demonstrating an interdigital plantar neuroma in the third web space (Morton's neuroma).

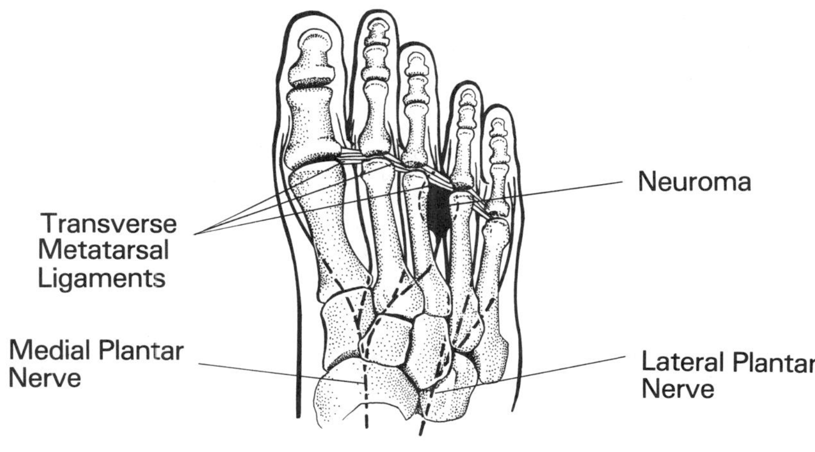

metatarsal area on weight-bearing. The patient often cannot relate a specific injury to the onset of pain.

Physical examination reveals point tenderness about the metatarsal shaft with swelling and edema. Initial radiologic evaluation may be negative for the first several weeks. A bone scan is often useful in revealing the source of the problem. Later radiographs will often reveal periosteal elevation at the fracture area, confirming the clinical suspicion (see Fig. 7-9).

Treatment consists of limitation of activities, the use of rubber-soled shoes or short leg plaster immobilization. Healing may take several months, and gradual return to activities is indicated.

Pain and deformity of the lesser toes can be classified according the joint at which the deformity occurs (see Fig. 7-10). A fixed flexion deformity of the distal interphalangeal joint of the toe, usually accompanied by a painful callosity of the distal interphalangeal joint, is called a mallet toe. A flexion deformity of the proximal interphalangeal joint with a painful callosity on the dorsum of the joint is called a hammertoe. The clawtoe is a flexion deformity at the proximal interphalangeal joint accompanied by an extension deformity at the metatarsophalangeal joint. Shoes with a wider toe box are the initial treatment for these painful lesser toe deformities. Soft donut type pads are also helpful. Gentle stretching exercises for the early deformity with local skin care can be successful.

Persistent deformity accompanied by pain should be referred for surgical correction. Fusion of the interphalangeal joints and division of the contracted tissue can often provide relief of the pain and deformity.

Figure 7-9. A typical stress fracture sequence of radiographs.

(A) Radiograph taken acutely in a patient whose chief complaint was pain about the second metatarsal shaft. The radiograph is essentially unremarkable. The patient was treated for a stress fracture. (B) Radiograph taken one month later confirming the stress fracture of the second metatarsal shaft.

Figure 7-9A

Figure 7-9B

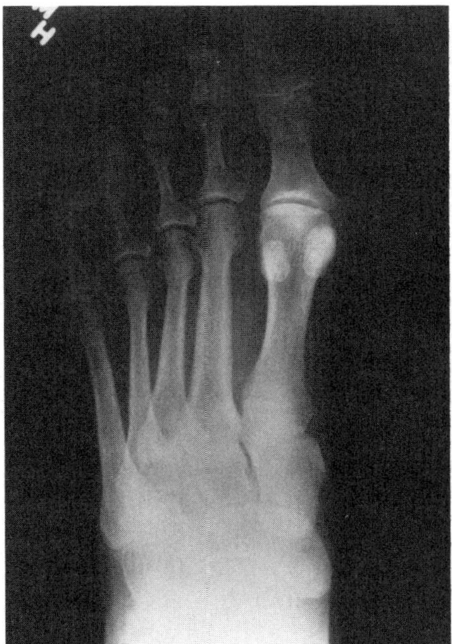

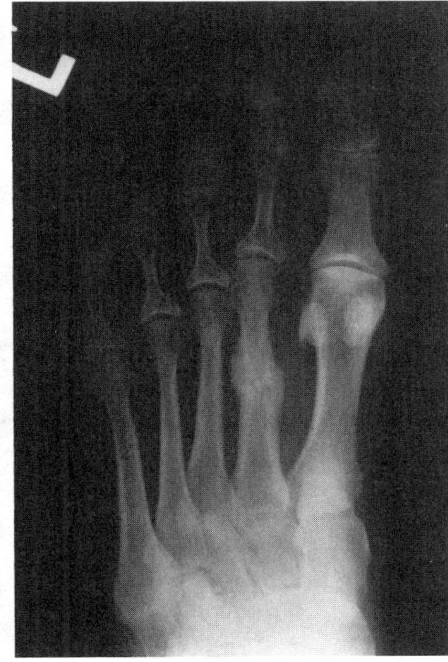

Figure 7-10. Deformities of the lesser toes consist of the claw, hammar, and mallet toe deformities. A painful callosity will often develop dorsally at the apex of the deformed joint.

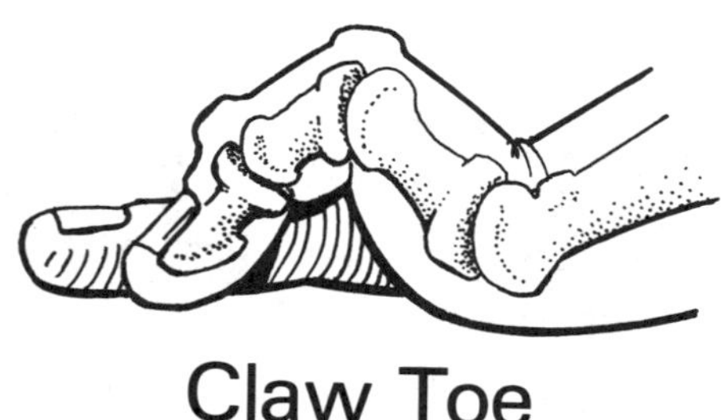

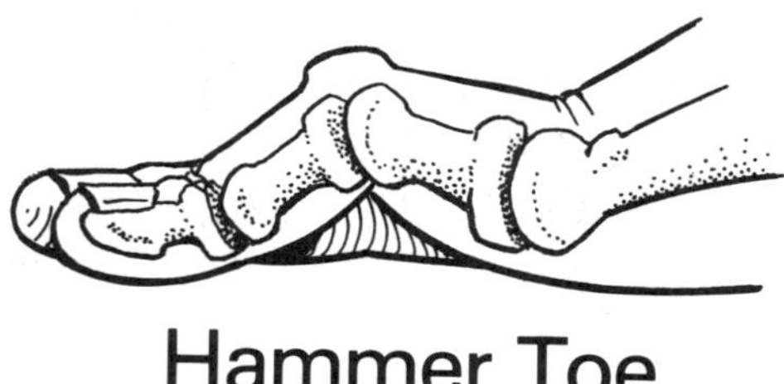

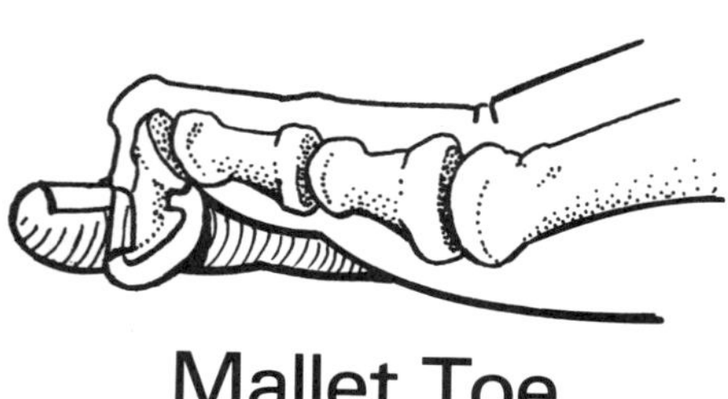

Bibliography

Mann R.A. (ed): <u>Surgery of the Foot</u>. St. Louis: C.V. Mosby, 1986.

Marcus R.E., Balourdas G.M., and Heiple K.G.: Ankle Arthrodesis by Chevron Fusion with Internal Fixation and Bone Grafting. <u>J. Bone Joint Surg.</u>, 1983; 65-A, 833-838.

Turek S.L.: The Foot and the Ankle, <u>In</u> Turek S.L. (ed): <u>Orthopaedics</u>. Philadelphia: J.B. Lippincott, 1984, pp. 1407-1482.

8

PEDIATRIC ORTHOPAEDICS
(Spine, Hips, Lower Extremities, and Feet)
By George H. Thompson, M.D.

Musculoskeletal problems in children and adolescents are common and the pediatrician or family practitioner is usually the first physician consulted for evaluation and treatment or possible referral for orthopaedic care. The majority of pediatric orthopaedic problems will involve the spine, hips, lower extremities, and feet. Upper extremity and hand abnormalities, other than trauma, occur less frequently. It is, therefore, important that the primary care physician have a basic understanding of the common disorders affecting these anatomical areas as well as the current concepts regarding management.

HISTORY

The key to an accurate diagnosis in a child with a musculoskeletal problem is a careful history. This is usually obtained from the parents, but the child, if old enough and cooperative, can also give useful information. Common presenting complaints include limp, deformity, swelling, pain, joint stiffness, and localized or generalized weakness. The location and duration of symptoms, antecedent factors such as trauma or vigorous physical activities, radiation of pain, neurologic symptoms, factors aggravating or alleviating symptoms, and previous evaluations or treatment must be ascertained.

The developmental history is important, especially in the diagnosis of neuromuscular disorders such as cerebral palsy or muscular dystrophy. The prenatal or pregnancy history includes maternal diseases or illnesses, vaginal bleeding, radiation exposure, ingestion of toxic substances or medications, and trauma. Birth history includes length of pregnancy, duration of labor, type of and any difficulty with delivery, birth presentation, birth weight, or problems with breathing (Apgar rating). The condition of the child during the neonatal period should be determined. This includes questions regarding breathing, oxygen therapy, muscle tone (flaccidity or rigidity), jaundice, exchange transfusions, and sucking or feeding habits. In older infants and young children, the presence of or delay in developmental milestones for posture, locomotion, dexterity, social activities, and speech are important.

PHYSICAL EXAMINATION

The examination of a child with an orthopaedic problem requires a careful evaluation of the musculoskeletal and neurologic system as well as a general physical examination

Observation

The first aspect of the musculoskeletal examination is inspection of the body. This is accomplished by observing the child undressed. If the child can stand, then the erect posture and alignment are observed. Symmetry of the trunk and extremities is assessed.

Palpation

The involved joint or area of the extremity or trunk should be palpated for tenderness, masses, soft-tissue swelling, or increased warmth. Abnormal joints should also be palpated for effusion, synovial thickening, increased temperature and areas of tenderness.

Range of Motion

The range of motion of the involved joint or joints should be recorded. If the opposite joint is normal, its range should also be recorded for comparison. It must be remembered that the range of motion of the joints changes from infancy through childhood and into adolescence. In-utero positioning produces soft-tissue contractures and torsional changes in the lower extremities that are frequently interpreted as abnormalities in infants and very young children. All normal newborns have 20 to 30 degree hip and knee flexion contractures. These typically decrease to neutral by four to six months of age. A newborn hip typically laterally rotates in extension to 80 to 90 degrees and has limited internal rotation to 0 to 10 degrees. Normally, there is approximately 45 degrees of medial and lateral rotation by one year of age. Overall hip rotation decreases by 15 to 20 degrees per decade during the first 20 years and then by five degrees per decade thereafter. Hip abduction at birth is typically 45 degrees on each side. This, too, decreases 10 to 15 degrees per decade during the first 20 years.

Gait

Human gait or locomotion is dynamic, complex, and repetitive. The gait cycle is the time between heel strike and the next heel strike of the same limb. The cycle is divided into two phases -- stance and swing. The normal developmental milestones for locomotion include independent sitting at six months of age, crawling at nine months, walking without assistance at 12 to 15 months, and running at 18 months. A normal one-year-old child has a wide base, rapid cadence with short steps, the elbows are kept flexed, and reciprocal arm motion is not present. Foot strike occurs without initial heel strike. By three years of age the gait is more mature. Base support is normal, the cadence slower but the step length is still slightly limited. The arms now have reciprocal movements. At six years of age the gait pattern is mature. Walking velocity, step length, and cadence are appropriately related.

Gait abnormalities require close observation. Common causes include pain (antalgic gait), lower extremity length inequality, neuromuscular diseases, or joint abnormalities.

SPECIAL TESTS

Diagnostic tests are usually necessary in the evaluation of pediatric musculoskeletal disorders. Routine radiographs are the most common procedure but occasionally other radiologic procedures, magnetic resonance imaging scans, ultrasound, and laboratory studies may be required.

Radiographic Procedures

Routine Radiographs

Routine radiographic evaluations are the first step in evaluating most pediatric orthopaedic abnormalities. These should always include an anteriorposterior (AP) and lateral view of the involved area. Comparison views of the opposite side, if uninvolved, may be helpful in difficult situations but are usually not necessary or ordered routinely. The specific type of radiographs for each anatomical area will be presented in the section on specific problems.

Technetium Bone Scans

Bone scans are particularly useful in assessing for occult lesions when routine radiographs are normal. Common indications for bone scans in children include: (1) early septic arthritis or osteomyelitis, (2) tumors, such as osteoid osteomas, (3) metastatic evaluation, (4) occult fractures, and (5) inflammatory disorders. Unfortunately, the radiation levels can be high, and bone scans should not be obtained unless absolutely necessary.

Computed Tomography (CT)

Coronal and axial cross-section studies with computed tomography can be beneficial in evaluating complex problems of the spine, pelvis, and feet. It allows a unique method of visualizing the bone anatomy and its relationship to contiguous structures that plain radiographs do not.

Magnetic Resonance Imaging (MRI)

Magnetic resonance imaging is relatively new although the technology and basic science knowledge has been known for many decades. Since it does not use ionizing radiation, the technique is presumed to be completely safe, and it does not produce biologically harmful effects. It produces excellent anatomical images of the musculoskeletal system, spinal cord, and brain. It is especially useful for soft-tissues. MRI can allow distinction between different muscles or muscle groups. Cartilage structures can be visualized and even different forms distinguished. Articular cartilage of the knee can easily be distinguished from the fibrocartilage of a meniscus. It also distinguishes the physiologic changes that occur in bone marrow with respect to age or disease.

In children, MRI scans can be very useful in the evaluation of (1) osteonecrosis or avascular necrosis of bone, especially the capital femoral epiphysis of the proximal femur, (2) bone and soft- tissue neoplasms, (3) intra-articular abnormalities of the knee joint, and (4) assessment for intraspinal pathology.

Ultrasound

Ultrasound evaluation is being increasingly utilized in pediatric orthopaedics. As with MRI scans, it uses no ionizing radiation and no contrast material is administered. It has no biological harmful effects, can be repeated as often as necessary, and the equipment is portable.

Scans can be obtained in any plane. More recently, Doppler studies of blood vessels and color flow mapping has been incorporated into ultrasound equipment. The disadvantages of ultrasound include: bone is not penetrated by sound wave, static images are difficult to interpret, and the results are heavily operator-dependent.

The major indications for ultrasound are (1) obstetric studies of the spine and extremities for evidence of neural tube defects (myelodysplasia) and skeletal dysplasias, (2) congenital instability and dislocation of the hip, (3) joint effusions, (4) occult neonatal spinal dysraphism, (5) foreign bodies in soft-tissues, and (5) popliteal cysts.

Laboratory Procedures

Only occasionally are hematological tests necessary in the evaluation of the pediatric musculoskeletal system. Common tests ordered include complete blood count (CBC), erythrocyte sedimentation rate (ESR) and rheumatologic studies such as rheumatoid factor, antinuclear antibodies and others. The most common indications for hematologic studies are septic processes and rheumatologic disorders.

SPINAL ABNORMALITIES

Abnormalities in the vertebral column are among the most common nontraumatic musculoskeletal problems of childhood and adolescents. A simplified classification of the common spinal abnormalities is presented in Table 8-1.

Scoliosis

Alterations in normal spinal alignment that occur in the anterior-posterior or frontal plane are termed scoliosis. The majority of scoliotic deformities are idiopathic (unknown causation). Others, however, can

Table 8-1. Classification of Spinal Deformities

```
SCOLIOSIS
    IDIOPATHIC
        Infantile
        Juvenile
        Adolescent
    CONGENITAL
        Failure of Formation
            Wedge Vertebrae
            Hemivertebrae
        Failure of Segmentation
            Unilateral Bar
            Bilateral Bar
        Mixed
    NEUROMUSCULAR
        Neuropathic Diseases
            Upper Motor Neuron
                Cerebral Palsy
                Spinocerebellar Degeneration
                    Friedrich's Ataxia
                    Charcot-Marie-Tooth
                Syringomyelia
                Spinal Cord Tumor
                Spinal Cord Trauma
            Lower Motor Neuron
                Poliomyelitis
                Spinal Muscular Atrophy
                Myelodysplasia
            Myopathic Diseases
                Duchenne Muscular Dystrophy
                Arthrogryposis
            Muscular Dystrophy
                Fiber Type Disproportion
    SYNDROMES
        Neurofibromatosis
        Marfan's
    COMPENSATORY
KYPHOSIS
    POSTURAL ROUNDBACK
    SCHEUERMANN'S DISEASE
    CONGENITAL KYPHOSIS
```

Adapted from the Terminology Committee of the Scoliosis Research Society be congenital or secondary to an underlying neuromuscular disorder or syndrome, or compensatory from a leg length inequality or intraspinal abnormality such as a tumor.

Idiopathic Scoliosis

Idiopathic scoliosis is the most common form of scoliosis. It occurs in healthy, neurologically normal children, and its exact etiology is unknown. The incidence is only slightly greater in females but they are more likely to progress and require treatment than males. Hereditary tendencies occur as approximately 20% of children with scoliosis have other family members with the same condition. Both autosomal and multifactorial traits have been suggested. Involved children tend to show subtle changes in proprioception and vibrating sensation. This suggests a possible neurologic basis.

Idiopathic scoliosis can be divided into three age groups: infantile (birth to three years), juvenile (four to 10 years), and adolescence (11 years and older). Idiopathic adolescent scoliosis is the most common cause of spinal deformity. It occurs in approximately 80% of children with scoliosis. Infantile scoliosis is very rare in the United States but more common in England. Juvenile scoliosis is not common, but many children with the diagnosis of adolescent scoliosis are actually juvenile in onset but not diagnosed until later.

Clinical Examination

A complete physical examination is required for any child or adolescent with a spinal deformity as the deformity may be indicative of an underlying disease process. The back is examined with the patient in the standing position and viewed from behind. The levelness of the pelvis is assessed first. Leg length inequality results in pelvic obliquity, and this can produce the clinical appearance of scoliosis. The top of the iliac crests are identified with the examiners hands, and any discrepancy in length will be manifested by a pelvic obliquity. When a pelvic obliquity is present, wooden blocks of various heights are placed beneath the foot on the short extremity until the pelvis is level. The height of the block determines the degree of leg length inequality. When the pelvis is level or has been leveled, the spine is examined for symmetry. The back is observed for areas of deformity, spinal curvature, and areas of tenderness. The shoulders and waist are evaluated for symmetry. Mobility with right and left lateral bending and rotation are determined. Next, the patient's palms are brought together and the patient is asked to bend forward with the hands directed between the feet. This maintains balance and symmetry of the trunk. Tangential view of the spine while standing behind (thoracic area) and in front (lumbar area) of the patient allows the observer to determine the symmetry of the back. The presence of a hump or asymmetry is the hallmark of a scoliotic deformity. The corresponding area opposite the hump is typically depressed. These humps and valleys are due to spinal rotation. Scoliosis represents a rotational malalignment of one vertebra on another. This results in rib rotation when the curve is in the thoracic area and paravertebral muscle rotation when in the lumbar region. On the convexity of the curve, the ribs are rotated posteriorly (hump) and in the concavity of the curvature, they are rotated anteriorly (valley). This rotation will also produce distortion anteriorly such as rib prominence or breast asymmetry.

When the trunk is viewed from the side with the patient still in the forward flexed position, the degree of roundback can be ascertained. A sharp, abrupt forward angulation in the thoracic or thoracolumbar region is indicative of a kyphotic deformity.

In a scoliosis patient, other areas of the body must be examined including the skin (hairy patches, nevi, lipomas, cafe´ au lait spots), extremities (skeletal dysplasia), heart (murmurs from Marfan's syndrome), and the neurologic system to determine whether the scoliosis is truly idiopathic or possibly secondary to an underlying syndrome such as a neuromuscular disorder.

Radiographic Evaluation

Initial radiographs of the spine include a posterior-anterior (PA) and lateral standing radiograph of the entire spine. This allows assessment for scoliosis, kyphosis, lordosis, congenital malformations, and if the iliac crests are visible, the skeletal maturity of the patient. The degree of curvature is measured from the most tilted or end vertebra of the curve superiorly and inferiorly using the Cobb method. In this method, a line is drawn across the proximal endplate of the superior end vertebra and the distal endplate of the inferior end vertebra and perpendicular lines erected. The angle at the intersection of the perpendicular lines determines the degree of curvature. The right thoracic curve is the most common curve type in idiopathic deformities. If two curves are present both should be measured. Curve flexibility can be determined by supine anterior-posterior (AP) right and left side bending radiographs. The same end vertebrae are used to measure the change in the deformity by the Cobb method.

Other radiographic procedures that may occasionally be indicated include computed tomography, myelography, tomography, and magnetic resonance imaging. The decision for these procedures should be made by the treating orthopaedic surgeon.

Warning Signs

Idiopathic scoliosis is a painless disorder. Any child with scoliosis and back pain requires a careful neurologic examination. Left thoracic curves and back pain have an increased incidence of intraspinal pathology such as a tumor. These children should be evaluated by an MRI scan.

Treatment

Treatment in idiopathic scoliosis is based on whether the curve is progressive or nonprogressive. No treatment is necessary for nonprogressive deformities. The possibility for progression varies with sex, skeletal age, curve location, and curve magnitude. Although the female-to-male ratio for the incidence of idiopathic adolescent scoliosis is approximately 1:1, the risk of progression is much higher for females. The treatment of progressive idiopathic adolescent scoliosis is by orthosis (braces) or surgery. Exercises alone are ineffective. Typically, progressive curves between 25 and 45 degrees in a skeletally immature patient are managed by orthoses. Curves greater than 45 degrees generally require surgery.

When orthotic management is being considered, the location of the curve is important. When the apical vertebra is at the eighth thoracic vertebra or higher, a Milwaukee brace with a neck ring to control the upper thoracic and cervical spine is necessary. When the apex is below this level, a molded plastic thoracic lumbar spinal orthosis (TLSO) may be utilized. It is important to realize that orthoses are only effective in controlling curve progression. They do not provide permanent correction of the deformity.

If surgery is necessary, a variety of techniques may be used, but most generally a posterior spinal fusion with some form of metallic instrumentation is involved. Harrington rod instrumentation and Cotrel-Dubousset instrumentation are the most commonly used forms of instrumentation in idiopathic deformities (see Fig. 8-1). Occasionally, anterior spinal fusion and instrumentation may be indicated especially in thoracolumbar and lumbar curves.

When to Consult

Because of the complexities involved in diagnosis, determining the risk of progression, and the various methods of management, any child or adolescent with an idiopathic scoliotic deformity should be referred for orthopaedic evaluation.

Congenital Scoliosis

Abnormalities of vertebral development during the first trimester often result in structural deformities of the spine that are evident at birth or become obvious in early childhood. Congenital scoliosis can be classified (see Table 8-1) as: (1) partial or complete failure of vertebral formation (wedge vertebrae or hemivertebrae), (2) partial or complete failure of segmentation (unsegmented bars), or (3) mixed. They may occur as single anomalies or in combination with other bone, neural or soft-tissue abnormalities of the axial or appendicular skeleton. Congenital genitourinary malformations occur in 20% of children with

Figure 8-1.

(A) Standing anterior-posterior radiograph of a 13-year-old girl with a progressive 48 degree right thoracic scoliosis between T6 and T12. The 35 degree left lumbar curve (T12 to L4) is flexible and compensatory. (B) Standing radiograph of the same girl 10 months following a posterior spinal fusion and Cotrel-Dubousset instrumentation from T3 and L1. The structural right thoracic curve has been reduced to 20 degrees (58% correction). The compensatory left lumbar curve resolved.

Figure 8-1A   Figure 8-1B

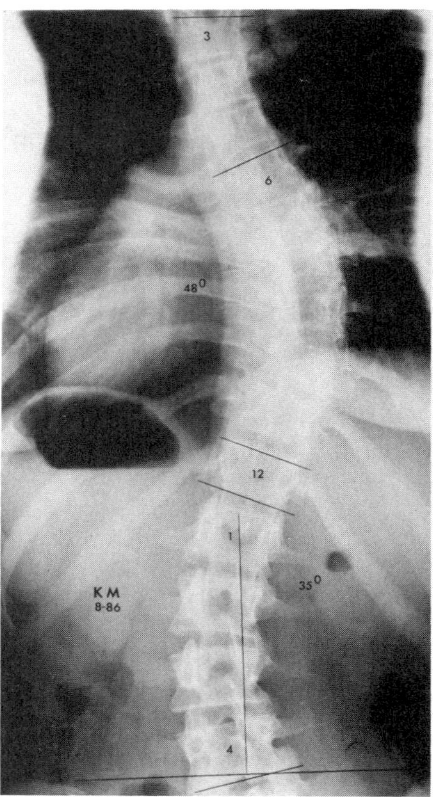
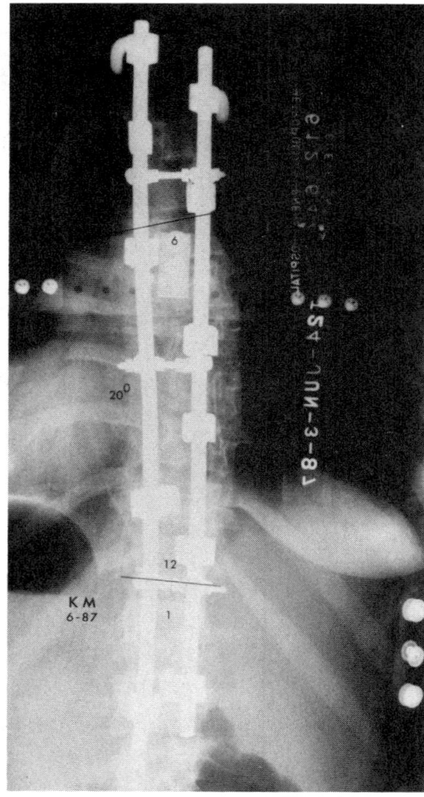

congenital scoliosis. Unilateral renal agenesis is the most common abnormality but 6% of children with associated genitourinary abnormalities may have a silent, obstructive uropathy. Renal ultrasound is performed in all patients to assess for possible genitourinary problems. Other procedures such as intravenous pyelography or MRI may be done if the ultrasound is abnormal. Congenital heart disease may be found in an additional 10% to 15% percent of involved children. Spinal dystrophic lesions occur in approximately 20% of patients with congenital scoliosis. These include tethered spinal cord, intradural lipomas, and diastematomyelia. These abnormalities are frequently associated with cutaneous lesions of the back such as hairy patches, skin dimples, hemangiomas, and abnormalities of the feet and lower extremities, such as cavus feet, calf atrophy, asymmetrical foot size, and neurologic changes. MRI scan is the procedure of choice for evaluation of possible spinal dysraphism. Congenital scoliosis also commonly occurs in association with syndromes, such as Klippel-Feil and VATER, and spinal dysraphism disorders, such as myelodysplasia (see Fig. 8-2). Thus, careful evaluation for other malformations must always be performed during the initial evaluation of a child with congenital scoliosis.

The risk for progression of spinal deformity in a child with congenital scoliosis is variable depending on the growth potential of the malformed vertebra. Defects such as a block vertebra have little growth potential and usually do not cause significant spinal deformity. Hemivertebrae may or may not cause significant deformity depending on location and nature of the defect. Unilateral unsegmented bars almost always produce progressive deformities. Overall, approximately 25% of patients with scoliosis will not demonstrate curve progression and do not require treatment. However, 75% of involved patients will demonstrate some progression and approximately 50% will require treatment. If progression occurs it almost always continues until the cessation of growth. Rapid progression can be expected during periods of rapid growth, before two and after 10 years of age. Early diagnosis and prompt treatment of progressive curves are the most essential elements in the care of congenital spinal deformity. Orthotic treatment is of limited value since these curves tend to be rigid. A posterior spinal fusion without instrumentation is the most common procedure. It is a

Figure 8-2. Standing anterior-posterior radiograph of an 11-year-old girl with lumbar level myelodysplasia and a progressive 69 degree right thoracic congenital scoliosis due to a unilateral unsegmented bar (see arrows). Note the large defect in the lumbar spine from her myelomeningocele.

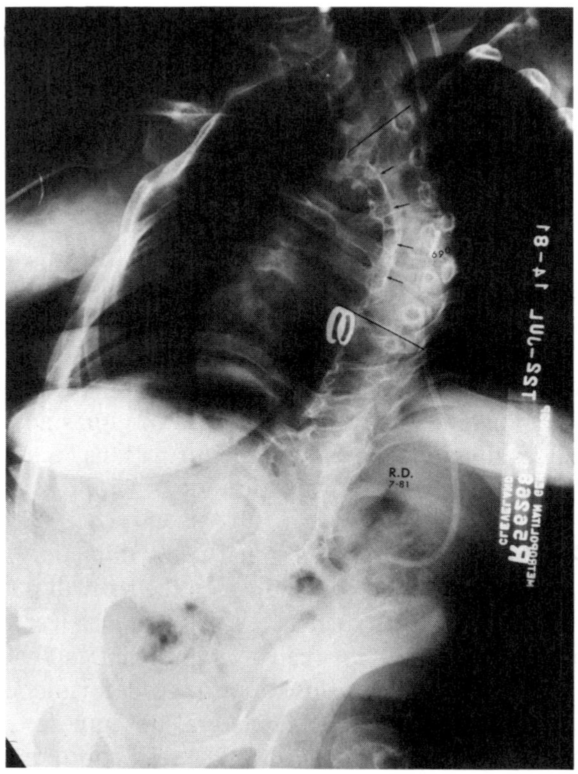

serious mistake to defer treatment of progressive spinal curvatures while awaiting further spinal growth.

When to Consult

Because of the high risk for curve progression in congenital scoliosis and the associated renal, cardiac, and intraspinal abnormalities, all children with congenital scoliosis should be referred for orthopaedic evaluation. If convenient, renal ultrasound evaluation of the urinary system can be performed while awaiting consultation. Also, providing the orthopaedist with information regarding the cardiac examination will be helpful.

Neuromuscular Scoliosis

Progressive spinal deformity is a common and potentially serious abnormality associated with many neuromuscular disorders of childhood and adolescence. The more common disorders with an increased incidence of scoliosis include cerebral palsy, Duchenne muscular dystrophy, spinal muscular atrophy, myelodysplasia, and arthrogryposis multiplex congenita. Progression is usually continuous once scoliosis begins. The magnitude of the deformity depends on the severity and pattern of weakness and whether the disease process is progressive. In non-ambulatory patients the curves tend to be long and sweeping, produce pelvic obliquity, involve the cervical spine, and alter pulmonary functions producing respiratory problems. As these curves progress, sitting balance can be lost, and affected individuals must use their arms to support an upright position thus further increasing their disability. It is, therefore, important that spinal alignment be part of the routine examination of a child with a neuromuscular disorder. Ambulatory patients have a much lower incidence of spinal deformity than the non-ambulatory or more severely involved patients. The standing or sitting forward bending test can be used in assessment for the symmetry of spinal alignment. Any asymmetry is an indication for radiographic evaluation. This should include a posterior-anterior and lateral standing or sitting radiograph of the entire spine. If the child or adolescent cannot sit unsupported then an anterior-posterior supine radiograph may be necessary.

The goal of treatment of neuromuscular scoliosis is to prevent progression and loss of function secondary to the spinal deformity. Nonambulatory patients are usually most comfortable, more independent, and have better respiratory function when they are able to sit erect without external support. Orthotic management or bracing is usually not effective in neuromuscular scoliosis. It may be effective in certain cases, particularly children, in slowing the rate of curve progression, allowing further spinal growth and delaying surgical intervention. Surgery will be necessary in most cases. The current instrumentation systems (Luque and Cotrel-Dubousset) are sufficiently strong and distribute the corrective forces such that postoperative immobilization is usually not necessary and the patient may be out of bed immediately after surgery (see Fig. 8-3).

When to Consult

Any child with a neuromuscular disorder should, if at all possible, be followed concomitantly by an orthopaedic surgeon experienced in the management of spinal deformities. Progression of these deformities can occur rapidly, and the spine should be assessed at each outpatient visit, preferably at six month intervals, especially in the older child and adolescent.

Syndromes

Children with syndromes are also at risk for spinal deformities. Common syndromes include neurofibromatosis and Marfan's syndrome. These children require careful periodic evaluation and prompt referral for orthopaedic evaluation at the first sign of a spinal deformity.

Compensatory Spinal Deformities

As stated previously, adolescents with a lower extremity length inequality may have a positive screening examination for scoliosis. With a pelvic obliquity the patient will stand erect and curve the spine in the opposite direction. The magnitude of the leg length discrepancy can be measured radiographically by a scanogram of the lower extremities. It is important to distinguish between a structural and compensatory spinal deformity. Any child with a lower extremity inequality should be referred for orthopaedic evaluation.

Kyphosis

The term kyphosis refers to a roundback deformity or to an increased angulation in the thoracic or thoracolumbar spine in the sagittal plane. Roundback deformities can either be postural or structural. The latter is termed Scheuermann's kyphosis. Kyphosis can also be congenital in origin.

Figure 8-3.

(A) Sitting anterior-posterior radiograph of a 10-year-old boy with lumbar myelodysplasia demonstrating a long sweeping 73 degree right thoracic paralytic spinal deformity between T5 and L1. Observe the absence of the posterior elements in the lumbar region due to the meningomyelocele. A ventriculoperitoneal shunt tube for hydrocephalus is visible.

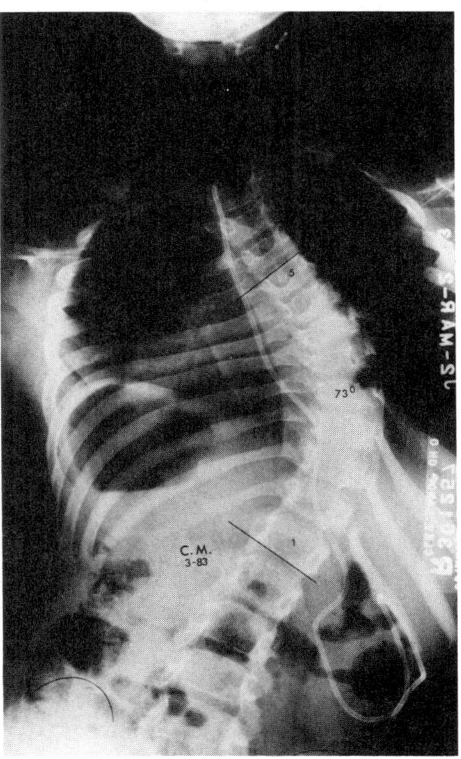

(B) Postoperative radiograph of the same boy following a combined anterior and posterior spinal fusion and Luque rod instrumentation from T3 to the sacrum. The curve has been reduced 49 degrees (33% correction), and there is improved spinal alignment.

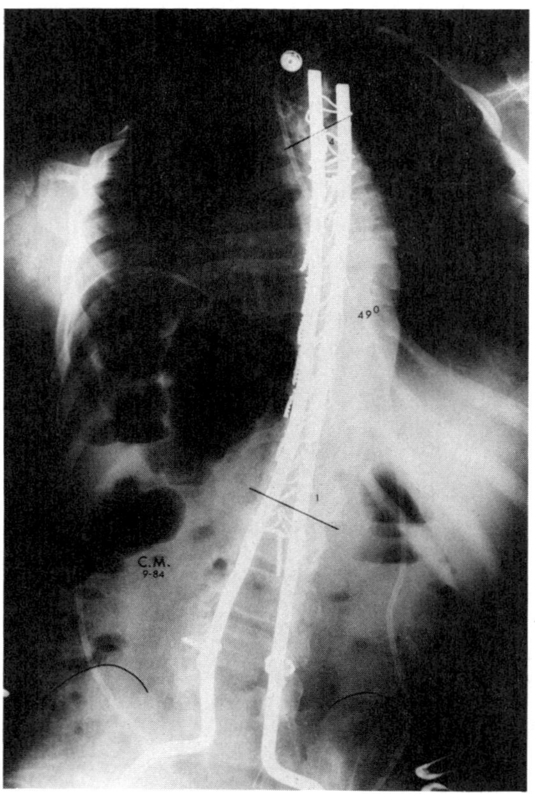

Postural Roundback

Postural kyphosis is secondary to bad posture. It is a common concern of parents. Postural kyphosis is diagnosed by the ability of the adolescent to voluntarily correct the roundback appearance in both the standing and prone position. Radiographically, no vertebral abnormalities are present. There may be some increase in the normal kyphosis of the thoracic region but a supine hyperextension film will show complete correction. The child is responsible for posture correction. Active treatment is not indicated. Orthopaedic referral is not routinely necessary for postural kyphosis.

Scheuermann's Disease

Scheuermann's disease is common and second only to idiopathic scoliosis as a cause of spinal deformity. It occurs equally among males and females. Its etiology is also unknown, but there are hereditary factors present but no definite pattern of inheritance. Kyphosis appearing in infants or young children is usually congenital in origin. The differentiation between postural kyphosis and Scheuermann's disease is determined by clinical and radiographic evaluation.

Clinical Examination

A patient with Scheuermann's disease cannot truly correct the kyphosis either in the standing position or in the prone, hyperextended position. When viewed from the side in the forward flexed position, patients with Scheuermann's disease will usually show an abrupt angulation in the mid to lower thoracic region. A patient with a postural roundback shows a smooth symmetric contour. In both conditions there is reversal of the normal lumbar lordosis. Approximately 50% of patients with Scheuermann's disease will have apical back pain especially in those patients with thoracolumbar kyphosis. A careful neurologic evaluation is necessary for all patients with kyphosis.

Radiographic Evaluation

Radiographic assessment for kyphosis is the posterior-anterior and lateral standing radiograph of the entire spine (see Fig. 8-4). The classic findings of Scheuermann's kyphosis include: (1) narrowing of disc space, (2) loss of the normal anterior height of the involved vertebra producing wedging of 5 degrees or more in three or more vertebrae, (3) irregularities of the endplates, and (4) Schmorl's nodes. The supine, hyperextension radiographs will demonstrate the degree of flexibility.

Figure 8-4. Standing lateral radiograph of a 14-year-old boy with a sever 92 degree T3 to T12 Scheuermann's kyphosis. Normal thoracic kyphosis is 20 to 40 degrees.

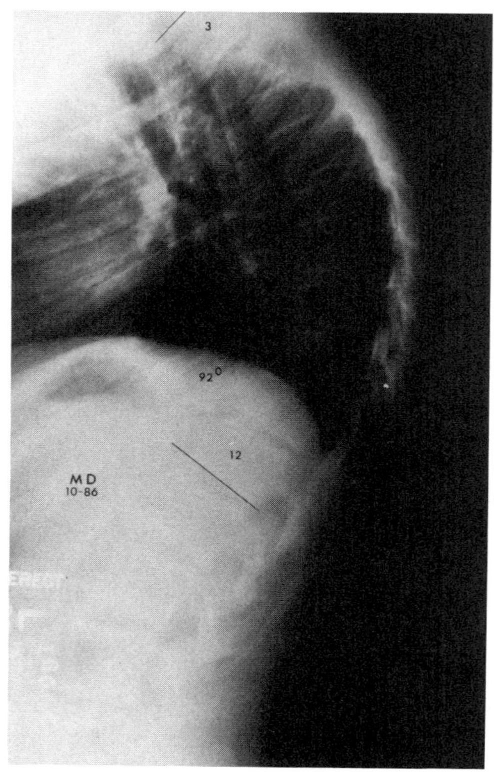

Treatment

Treatment for Scheuermann's kyphosis is similar to scoliosis and is dependent on the skeletal age of the patient, the degree of deformity, and the presence or absence of pain in the apical region. Nonoperative treatment consists of either corrective plaster casts or an orthosis. Thoracic kyphosis usually requires a Milwaukee brace while an underarm hyperextension TLSO can be used for thoracolumbar kyphosis. Permanent correction of the kyphotic deformity can be achieved with nonoperative management.

Surgical treatment in Scheuermann's disease is rarely necessary. It is indicated only for those patients who have completed growth, who have a significant deformity, or who have chronic pain in the apical region. When these indications are met, both an anterior and posterior spinal fusion are usually necessary. The anterior procedure consists of excision of the discs in the apical area of the curvature. This provides increased spinal flexibility as well as placing the arthrodesis under compression. The latter minimizes the risk for pseudoarthrosis. The correction of the deformity is achieved posteriorly with some form of instrumentation. This can either be Harrington compression instrumentation, Luque rod, or Cotrel-Dubousset instrumentation.

When to Consult

As with scoliosis, all patients with kyphosis should be referred for orthopaedic evaluation.

Congenital Kyphosis

Congenital kyphosis or kyphotic deformity is due to vertebral malformations. There are two basic types: (1) congenital failure of formation of all or part of the vertebral body but with preservation of the posterior elements, and (2) failure of anterior segmentation of the spine (anterior unsegmented bar). The more severe deformities are usually recognized at birth and rapidly progress thereafter. The less obvious deformities may not appear until years later. Once the progression begins it does not cease until the end of growth. The most important factor regarding congenital kyphosis is that a progressive deformity in the thoracic spine can result in paraplegia. This is usually associated with the failure of vertebral body formation.

Treatment of congenital scoliosis, when necessary, is operative. Orthotic management is ineffective.

When to Consult

All patients with congenital kyphosis should be referred to the orthopaedic surgeon for evaluation because of the risk of progression and possible paraplegia.

Spondylolysis/Spondylolisthesis

Spondylolysis is a defect in the pars interarticularis without forward slippage of one vertebra on another. Spondylolisthesis refers to the forward slippage or displacement of one vertebra in relation to another. Isthmic spondylolisthesis is the most common type seen in children and adolescents. It occurs in approximately 5% of the general population. Studies have shown that the lesions are not present at birth but occur in 5% of children by six years of age. Children involved in certain sports, such as gymnastics, have an even higher incidence of spondylolysis. This has been attributed to repetitive hyperextension stresses.

Spondylolisthesis is classified according to the degree of slippage of one vertebra on the other: grade 1 (less than 25% slippage), grade 2 (25% to 50% percent slippage), grade 3 (50% to 75% percent slippage), grade 4 (75% to 100% slippage), and grade 5 (complete displacement). The most common location for spondylolisthesis is the fifth lumbar vertebra on the sacrum (first sacral vertebra).

Clinical Examination

Physical examination for spondylolysis or spondylolisthesis is similar to that for any disorder of the spine. This includes general spinal alignment, posture, presence or absence of scoliosis or kyphosis, and areas of tenderness. A palpable "step off" at the lumbosacral area or a vertically oriented sacrum are findings indicative of severe spondylolisthesis. Complete neurological examination should also be performed as nerve root involvement can occur, especially with severe displacement.

Radiologic Evaluation

Radiologic evaluation should include a standing posterior-anterior and lateral view of the entire spine with oblique radiograph of the lumbar spine. Myelography and magnetic resonance imaging scans may be required in patients with neurological signs or symptoms.

Treatment

Treatment of spondylolysis is rarely required. Children and adolescents with asymptomatic spondylolysis require periodic evaluation during growth to assess for possible slippage. Painful spondylolysis may benefit from orthotic management. If this does not relieve pain then surgical intervention with a in situ posterior spinal fusion may be required. Adolescents with spondylolisthesis may require treatment. This depends on age of the patient, type of defect, degree of the slippage, and associated malalignment in the involved area. Grade 1 spondylolisthesis usually does not require treatment unless there is chronic pain. Conservative management may be tried initially and if this fails then surgical intervention may be necessary. Grade 2 usually require a spinal fusion because of the high risk for further progression. Grade 3 and grade 4 spondylolisthesis almost always require fusion to prevent further deformity.

When to Consult

It is important that patients with spondylolysis or spondylolisthesis be referred to an orthopaedic surgeon for discussion of possible etiologies, the factors for progression, and possible treatment.

Disc Space Infection

This disease is usually regarded as an osteomyelitis of the vertebral endplates that secondarily invades the disc without producing an acute osteomyelitis of the vertebral body. The most common organism producing this type of infection is <u>Staphylococcus aureus</u>. It can occur at any age. Children may present with back pain, but it may also present as abdominal or pelvic pain.

Clinical Examination

The physical findings in a child with a disc space infection are usually quite characteristic. The child typically maintains the spine in a straight, stiff or splinted position and will refuse to flex the lumbar spine. The normal lumbar lordosis is reversed and there may be paravertebral muscle spasms. However, in comparison with other forms of osteomyelitis, there are a few systemic symptoms such as fever or an elevated white blood cell count. The sedimentation rate is typically elevated.

Radiographic Evaluation

The radiographic features will vary according to the interval between the onset of symptoms and delay in diagnosis. Anterior-posterior, lateral, and oblique radiographs of the lumbar spine or thoracic spine depending on the location of symptoms are usually necessary to make the necessary diagnosis. Characteristically there is narrowing of the disc space with irregularity of the adjacent vertebral body endplates. Lateral tomograms are occasionally necessary in order to demonstrate the abnormalities. In very early cases bone scan or magnetic resonance imaging scans may be helpful in making the diagnosis, as they may be positive before routine radiographic changes are present.

Treatment

The treatment of disc space infection in children is usually by antibiotic therapy. Blood cultures may be helpful in establishing a precise organism. Aspiration needle biopsy of the spine is reserved for children who do not respond to initial treatment with anti-staphylococcal antibiotics. Immobilization of the spine may be used on a symptomatic basis. However, most children will have their symptoms rapidly resolve with intravenous antibiotics. The current recommendation for antibiotic therapy is oxacillin or cephalosporin in standard doses for osteomyelitis. Intravenous antibiotics are continued for one to two weeks and followed by oral antibiotics for an additional four weeks.

When to Consult

It is best to refer all children with disc space infection to an orthopaedic surgeon for evaluation and treatment. Although it is rare to develop a chronic osteomyelitis, occasionally a needle biopsy or even an open biopsy may be necessary to establish a precise diagnosis in difficult cases.

Back Pain in Children

Back pain in children is unusual and should be viewed with concern. In contrast to adults, where back pain is frequently mechanical or psychologic in origin, back pain in children is almost always due to organic causes, especially in the pre-adolescent. Back pain lasting more than a few days requires careful investigation. Hensinger has reported that approximately 85% of children with back pain for more than two months will have a specific diagnosable lesion -- 33% post-traumatic (occult fracture, spondylolysis), 33% developmental (kyphosis, scoliosis), and 18% infection or tumor. Only in the remaining 16% will the diagnosis be nonspecific.

Clinical Examination

When confronted with a child with back pain, a careful history and physical evaluation are mandatory. The history should include the onset and duration of symptoms, antecedent factors, general health, family history, location, character and radiation of pain, and neurologic symptoms such as muscle weakness, sensory changes, bowel or bladder dysfunction. Physical examination includes a complete musculoskeletal and neurologic evaluation. Spinal alignment, mobility, muscle spasm, and areas of tenderness are evaluated and recorded. Muscle strength, sensory assessment such as pain and light touch, deep tendon reflexes, and pathologic reflexes such as the Babinski sign are tested. The danger signs in childhood back pain include: (1) persistent or increasing pain, (2) systemic symptoms such as fever, malaise or weight loss, (3) neurologic symptoms or findings, (4) bowel or bladder dysfunction, (5) young age, especially under four years (suspect tumor), and (6) painful, left thoracic spinal curvatures.

Radiographic Evaluation

Plain radiographs are the first diagnostic procedure in the evaluation of pediatric back pain. Usually posterior-anterior and lateral standing films are obtained with right and left oblique views of the involved area. However, other radiographs may be necessary depending on the location of the pain and the differential diagnoses. Other radiographic procedures commonly used in evaluation of back pain include: (1) technetium bone scans, (2) computed tomography (CT scan), (3) laminograms, (4) metrizamide myelography (see Fig. 8-5), and (5) magnetic resonance imaging (MRI scan). MRI scans are especially useful when intraspinal pathology is suspected.

Laboratory Evaluation

Laboratory studies such as complete blood count, erythrocyte sedimentation rate, and tests for the juvenile forms of arthritis (JRA and ankylosing spondylitis) may be necessary in certain cases. Cerebrospinal fluid should be evaluated if myelography is performed.

Differential Diagnosis

The differential diagnosis in pediatric back pain is extensive and presented in Table 8-2.

Table 8-2. Differential Diagnosis of Pediatric Back Pain

CONGENITAL
- Diastematomyelia
- Cervical Spine Anomalies

DEVELOPMENTAL
- Scoliosis (Left Thoracic)
- Kyphosis (Lumbar or Dorsolumbar
    Scheuermann's Disease)

TRAUMATIC
- Occult Fractures
- Spondylolysis - Spondylolisthesis
- Herniated Disc
- Slipped Vertebral Apophysis
- Upper Cervical Spine Instability

INFECTIOUS
- Disc Space Infection
- Vertebral Osteomyelitis
- Tuberculosis

SYSTEMIC DISEASES
- Chronic Infection
- Storage Diseases
- Juvenile Osteoporosis

JUVENILE ARTHRITIS
- Rheumatoid Arthritis
- Ankylosing Spondylitis

NEOPLASTIC (BENIGN AND MALIGNANT)
- Benign
    - Eosinophilic Granuloma
    - Osteoid Osteoma
    - Osteoblastoma
    - Aneurysmal Bone Cyst
- Malignant (Rare)
    - Osteogenic Sarcoma
    - Metastatic

PSYCHOGENIC

When to Consult

Treatment of the specific causes of pediatric back pain is as diverse as the differential diagnosis. It is important to obtain orthopaedic consultation for the evaluation and treatment of any child or adolescent with back pain.

Figure 8-5. Myelogram demonstrating an intraspinal lesion in the upper thoracic (T1 to T5) region. An open biopsy was performed and the lesion was a malignant glioblastoma multiforme.

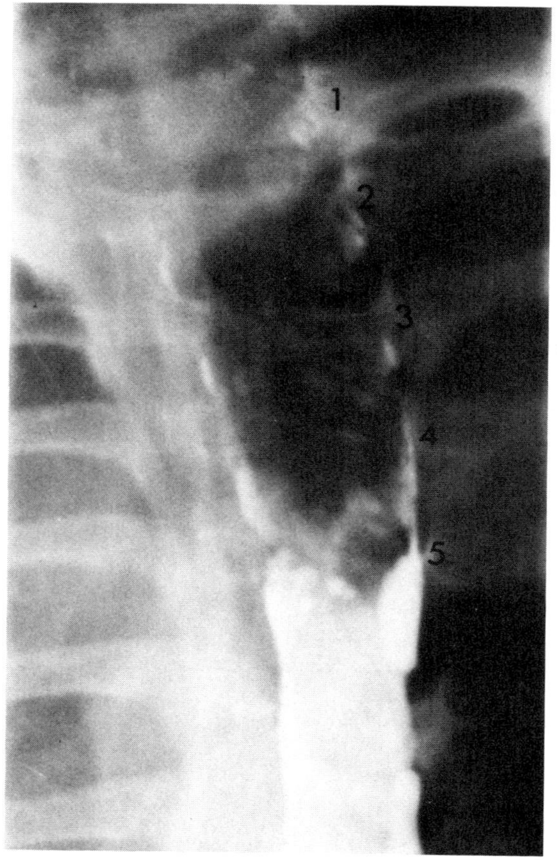

HIP DISORDERS

There are five common pediatric hip disorders. These include (1) congenital dislocation of the hip (CDH), (2) septic arthritis and osteomyelitis, (3) transient monoarticular synovitis, (4) Legg-Calvé-Perthes disease (LCPD), and (5) slipped capital femoral epiphysis (SCFE).

Congenital Dislocation of the Hip

Congenital dislocation of the hip usually occurs in the neonatal period. The hips at birth are usually not dislocated, but rather "dislocatable". Dislocations tend to occur following delivery and thus, are postnatal in origin. The exact time when dislocations occur is controversial. Since they are not truly congenital in origin, the alternate term of development dysplasia of the hip (DDH) is being considered as a replacement. Congenital dislocation of the hip is classified into two major groups: typical, in a neurologically normal infant, and teratologic, in which there is an underlying neuromuscular disorder (myelodysplasia or arthrogryposis multiplex congenita) or syndrome complex. Teratologic CDH can occur in utero. This discussion will concentrate only on typical CDH as it is the most common form.

Etiology

The etiology of CDH is multifactorial with both physiologic and mechanical factors. The physiologic factors include: (1) positive family history (20%), (2) generalized ligamentous laxity, (3) maternal estrogen and other hormones associated with pelvic relaxation, and (4) female predominance (9:1). Mechanical factors include: (1) primigravida, (2) breech presentation, and (3) postnatal positioning.

The positive family history and the generalized ligamentous laxity are related etiological factors. The majority of children with CDH have generalized ligamentous laxity (an autosomal dominant trait), and this predisposes to hip instability. Maternal estrogens and other hormones associated with pelvic relaxation also results in further, although temporary, relaxation of the newborn hip joint.

Approximately 60% of children with typical CDH are first-born and 30% to 50% developed in the breech position. The frank breech position with the hips flexed and the knees extended is the position of highest risk. In the breech position, the fetal pelvis is in the maternal pelvis resulting in extreme hip flexion and limitation of hip motion. Increased hip flexion results in stretching of the already lax capsule and ligament teres. It also produces posterior uncoverage of the femoral head. Decreased hip motion leads to a lack of normal development of the cartilaginous acetabulum. The sex ratio of infants with CDH who developed in a breech presentation declines to 2:1 female. This decline substantiates the importance of the mechanical factors of the breech position in the development of CDH.

There is also an association of congenital muscular torticollis (14% to 20%) and metatarsus adductus (1% to 10%) with CDH. The presence of either of these two conditions requires a careful examination of the hips.

Postnatal factors are also important determinants in the development of CDH. Maintaining the hips in the position of adduction and extension is a major factor leading to dislocation. This is primarily a cultural trait associated with the use of cradle boards and the binding of the infant's lower extremities. This accounts for the increased incidence among certain North American tribes and in Scandinavian countries. There are also seasonal variations as the incidence of CDH increases during the winter. This is due to wrapping of the infant's lower extremity for warmth. Placing the extremities in the position of extension and adduction puts the unstable hip under pressure due to the normally present hip flexion and abduction contractures. The femoral head, as a consequence, can be displaced from the acetabulum over several days or weeks.

Pathoanatomy

Since hips are not dislocated at birth, the components of the hip joint excluding the hip capsule and ligament teres are relatively normal.

There may be some minor variations in the cartilaginous anlage of the acetabulum, especially if the child had developed in a breech position. If a dislocation is allowed to occur and is unrecognized, then the usually described pathological abnormalities of acetabular dysplasia and maldirection, excessive femoral anteversion (torsion), and hip muscle contractures will develop. It must be emphasized that these are secondary changes occurring with growth in the presence of untreated dislocation.

Clinical Examination

Common physical findings in infants with CDH include: (1) Barlow test (unstable hip), (2) Ortolani test (dislocated hip), (3) limitation of hip abduction, (4) asymmetrical thigh skin folds, (5) uneven knee levels (Galeazzi sign), and (6) the absence of normal knee flexion contracture.

The Barlow test is the most important maneuver in examining the newborn hip. This is a provocative test that attempts to dislocate the unstable hip. This test is performed by stabilizing the pelvis with one hand and then flexing and adducting the opposite hip and applying a posterior force. If the hip is dislocatable, it is usually readily felt. Following release of the posterior pressure, the hip will usually spontaneously relocate. It has been estimated that only one in 100 newborns have clinically unstable hips (subluxation or dislocation) while only one in 800 to 1000 infants eventually develop a true dislocation. The Ortolani test is a maneuver to reduce a recently dislocated hip. It is most likely to be positive in infants that are one to two months of age since adequate time must have past for the true dislocation to have occurred. In performing this test, the thigh is flexed and abducted and the femoral head is lifted anteriorly into the acetabulum. If reduction is possible, the relocation will be felt as a "clunk" not a "click". After two months of age, manual reduction of a dislocated hip is usually not possible because of the development of soft-tissue contractures.

Limitation of hip abduction is indicative of soft-tissue contractures and may indicate CDH. Conversely, hip abduction contractures may indicate dysplasia of the contralateral hip. An asymmetrical number of thigh skin folds and apparent shortening of an extremity when the supine infant's feet are placed together on the examining table with the hips and knees flexed (Galeazzi sign) indicates CDH with proximal displacement of the femoral head.

A common source of referral to orthopaedic surgeons' offices is the presence of hip clicks in infants. Hip clicks per se are usually not pathological and are secondary to: (1) breaking the surface tension across the hip joint, (2) snapping of gluteal tendons, or (3) patellofemoral motion, or (4) femorotibial (knee) rotation.

In older or walking children, complaints of limping, waddling, increased lumbar lordosis (swayback), toe-walking and in-toeing may be associated with an unrecognized CDH.

Radiographic Evaluation

Ultrasonography is becoming an increasingly popular method for initial evaluation and for accessing the results after treatment in newborns and infants with CDH. Hip stability as well as acetabular development can accurately be assessed by an experienced ultrasonographer. Ultrasonography avoids the use of ionizing radiation but results are very operator dependent.

Radiographic evaluation, when necessary, of a typical CDH is made from standard anterior-posterior and Lauenstein (frog) lateral radiographs of the pelvis. The ossific nucleus of the femoral headdoes not appear until four to six months of age and it may be further delayed in CDH. Line measurements are usually made in order to determine the relationship of the femoral head to the acetabulum. The most commonly employed measurements include: (1) acetabular index, (2) quadrant assessment, (3) Shenton's line, and (4) the center edge angle of Wiberg. Arthrography, computed tomography, and magnetic resonance imaging scans may be beneficial in difficult cases especially older infants.

Treatment

The treatment of congenital dislocation of the hip is very individualized and primarily dependent upon the patients's age at diagnosis.

Birth

When an unstable hip is recognized at birth, maintenance of the hip in the position of flexion and abduction ("human" position) for one to two months is usually sufficient. This position maintains reduction of the femoral head and allows for tightening of the ligamentous structures as well as for stimulation of normal growth and development of the femoral head and acetabulum. Methods that can be used to maintain the hip in this position include double or triple diapers, Pavlik harness, Friejka splint, and a variety of abduction orthoses. Double and triple diapers tend to be the primary method of treatment in early infancy as the latter devices usually do not fit satisfactorily. Treatment is usually continued until there is clinical stability of the hip and the radiographic measurements are within normal limits and symmetrical.

One to Six Months

During this age a true dislocation of the hip will usually develop. As a consequence, treatment is directed toward reduction of the femoral head into the acetabulum. The Pavlik harness is the major mode of treatment in this age group. The harness attempts to place the hips in the human position by flexing the hips more than 90 degrees (preferably 100 to 110 degrees) and maintaining full but gentle abduction. This redirects the femoral head towards the acetabulum. Usually, spontaneous relocation of the femoral head will occur within three to four weeks. The Pavlik harness is approximately 95% successful in dysplastic hips and 80% in true CDH. If reduction is achieved, then the Pavlik harness is maintained until the acetabular index and other parameters have returned to normal. If a spontaneous reduction does not occur, then a surgical closed reduction is attempted. This consists of: (1) preliminary skin traction for one to three weeks in order to bring the femoral head opposite the acetabulum, (2) percutaneous adductor tenotomy, (3) closed reduction, and (4) application of a hip spica cast in, again, the "human" position. Treatment is continued until the radiographic parameters are normal and symmetrical.

Six to 18 Months

In the older infant, surgical closed reduction is the major method of treatment. If the reduced hip shows significant residual instability, an open reduction may be indicated.

18 Months to 8 Years

Following 18 months of age the progressive deformities are now so severe that open reduction followed by pelvic (innominate) or femoral osteotomy to redirect the acetabulum or femoral head becomes necessary. Following osteotomy, the child is maintained in a spica cast for six to eight weeks to allow for healing. Thereafter, the child may be allowed to gradually return to full activities. Implanted metal is removed shortly after healing to prevent incorporation into the growing bone. It should be mentioned that 18 months of age is not an arbitrary age for osteotomies. It has been demonstrated that approximately 25% of children who have a closed reduction performed between nine and 12 months of age, 50% between 12 and 18 months and 75% between 18 and 36 months will have residual acetabular dysplasia requiring osteotomy at a later date. Residual acetabular dysplasia can be satisfactorily managed with a rotational pelvic osteotomy such as a Salter innominate osteotomy from childhood into mid-adult life.

Complications

The most important and severe complication of CDH is osteonecrosis (avascular necrosis) of the capital femoral epiphysis (CFE). This is an iatrogenic complication. Reduction of the femoral head under pressure produces cartilaginous compression and this can result in occlusion of the intra-articular, extra-osseous epiphyseal vessels and produce CFE infarction, either partial or total. Revascularization follows but abnormal growth and development may occur, especially if the growth plate is severely damaged. The hip is most vulnerable to this complication prior to the development of the ossific nucleus (four to six months). The techniques of appropriate management as outlined are designed to minimize this complication. Utilizing these techniques, the incidence of avascular necrosis will be approximately 5%.

Other potential complications in CDH include redislocation, residual subluxation or acetabular dysplasia, and postoperative complications such as wound infections.

When to Consult

Any infant or child with a suspected CDH should be referred to an orthopaedic surgeon as soon as possible. It is appropriate to place newborns or neonates in double or triple diapers pending consultation.

Septic Arthritis and Osteomyelitis

Infection of the hip joint is a surgical emergency because of the risk of avascular necrosis of the capital femoral epiphysis. Hematogenous infection of the synovium without bone involvement is termed septic arthritis while infection of the femoral neck (metaphysis) is osteomyelitis.

Each disorder has a different organism as the most common etiologic organism depending on the age of the patient. In septic arthritis, Staphylococcus aureus is most common in children over five years of age. In children between six months and five years of age, Hemophilus influenzae is a common cause. In the neonate, group B streptococcus and gram negative organisms are also common etiologic agents. In osteomyelitis, Staphylococcus aureus is the most common organism in all age groups.

Clinical Examination

Neonates with an infected hip may only show irritability, especially with diaper change, and refuse to eat. They typically do not have fever or a significantly elevated white blood count. This lack of systemic response is due to the immaturity of their immune system. This impairs both their cellular and hormonal immunity and results in a decrease in immune and inflammatory responses to infection.

Older infants and children with infection of the hip joint usually exhibit all of the clinical signs of sepsis including elevated temperature, white blood cell count and erythrocyte sedimentation rate. The hip joint is usually not swollen but may be tender to palpation and with motion. Classically the hip is held in flexion, abduction and external rotation to unwind the hip capsule and allow it to hold the greatest volume of intracapsular fluid. This is an involuntary attempt to decompress the hip. Early on the child may walk with a limp, but later will usually refuse to walk at all.

Radiographic Evaluation

Anterior-posterior and frog lateral radiographs of the pelvis are obtained. This will allow comparison of both the involved and uninvolved hips. Early in a septic process the radiographs are usually normal. There may be occasional widening of the medial joint space. It is usually 10 to 14 days before there is radiographic evidence of bone destruction in osteomyelitis (see Fig. 8-6). Technetium bone scans and magnetic resonance imaging may be beneficial in early cases.

Treatment

Diagnosis of septic arthritis and osteomyelitis is made by arthrocentesis or aspiration of the hip joint. This can be difficult and must always be done under a fluoroscopic control. If no fluid is obtained from the hip joint, an arthrogram is obtained documenting that the hip joint had been aspirated. If cloudy fluid with an elevated white blood cell count is obtained, surgical drainage is necessary. It is not necessary to await culture results before draining an infected hip. The hip joint should never be treated by multiple aspirations and irrigations because of the dangers of avascular necrosis as a result of increased joint fluid pressure from the infection. The hip may be drained by either an anterior or posterior approach. Drilling the femoral neck is controversial as there is easy drainage of an osteomyelitic process through the haversian canals into the hip joint itself. Broad spectrum intravenous antibiotics are utilized pending results of culture and sensitivity tests.

The antibiotics selected will be based on the patients age and suspected organism. Depending on the degree of irritability and duration of symptoms, the hip joint may need to be immobilized for several days to allow for the inflammation to subside and to decrease the risk for a pathologic dislocation of the hip. Once acute inflammation has subsided, motion should be allowed so that nutrition to the overlying articular cartilage can be obtained. Joint motion also helps to prevent fibrosis and loss of motion.

When to Consult

Any child with a suspected septic process involving the hip must have an immediate orthopaedic evaluation. Early diagnosis and prompt surgical drainage are the major factors in achieving long-term satisfactory results.

Figure 8-6. Anterior-posterior radiograph of the pelvis of a two-year old infant with osteomyelitis of the left femoral neck. There is marked bone destruction beneath the physeal plate of the capital femoral epiphysis.

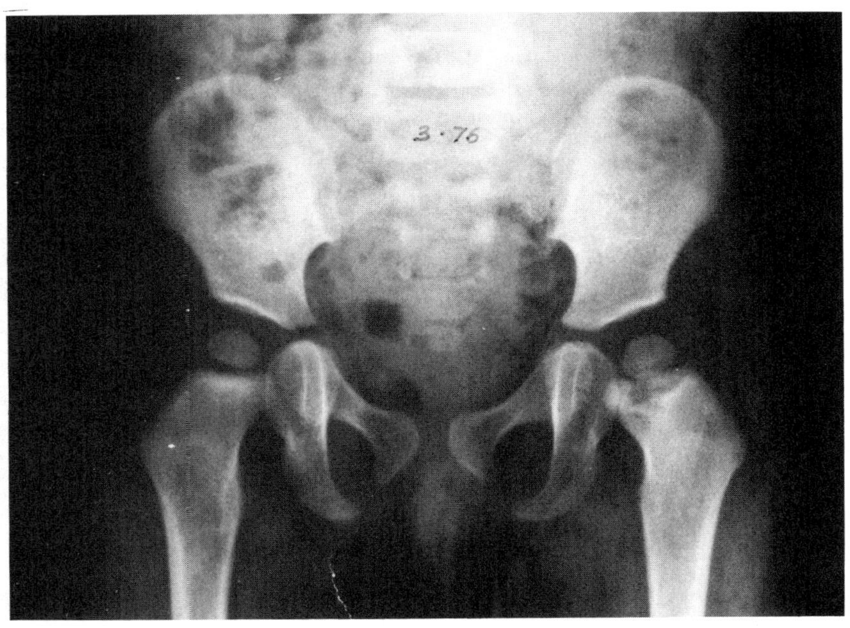

Transient Monoarticular Synovitis

Transient synovitis of the hip is one of the most common cause of limping in a normal children. It is characterized by acute onset of monoarthritic hip pain, limp, and mild restriction of hip motion, especially abduction and medial rotation. Septic arthritis and osteomyelitis of the hip must be excluded before this diagnosis can be confirmed. The etiology of transient synovitis remains uncertain. Possible etiologies include: (1) active or recent systemic viral syndrome, (2) trauma, and (3) allergic hypersensitivity. Approximately 70% of involved children will have had a nonspecific upper respiratory infection seven to 14 days prior to the onset of hip symptoms. Biopsy specimens from the hip joint of patients with transient synovitis have demonstrated synovial hypertrophy secondary to nonspecific inflammatory reaction. Hip joint aspirations have been negative although a synovial effusion from one to three millimeters is not uncommon.

Clinical Examination

Transient monoarticular synovitis can occur in all age groups but the average age of onset is six years with the most being three to eight years of age. There is an acute onset of symptoms. The pain is usually felt in the groin, anterior thigh, or knee. It must be remembered that any child with nontraumatic anterior thigh or knee pain must be carefully evaluated for hip pathology as this is the site of referred pain. These children are usually ambulatory and the hip is not held in the flexed, abducted and laterally rotated position unless a significant effusion is present. However, they walk with an antalgic or painful gait (limp) on the involved side. Children are usually afebrile or have a low grade fever of less than 38 degrees centigrade.

Laboratory values are usually within normal limits but occasionally a slight elevation in the white blood cell count and sedimentation rate may be seen.

Radiographic Evaluation

Anterior-posterior and frog lateral radiographs of the pelvis are obtained. This, again, allows comparison of the involved and uninvolved hips. These radiographs will usually be normal. Occasionally, ultrasound of the hip may be useful in demonstrating a hip joint effusion. Bone scans may also be of value.

Treatment

Treatment for monoarticular synovitis of the hip is symptomatic. Bed rest and non-weight-bearing until the pain resolves followed by limited activities thereafter are the treatments of choice. Most children are maintained at bed rest for approximately seven days. They are then maintained on limited activities for one to two additional weeks. This sometimes is difficult as children want to return to normal activities when their symptoms resolve. However, if the child is allowed to return to normal activities too early, then exacerbation of symptoms can occur.

When the diagnosis of transient monoarticular synovitis is in doubt, hip aspiration may be necessary. The fluid that is aspirated will show a very low white blood cell count and will be culture negative.

When to Consult

Many physicians feel comfortable diagnosing and managing transient monoarticular synovitis of the hip especially if the child is afebrile. However, when the diagnosis in is in doubt, such as when fever is present or there is a significant loss of motion, then an urgent orthopaedic evaluation is necessary.

Legg-Calve´-Perthes Disease (LCPD)

Legg-Calve´-Perthes disease (LCPD) is idiopathic (unknown causation) osteonecrosis or avascular necrosis of the capital femoral epiphysis (CFE) and the associated complications thereof occurring in an immature growing child. It is currently accepted that this disorder is caused by an interruption of the CFE blood supply. It is primarily a disorder of males (4-5:1) and is bilateral in approximately 20% of involved children. It has been consistently observed that children with LCPD have delayed bone ages, disproportionate growth, and mild short stature.

Pathogenesis

The pathogenesis and pathology of LCPD is relatively well understood at this time. Initially, there is an ischemic episode that renders most, if not all, the CFE avascular. Endochondral ossifications in the preosseous cartilage and growth plate ceases temporarily while the articular cartilage, being nourished by synovial fluid, continues to grow. A widened medial cartilage (joint) space and a small ossific nucleus in the involved hip are seen on the radiographs at this time. Revascularization of the structurally intact epiphysis occurs from the periphery as new capillaries recanalize the previous vascular channels. Resumption of endochondral ossification within the epiphysis begins peripherally and progresses centrally. With the ingrowth of capillaries, osteoclasts and osteoblasts cover the surface of the avascular subchondral cortical bone and the central trabecular cancellous bone. Deposition of new immature woven bone on the avascular bone produces a net increase in bone mass per unit area, which accounts for the increased radiodensity seen in the early stages. The deposition of new woven bone and resorption of avascular bone occur simultaneously. In the subchondral area, resorption exceeds new bone formation because of the greater volume of avascular cortical bone. A critical point is reached when the subchondral area becomes weak biomechanically and susceptible to a pathologic fracture. Up to this point, the disease process is clinically silent and the involved child asymptomatic. The continuation of this "potential" LCPD or the development of the "true" LCPD depends on whether a subchondral fracture occurs. If a fracture does not occur then the subchondral area eventually regains its normal strength and a head-within-a-head appearance is visible radiographically. This represents a growth arrest line of the size of the ossific nucleus at the time of the initial infarction. If a subchondral fracture occurs then the typical clinical course of "true" LCPD will occur. The subchondral fracture is painful and heralds the clinical onset of the disease process.

Clinical Examination

The clinical onset of LCPD typically occurs between the ages of two to 12 years with a mean age of seven years. Most children present with mild or intermittent pain in the anterior thigh and/or limp. The classic presentation has been described as a "painless limp". The pertinent early physical findings include: (1) antalgic (painful) gait, (2) muscle spasm and mild restriction of motion, especially abduction and medial rotation (Fig. 8-7), (3) proximal thigh atrophy, and (4) mild shortness of stature.

Radiographic Evaluation

The radiographic characteristics of LCPD can be divided into five distinct stages representing a continuum of the disease process: (1) cessation of CFE growth, (2) subchondral fracture, (3) resorption (fragmentation), (4) reossification, and (5) healed or residual stage.

In 1971, Catterall proposed a four-group classification. This was based on the radiographic appearance of the femoral head at the time of maximum epiphyseal resorption. This classification has been extremely useful in the retrospective analyses of the results of treatment. However, it has limited prognostic value in the early phases of the disease process. In 1984, Salter and Thompson introduced a simplified two-group classification based on the subchondral fracture and correlated it with a statistical analysis of long-term results. This classification is dependent upon early diagnosis.

Catterall Classification

The major radiographic characteristics of Catterall's four groups are as follows: (Group 1) involvement is limited only to the anterior aspect of the CFE. The posterior, medial and anterior portions are uninvolved, (Group 2) the anterior and only a portion of posterior aspect of the CFE

Figure 8-7. Prone hip rotation in extension demonstrates decreased medial rotation of the left hip in an eight-year-old boy with Legg-Calve'-Perthes disease.

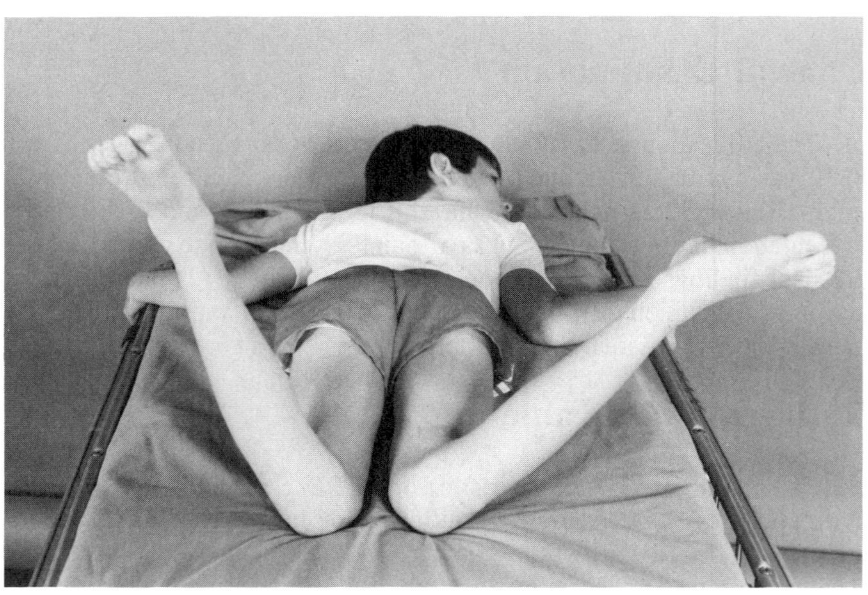

are involved. The medial and lateral portions are uninvolved and continue to support the epiphysis, (Group 3) the anterior, posterior, and lateral aspects of the CFE are now involved. The loss of the lateral margin predisposes to epiphyseal collapse and deformity. This group is the most common type accounting for approximately 65% of all cases, (Group 4) this group is characterized by whole-head involvement and has the worst prognosis for residual deformity.

Salter-Thompson Classification

Based on long-term studies, Salter and Thompson recognized that there were only two statistically significant groups and developed a simplified classification. This classification consists of group A (Catterall groups 1 and 2) in which less than one-half of the CFE is involved and group B (Catterall groups 3 and 4) with more than one-half involvement. The determining factor is the presence (group A) or absence (group B) of an intact, viable lateral aspect of the CFE. When present, the intact lateral portion acts as a supporting column that shields the epiphysis from stress and minimizes the possibility of epiphyseal collapse and subsequent deformity. Its absence indicates a potentially poor prognosis.

Radiographic assessment is necessary during the disease process to determine the disease progression, sphericity of the femoral head, the possibility of CFE collapse and extrusion, and the response to treatment. Plain radiographs are usually adequate but occasionally additional procedures such as arthrography, radionuclide bone scans, and magnetic resonance imaging (MRI) may be useful (see Figs. 8-8). Bone scans and MRI scans are extremely accurate in recognizing potential LCPD, but they are of limited value in assessing the extent of CFE involvement or following the progression of the disease process. The MRI scan also demonstrates the contours of the femoral head and can be valuable in determining sphericity.

Prognosis

The prognosis for LCPD is two-fold. The short-term prognosis concerns femoral head deformity at the completion of the healing stage. The long-term prognosis involves the potential for osteoarthritis of the hip in adulthood. The six prognostic factors for the short-term prognosis are: (1) sex, (2) age at clinical onset, (3) extent of CFE involvement, (4) femoral head containment, (5) hip range of motion, and (6) premature growth plate closure. The prognostic factors for the development of late degenerative arthritis include (1) femoral head deformity and (2) age at clinical onset. Older children with significant residual femoral head deformity are at risk for the development of degenerative arthritis. The incidence is essentially 100% in children who are 10 years of age or older at onset who have residual femoral head deformity. This is compared with a negligible risk in children five years or less and 38% when onset occurs between six and nine years.

Figure 8-8.

(A) Anterior-posterior radiograph of the pelvis of a six-year-old boy with non-traumatic pain in the left anterior thigh and knee region. Observe the slight decrease in height and width of the left capital femoral epiphysis suggestive of very early Legg-Calve'-Perthes disease.

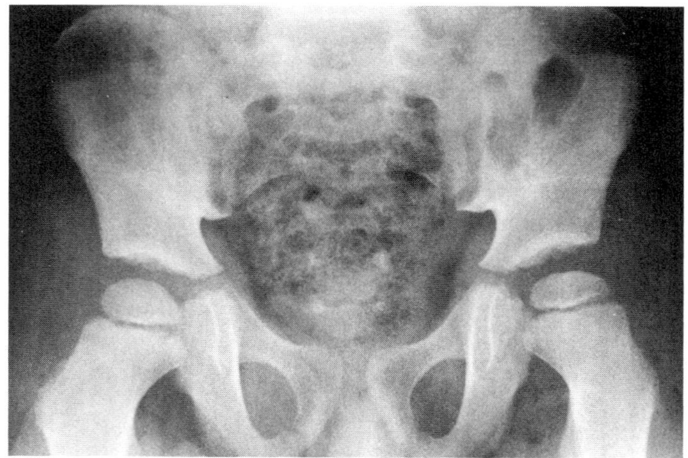

(B) Magnetic resonance imaging confirmed the avascularity and the diagnosis of Legg-Calve'-Perthes disease of the left capital femoral epiphysis.

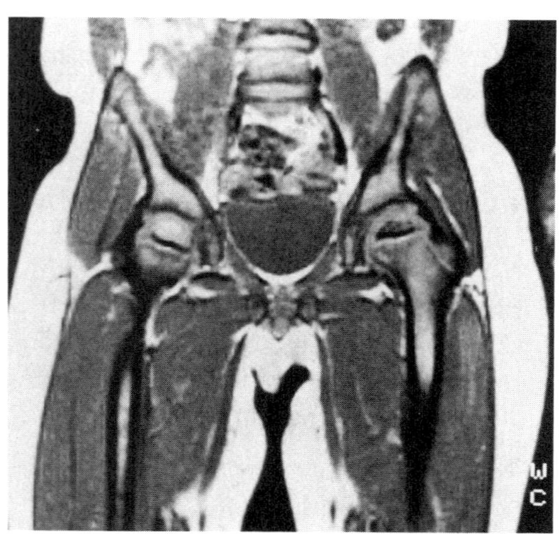

(C)   Six months later there are typical radiographic changes of Legg-Calve'-Perthes disease.

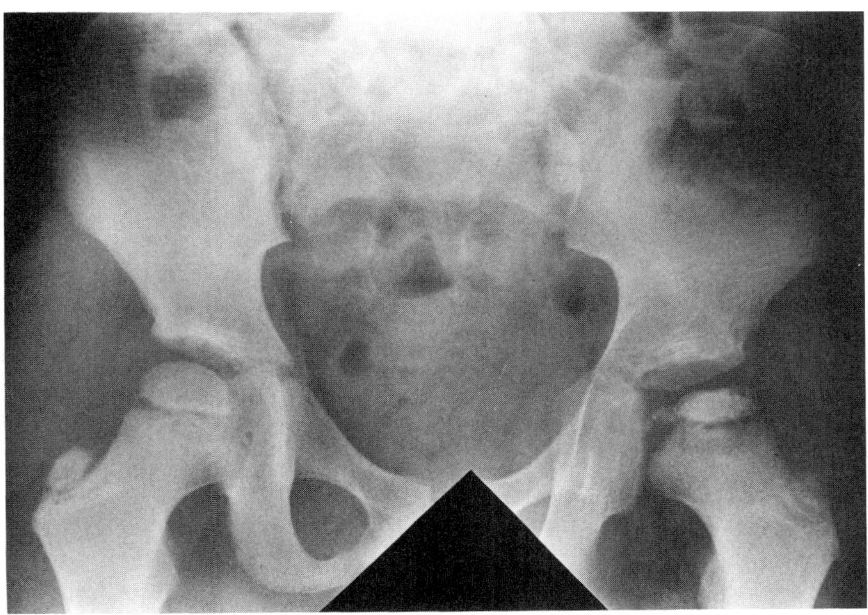

Treatment

LCPD is a local, self-healing disorder. Prevention of femoral head deformity and secondary osteoarthritis are the only justifications for treatment. There are four basic treatment goals: (1) elimination of hip irritability, (2) restoration and maintenance of a good range of hip motion, (3) prevention of CFE collapse, extrusion or subluxation, and (4) attainment of a spherical femoral head at healing. Current treatment methods utilize the concept of containment. In this concept, the femoral head is contained within the acetabulum so that the latter acts as a mold for the reossifying CFE. This may be accomplished by non-surgical containment using abduction casts and orthoses or by surgical containment with proximal femoral varus osteotomy, with or without derotation, and pelvic osteotomies to redirect the acetabulum and thereby contain the femoral head in the position of weight-bearing. All children with Legg-Calve´-Perthes disorder must be under the care and supervision of an orthopaedic surgeon.

Methods of Treatment

The currently accepted forms of management can be divided into four broad categories: (1) observation, (2) intermittent symptomatic treatment, (3) definitive early treatment to prevent deformity, and (4) surgical treatment of existing deformity.

Observation

Expectant observation is appropriate for all children under six years of age at clinical onset regardless of the extent of CFE involvement. However, these children must be followed closely, both clinically and radiographically.

Intermittent Symptomatic Treatment

Temporary or periodic treatment with bedrest or abduction stretching exercises to maintain mobility can be used in conjunction with observation. Recurrent episodes of hip irritability with temporary decrease in motion commonly occur during the phases of subchondral fracture and fragmentation and the child may benefit from symptomatic treatment.

Definitive Early Treatment

Non-surgical or surgical containment of the femoral head in the course of the disease is indicated when: (1) the age at clinical onset is six years or older (possibly five years in girls), (2) there is Catterall group 3 or 4 or Salter-Thompson group B CFE involvement, or (3) there is a loss of containment, as manifested by extrusion of the femoral head as seen on anterior-posterior weight-bearing radiographs.

Abduction casts (Petrie) or orthoses are commonly used to contain the femoral head within the acetabulum. Containment is continued only until there is early radiographic subchondral reossification. Since this usually occurs 12 to 17 months after clinical onset, non-surgical containment methods can be limited to 18 months or less with no adverse effect on the outcome. Currently, the Atlanta Scottish Rite Hospital orthosis is the most widely used because it allows reciprocal motion and ambulation without crutches or external support. The published long term results of nonsurgical containment indicate 75% to 90% satisfactory results.

The selection of pelvic or femoral osteotomy for surgical containment is based on the philosophy and technical expertise of the surgeon. The long-term results of surgical containment also demonstrate 75% to 90% satisfactory results.

Late Surgical Management for Deformity

If significant femoral head deformity prevents reduction of the femoral head into the acetabulum, an alternative method must be considered. Several surgical procedures at least partially correct the various existing deformities and thereby alleviate the associated symptoms. These include: (1) muscle release and abduction casts followed by either pelvic or proximal femoral osteotomy when appropriate containment has been obtained, (2) combined pelvic and femoral osteotomy, (3) partial excision of the femoral head; (4) proximal femoral valgus osteotomy, (5) greater trochanteric advancement, and (6) Chiari osteotomy.

Because of the complexities and controversies surrounding LCPD, all children with this disorder should be under the supervision of an orthopaedic surgeon.

Slipped Capital Femoral Epiphysis

Slipped capital femoral epiphysis (SCFE) is the most common adolescent hip disorder. Recent studies suggest an incidence of one to three per 100,000. Its etiology is unknown. An endocrine basis has been suggested because SCFE is frequently accompanied by abnormalities of growth. It typically occurs in adolescents who are either obese and have delayed skeletal maturation or in tall, thin individuals who have had a recent growth spurt. In the obese children, a low level of sex hormones has been postulated while in tall, thin children, an overabundance of growth hormone is implicated. It is known that sex hormones, as well as growth hormones, alter the rate of proliferation of the cartilage cells in the growth plate (physis) and the rate of skeletal growth. SCFE can also occur as a complication of an underlying endocrine disorder such as hypothyroidism, pituitary disorders, pseudohypoparathyroidism and others. When a SCFE occurs prior to puberty a hormonal abnormality or systemic disorder should be suspected. SCFE also tends to occur more frequently in the spring and this has been attributed to decreased vitamin D intake from being indoors during the winter. Slippage occurs through the zone of cell columns as the columns of cartilage cells are disorganized and grouped into clusters. The cartilage matrix appears to be less cohesive. Recent studies of the histopathology of SCFE indicated mechanical factors as the ultimate cause of slippage. Thus, the initial growth plate abnormality is most likely secondary to endocrine changes during early adolescence but the slippage itself is probably mechanical. Obesity produces high shear forces across the weakened and obliquely oriented growth plate.

Radiographic Evaluation

Anterior-posterior and Lauenstein (frog) lateral radiographs of the pelvis are used for assessment of the hips. Both hips must be evaluated simultaneously for comparison purposes. The earliest sign of SCFE is widening of the growth plate without slippage. This is considered a pre-slip condition. As slippage occurs, the capital femoral epiphysis stays in the acetabulum, and the femoral neck rotates predominantly posteriorly although occasionally superiorly resulting in a varus, retroverted femoral head and neck. The degree of slippage between the epiphysis and the femoral neck can be classified into mild (0% to 33%), moderate (34% to 50%) and severe (more than 50%) categories by radiographic measurement techniques (see Fig. 8-9). Slippage resulting in a valgus deformity is rare except in metabolic disorders such as renal osteodystrophy, Marfan syndrome, and as a sequelae irradiation therapy.

Classification

SCFE is classified into four distinct clinical groups: (1) pre-slip, (2) acute, (3) acute-on-chronic, and (4) chronic.

Pre-Slip

The growth plate is wide but slippage has not occurred. There may be mild discomfort, but the physical examination is usually normal. Pre-slips are frequently seen in the opposite hip of an adolescent with a previous SCFE.

Acute SCFE

In acute SCFE there are usually no or only mild antecedent symptoms such as pain or limp for less than three weeks duration. Slippage occurs suddenly, with or without significant trauma, and the pain is so severe that the child is usually unable to stand or bear weight on the involved extremity. This is not considered a type I epiphyseal injury, as there is a pre-slip condition prior to the acute slip.

Acute-on-Chronic SCFE

In the acute-on-chronic SCFE, the epiphysis slips acutely on an existing chronic slip. These adolescents have had previous symptoms (pain, limp, out-toed gait) for several months or longer. Trauma is a potential underlying factor that results in the sudden slippage.

Chronic SCFE

Chronic SCFE is the most common type. There is usually a several month history of the previously described symptoms. The symptoms typically worsen as the slip progresses. However, since there is continuity between the femoral neck and capital femoral epiphysis, the

Figure 8-9.

(A) Anterior-posterior radiograph of the pelvis of an obese 12-year-old boy with non-traumatic left anterior thigh and knee pain. The height of the left capital femoral epiphysis is slightly less than on the right indicative of either slight hip flexion or slippage.

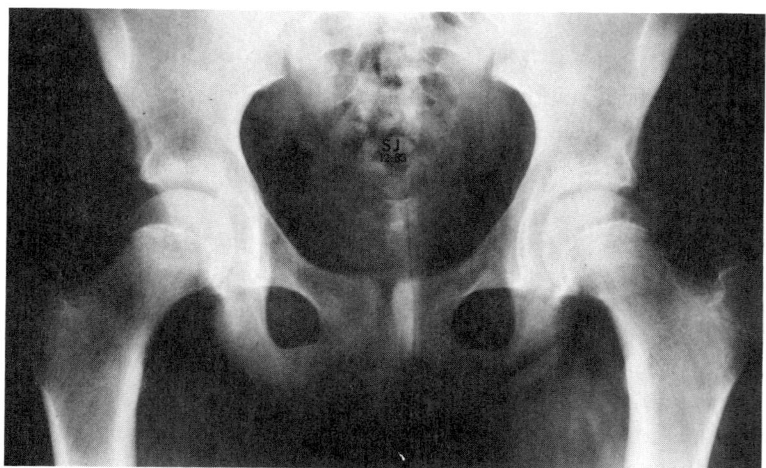

(B) The frog lateral radiograph demonstrates a mild left slipped capital femoral epiphysis.

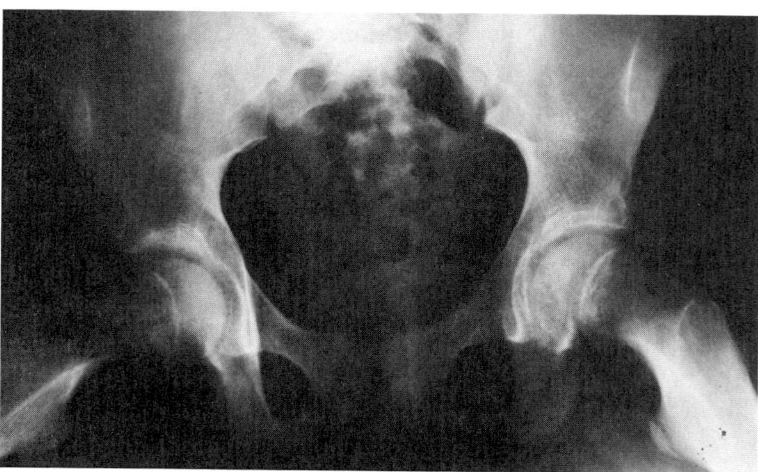

symptoms are not severe, and the child is able to walk, albeit with a mildly antalgic, externally rotated gait.

Clinical Examination

The physical findings in SCFE depend on the degree of slippage and the classification. In the acute or acute-on-chronic slip, the physical examination is limited due to pain with any attempted hip motion. In the chronic SCFE, the patient will have an antalgic gait and the affected extremity is externally rotated. Hip range of motion will demonstrate a lack of medial rotation and increased lateral rotation. Also, as the hip is flexed it will become progressively laterally rotated. Limitation of flexion and abduction may also be present due to a varus deformity of the proximal femur.

20% of patients will complain of only knee pain although they will have decreased hip rotation on physical examination. Adolescents, especially those who are obese, with non-traumatic knee pain (referred pain) should be carefully evaluated for slipped capital femoral epiphysis.

Treatment

The goals of treatment for SCFE are to prevent further slippage and minimize complications. This is accomplished by performing an epiphysiodesis of the capital femoral epiphysis. The technique selected depends on the classification and the severity of the slippage. The current methods include: (1) in situ internal fixation with pins or screws (single or multiple), (2) open bone graft epiphysiodesis, (3) closed bone graft epiphysiodesis, (4) osteotomies of the femoral neck or subtrochanteric regions to realign the proximal femur, and (5) hip spica cast immobilization.

Complications

The two serious complications in SCFE are osteonecrosis and chondrolysis. Osteonecrosis occurs as a result of injury to the retinacular vessels. This can be due to forced manipulation of an acute slip, compression from intracapsular hematoma, or direct injury during surgery. Partial forms of osteonecrosis may also occur following internal fixation due to disruption of the intra-epiphyseal blood vessels. Chondrolysis occurs when there is destruction of the articular cartilage of the hip joint. The etiology of this complication is unclear but has been demonstrated to be associated with more severe slips, black population, pins or screws protruding out of the femoral head, and females.

When to Consult

All children and adolescents who are suspected of having a SCFE require an immediate evaluation and treatment by an orthopaedic surgeon. They should be made non-weight-bearing on the affected extremity and use crutches pending consultation. Early treatment will prevent further slippage, prevent a chronic SCFE from becoming acute-on-chronic, minimize residual deformity, and prevent complications.

LOWER EXTREMITIES

Torsional (in-toeing and out-toeing) and angular (physiologic bowlegs and knock-knees) variations of the lower extremities in young children are among the most common reasons for parents to seek advice from their physicians. Most do not require active treatment as they will improve and resolve with normal growth and development. However, the physician must understand the etiology and natural history in order to adequately reassure the concerned family.

Torsional Variations

Table 8-3 delineates the common causes for in-toeing and out-toeing.

Table 8-3. Common causes for in-toeing and out-toeing.

In-Toeing	Out-Toeing
Medial femoral torsion	Lateral femoral torsion
Medial tibial torsion	Lateral tibial torsion
Metatarsus adductus	Calcaneovalgus feet
Talipes equinovarus (clubfoot)	Hypermobile pes planus (flatfeet)

Before beginning a discussion of torsional variations, it is imperative to have an understanding of the effects that in utero positioning has on the developing lower extremities. In the typical in utero position, the hips are flexed, abducted, and laterally rotated; the knees are flexed and lower legs medially rotated; and the feet are in slight equinus, supination and in contact with the posterolateral aspect of the opposite thigh. This position, therefore, produces: (1) hip flexion, abduction and lateral rotation contractures, (2) knee flexion contractures and medial tibial torsion, and (3) mild supination of the feet. These clinical features are commonly seen in the musculoskeletal examination of the newborn infant. These physical findings are frequently interpreted as abnormalities rather than normal physiological changes.

In-Toeing

Medial Femoral Torsion

Medial or internal femoral torsion is the most common cause of in-toeing in children two years of age or older. It occurs more commonly in girls than boys (2:1). The vast majority of children with this condition have the common autosomal dominant condition - generalized ligamentous laxity. The etiology of femoral torsion is controversial. Some feel that it is congenital (persistent infantile femoral anteversion) while others feel that it is acquired secondary to abnormal sitting habits.

Clinical Examination

The clinical features of medial femoral torsion include an in-toed gait. However, while watching the undressed child walk, it will be observed that the entire lower leg is medially rotated. Clinical examination demonstrates 80 to 90 degrees of medial rotation of the hip in the extended position. Lateral rotation, as a consequence, is limited to 0 to 10 degrees. There will be features of generalized ligamentous laxity including elbow and finger hyperextension, knee recurvatum, and hypermobile pes planus. These children sit almost exclusively in the "television" or "W" style position. It is felt that this position allows the lower leg to act as a lever thereby producing the torsional change in the "biologically plastic" femur. This condition has also been called femoral anteversion, implying an abnormality of the proximal femur. However, it is actually a torsional abnormality throughout the femoral shaft that results in a change in the normal alignment between the hip and knee.

Radiographic Evaluation

Radiology for medial femoral torsion is not routinely necessary. An anteroposterior radiograph of the pelvis is usually normal but there may be an appearance of a relatively vertical femoral neck or coxa valga. However, if the radiograph is repeated with the legs in 15 degrees of abduction and maximum internal rotation the femoral neck angles are typically normal. Computed tomography scans of the hip and knee can be used to radiographically measure the degree of torsion.

Treatment

Treatment is primarily observation. It was previously felt that medial femoral torsion was associated with bunions, back pain, degenerative osteoarthritis, and depressed athletic ability. However, this is no longer accepted. Correction of abnormal sitting habits will usually allow this torsional variation to resolve with normal growth and development. However, it can take one to three years for complete correction to occur depending on the age of the child at correction of sitting habits. Nighttime orthosis and daytime twister cables are of no value and may produce a compensatory lateral tibial torsion. The combination of medial femoral and compensatory lateral tibial torsion produces a genu valgum deformity. This can eventually result in patellofemoral malalignment with patella subluxation or dislocation and pain.

Children over 10 years of age and young adolescents may not have enough remaining musculoskeletal growth for spontaneous correction to occur. After these children have been followed for one to two years without documentation of improvement and when there is a significant cosmetic or functional disability, then surgical intervention can be considered. The surgical procedures advocated include proximal femoral varus derotation osteotomy and simple derotation osteotomy of either the proximal or distal femur. Sufficient derotation is performed to allow for equal medial and lateral rotation of the hip in the extended or functional position.

When to Consult

Since correction of abnormal sitting habits is difficult to achieve in preschool-aged children, most involved children continue to have in-toeing until six or seven years of age. Once in school there is a normal transition from floor to chair-sitting activities and, as a consequence, femoral torsion begins to improve. Medial femoral torsion persisting after age seven years may ultimately require surgical correction and such cases should be referred orthopaedic specialist.

Medial Tibial Torsion

Medial or internal tibial torsion is the most common cause of in-toeing in children under two years of age and is secondary to in utero positioning. This condition is commonly seen during the second year of life and may be associated with metatarsus adductus.

Clinical Examination

The degree of tibial torsion can be measured by the supine or prone thigh-foot angle. In both tests, the knee is flexed to 90 degrees to neutralize the normal tibiofemoral rotation and the foot placed in a neutral or simulated weight-bearing position. The long axis of the foot is compared with the long axis of the thigh (prone test) or tibia (supine test). An inwardly rotated foot is assigned a negative value and represent medial tibial torsion. It is important that the measurements be recorded on each visit to document improvement. Radiographic measurements are usually of no value in assessment of medial tibial torsion.

Treatment

Treatment of medial tibial torsion is primarily conservative. This is a physiologic condition and spontaneous resolution with normal growth and development can be anticipated. However, significant improvement usually does not occur until the child begins to pull-to-stand and to ambulate. Thereafter, it may take six to 12 months for complete correction to occur. If there has been no documented improvement by two years of age, then the use of a nighttime orthosis, such as a Denis-Browne splint, may be considered. The effectiveness of night splints is controversial due to a lack of prospective studies. Persistent medial tibial torsion in an older child or adolescent may require surgical derotation. However, this rarely occurs.

When to Consult

Medial tibial torsion persisting after two years of age and without documentation of improvement with growth should be referred for an orthopaedic evaluation

Out-Toeing

Lateral Femoral Torsion

Lateral femoral torsion, also known as femoral retroversion, is a very uncommon disorder that is usually associated with a slipped capital femoral epiphysis. However, it can occur as idiopathic abnormality and is manifested by excessive lateral rotation of the hip and limited medial rotation.

Lateral Tibial Torsion

Lateral or external tibial torsion is relatively common and is almost always associated with a calcaneovalgus foot.

Angular Variations

Physiologic Bowlegs (Genu Varum)

Physiologic bowlegs are a common torsional combination secondary to in utero positioning. The tight posterior hip capsule produces a lateral rotation contracture of the hip. When it is combined with medial tibial torsion below the knee, it gives the clinical appearance of a genu varum deformity. Mild lateral tibial bowing may occur simultaneously and this too is from in utero positioning. Because bowlegs are a physiologic condition, spontaneous resolution with normal growth and development can be anticipated. It follows the same clinical course as does medial tibial torsion. Significant improvement usually does not occur during the first year of life. The typical infant has 15 degrees of genu varum or bowleg configuration. This decreases to approximately 10 degrees by one year of age and is neutral by two years. Medial tibial torsion is the major component of physiologic bowlegs. Treatment, if necessary, will be for persistent tibial torsion.

Radiographic evaluation is not necessary for bowlegs unless a pathologic form is suspected such as tibia vara (Blount's disease), metabolic abnormalities, or skeletal dysplasia.

The major disorder that must be differentiated from physiologic bowlegs is infantile tibia vara or Blount's disease. This can be difficult in children under two years of age. Factors associated with Blount's disease include: (1) black race, (2) obesity, (3) progressive deformity, and (4) asymmetry. Radiographically, the changes typical of Blount's disease do not occur until after two years of age (see Fig. 8-10). However, the radiographic tibia metaphyseal-diaphyseal angle may be helpful in distinguishing between these two disorders.

Figure 8-10. Anterior-posterior radiograph of the left knee of a four-year-old obese black girl with unilateral genu varum. There is a medial slope to the epiphysis and metaphysis as well as metaphyseal beak characteristic of infantile tibia vara (Blount's disease).

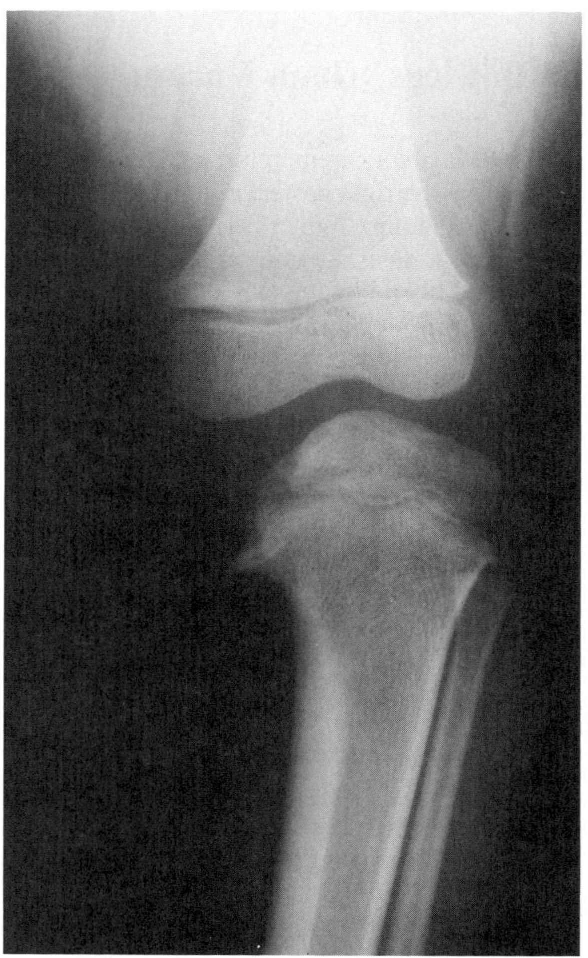

When to Consult

A symmetrical genu varum deformity persisting after two years of age should be evaluated by an orthopaedic surgeon. Asymmetrical and progressive deformities should be referred earlier.

Physiologic Knock-Knees (Genu Valgum)

As the spontaneous correction of physiologic bowlegs continues there is typically an over-correction, of variable degree, into mild genu valgum or knock-knee. This physiologic angular variation is commonly seen between three and four years of age. This, too, resolves spontaneously with the normal knee ligament being obtained between six and seven years. Orthotic management is rarely indicated. Persistent and excessive genu valgum after 10 years of age may require surgical treatment such as medial physeal stapling or distal femoral osteotomy.

When to Consult

The vast majority of physiologic genu valgum deformities will resolve spontaneously. Only those that are excessive (greater than 15 degrees), asymmetrical, or progressive require orthopaedic evaluation.

FOOT ABNORMALITIES

The most common of the pediatric foot disorders include: (1) metatarsus adductus, (2) calcaneovalgus feet, (3) talipes equinovarus (clubfeet), (4) hypermobile pes planus, and (5) peroneal spastic flatfeet.

Metatarsus Adductus

Congenital metatarsus adductus is a common problem of infants and young children. It is also known as metatarsus varus if the forefoot is supinated as well as adducted. It occurs equally in males and females and is bilateral in approximately 50% of patients. Metatarsus adductus has hereditary tendencies and tends to be more common in first born than in later children due to increased molding effect from the primigravida uterus and abdominal wall. There may be an association with acetabular dysplasia. Approximately 10% of children with metatarsus adductus will have acetabular dysplasia. Thus, careful examination of the hips is necessary in an involved child.

Clinical Examination

Clinically, the forefoot is adducted and occasionally supinated. The hindfoot and midfoot are normal. The lateral border of the foot is convex and the base of the fifth metatarsal appears prominent. The medial border of the foot is concave. There is usually an increased interval between the first and second toes with the great toe being held in a greater varus position. Ankle dorsiflexion and plantar flexion are normal. Forefoot flexibility can vary from flexible to rigid. This is assessed by stabilizing the hindfoot and midfoot in a neutral position and applying pressure over the first metatarsal head with the other. In the walking child with an uncorrected metatarsus adductus deformity an in-toed gait is noted. Abnormal shoe wear is also commonly seen.

Radiographic Evaluation

Routine radiographs of the foot are not necessary for metatarsus adductus. Anterior-posterior weight-bearing radiographs will demonstrate adduction of the metatarsals at the tarsometatarsal articulation and an increased intermetatarsal angle between the first and second metatarsals. The lateral four metatarsals appeared to have increased closeness and occasionally overlap at their base. The anterior-posterior and lateral talocalcaneal angles are usually normal.

Treatment

Treatment of metatarsus adductus deformities is primarily conservative. The feet may be classified into three groups depending on forefoot flexibility. Type I deformities are feet that are flexible and can be placed into the overcorrected (abducted) position. Voluntary correction can usually be elicited by stimulating the peroneal musculature by stroking the lateral border of the foot. These feet usually require no treatment and may be observed. Type II deformities represent feet that correct to the neutral position both passively and actively. These feet may benefit from a trial of modified or corrective shoes such as straight or reversed last shoes. These shoes are worn full-time (22 hours per day) and reevaluated in four to six weeks. If improved, the treatment can be continued. If no improvement occurs, then serial plaster casts are necessary. Type III deformities are rigid and do not correct. These feet are treated with serial casts. The forefoot is manipulated prior to each cast application to stretch the medial soft-tissue contractures. Short leg walking casts are applied with the hindfoot held in the neutral position and the forefoot abducted. The casts are changed at one to two week intervals. Usually, complete correction can be obtained in four to six weeks depending on the age of the child and the severity of deformity. The best results are obtained when casting is initiated before eight months of age. Once correction has been achieved, outflared or straight last shoes may be used for an additional one to two months to maintain correction. Mild hallux varus deformity may persist for several years following conservative correction and may be of concern to the parents. However, this deformity will eventually disappear with the wearing of shoes.

Metatarsus adductus deformities persisting or presenting after four years of age usually requires surgical intervention. Children four to six years of age with a fixed deformity, unresponsive to serial casts, may be considered for soft-tissue release. The treatment may consist of a medial release, which consists of release of the tendinous portion, of the abductor hallucis muscle and capsulotomies of the first metatarsal-medial cuneiform and the medial cuneiform-navicular joints, or capsulotomies of all the tarsometatarsal articulations. Serial casting is then carried out until forefoot correction has been obtained. This usually requires two to three months. Children seven years of age or older usually do not benefit from the soft-tissue release and require base of the metatarsal osteotomies to achieve satisfactory correction.

When to Consult

Type I metatarsus adductus in infants can be observed. Type II and type III metatarsus adductus deformities should be referred for orthopaedic consultation.

Calcaneovalgus Feet

The calcaneovalgus foot is a relatively common finding in the newborn and appears to be secondary to in utero positioning. This condition is manifested by a hyperdorsiflexed foot with varying degrees of eversion, abduction, and lateral rotation. It is almost always associated with lateral tibial torsion. These variations are usually unilateral but occasionally may be bilateral. In utero, the plantar surface of the foot was against the wall of the uterus forcing it into a hyperdorsiflexed, abducted, and laterally rotated position. The position also produces lateral tibial torsion. When these two conditions are combined with the normal newborn lateral rotation of the hip (tight posterior capsule), it results in a lower extremity that appears excessively laterally rotated.

Clinical Examination

The infant typically presents with an out-toed position of the involved extremity. The dorsum of the foot can easily be brought into contact with the anterior aspect of the tibia and the forefoot will have an abducted appearance. This should not be confused with the neonatal maturity classification of Dubowitz. Lateral tibial torsion (20 to 30 degrees) is a common associated finding. The foot and ankle are typically quite flexible and there is usually normal or almost normal plantar flexion.

There are three conditions that must be distinguished from the calcaneovalgus foot: (1) vertical talus, (2) posteromedial bow of the tibia, and (3) neuromuscular abnormalities with paralysis of the gastrocnemius muscle. The differentiation can usually be made clinically during the clinical examination of the foot, lower leg, and neurologic system. Occasionally, radiographs will be required.

Radiographic Evaluation

Simulated weight-bearing anterior-posterior and lateral radiographs of the feet may be necessary to differentiate between the calcaneovalgus foot and a congenital vertical talus. In a calcaneovalgus foot, the radiographs are either normal or there is an increased hindfoot valgus. In the congenital vertical talus, the hindfoot is in equinus and the midfoot and forefoot are dorsally displaced (rocker bottom).

Treatment

In the typical calcaneovalgus foot no treatment is necessary. The hyperdorsiflexion of the foot will resolve during the first three to six months of life. Occasionally resistant feet may require passive stretching, taping, or casting into the plantar flexed position. The lateral tibial torsion, however, will persist and follow the same natural history as medial tibial torsion. Spontaneous improvement will not occur until the child begins to pull to stand and walk independently. It will take approximately six to 12 months thereafter for complete correction to occur. The majority of infants with calcaneovalgus feet and lateral tibial torsion will have normally aligned feet and lower extremities by two years of age.

When to Consult

All infants with calcaneovalgus feet require orthopaedic evaluation for differential diagnosis.

Talipes Equinovarus (Clubfoot)

A clubfoot represents a deformity not only of the foot but the entire lower leg. It can be classified into three groups: (1) congenital, (2) teratologic, and (3) positional. The congenital clubfoot is usually an isolated abnormality while the teratologic form is associated with a neuromuscular disorder such as myelodysplasia, arthrogryposis multiplex congenita, or a syndrome complex. Positional clubfoot is a normal foot that has been held in a deformed position in utero.

Etiology

The etiology of clubfoot is unknown. There are inheritance factors, and these are currently considered multifactorial with a major influence from a single autosomal dominant gene. Recent biopsy studies of the extrinsic muscles of the calf by Handelsman and Badalamente have indicated a probable neuromuscular etiology. They found fiber type disproportion and increased neuromuscular junctions within these muscles. Electron microscopy abnormalities were also present. These findings are in contrast to previous etiological theories where deformity of the talus was felt to be the primary abnormality. While the talus is certainly deformed with medial deviation of the head and neck, this is currently considered to be a secondary deformity.

Pathoanatomy

The pathoanatomy in clubfoot deformities is complex. Abnormalities include: (1) lateral rotation of the talus in the ankle mortise, (2) posterior deviation of the lateral malleolus, (3) medial dislocation of the navicular, (4) talar head and neck deformity, (5) supination of the calcaneus, and (6) soft-tissue contractures.

Clinical Examination

The congenital form of clubfoot, which constitutes approximately 75% of all cases, is characterized by: (1) the absence of other congenital abnormalities, (2) variable rigidity of the foot, (3) mild calf atrophy, and (4) mild hypoplasia of the tibia, fibula and bones of the foot. It occurs more commonly in males (2:1) and is bilateral in 50% of cases. The probability for the deformity to occur at random is approximately 0.1% but within involved families the probability is approximately 3% for subsequent siblings and 20% to 30% for offspring of involved parents.

Examination of the infant clubfoot demonstrates hindfoot equinus, hindfoot varus, forefoot adduction, and variable rigidity. All of these findings are secondary to the medial dislocation of the talonavicular joint. When this joint is subluxated experimentally in a fresh cadaver specimen the clinical and radiographic appearance of a congenital clubfoot is reproduced, including functional rigidity.

In the older child, the calf and foot atrophy are more obvious than in the infant regardless of how well corrected or functional the foot. These findings are due to the etiologic aspects of clubfoot, not the method of treatment.

Radiographic Evaluation

Anterior-posterior and lateral standing or simulated weight-bearing radiographs are used in the assessment of clubfeet. Non-weight-bearing radiographs are useless. Many authors have recommended a maximum dorsiflexion lateral view, but in the untreated clubfoot, the lateral weight-bearing view is essentially a maximum dorsiflexion view. Multiple different radiographic measurements can be made. The measurements that have been demonstrated to be most beneficial in infancy and young children include: (1) the anterior-posterior talocalcaneal angle, (2) the lateral talocalcaneal angle, and (3) the talocalcaneal overlap (see Fig. 8-11). The navicular, which is the primary site of deformity, does not ossify until three years in the female and four years in the male. Thus, line measurements are necessary in order to determine the position of the unossified navicular.

Treatment

Conservative and surgical methods are utilized in the treatment of clubfoot deformities. All infants with clubfeet must be referred for orthopaedic consultation.

Figure 8-11.

(A) Simulated weight-bearing anterior-posterior radiograph of the left foot of a nine-month-old infant with a clubfoot. There is a parallelism of the hindfoot and metatarsus adductus.

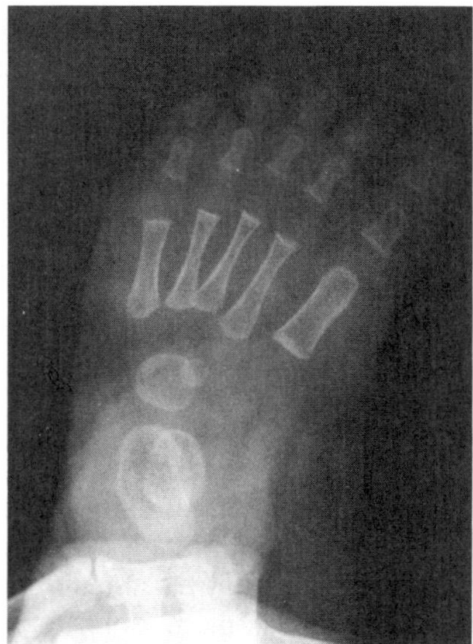

(B) The lateral radiograph also shows hindfoot parallelism as well as equinus.

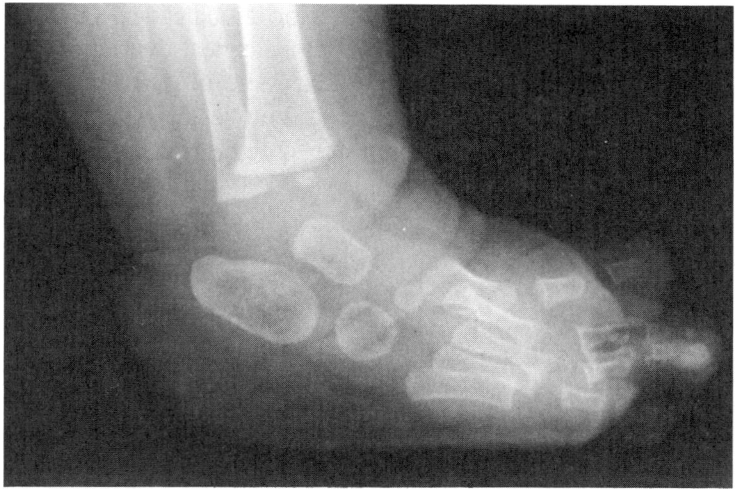

Conservative Management

Conservative methods of treatment include taping, malleable splints, and serial plaster casts. Taping and malleable splints are particularly useful in premature infants until they obtain an appropriate size for casting. Serial plaster casts are the major method of treatment. Before the cast is applied, the foot should receive gentle manipulation into the corrected position. The cast is then applied and changed at one to two week intervals. The manipulation technique consists of forefoot traction to disengage the dislocated navicular followed by forefoot abduction to reduce it on the head of the talus. Following correction of the midfoot and forefoot, the equinus is corrected by gently dorsiflexing the foot. Complete correction, both clinically and radiographically, should be achieved by three months of age. If this is accomplished, then holding casts are used for an additional three to six months followed by nighttime bivalved casts or outflared shoes until the child is walking well. Failure to achieve clinical and radiographic correction by three months of age is an indication for surgical treatment. Further attempts at conservative management may result in articular damage and a midfoot breech (rocker-bottom deformity).

Surgical Management

Surgical treatment includes soft-tissue releases, tendon transfers, bone procedures, including arthrodeses and combinations thereof.

The initial method of surgical treatment is a complete soft-tissue release utilizing either the posteromedial (Turco) or posteromedial plantar release. The timing for the initial surgery is controversial as many surgeons prefer early surgery (three to six months) while others prefer to wait until nine to twelve months of age. Those who advocate early surgery feel the percentage of foot growth during the first year of life is considerable and that by correcting the foot early, more remodeling in the corrected position occurs resulting in a more stable congruous alignment. Those who prefer to wait feel that anesthesia is safer, the structures to be released are larger and easier to deal with, and that early weight-bearing on the corrected foot helps to maintain correction. Most surgeons prefer to delay surgery.

The posteromedial or posteromedial plantar release consists of a one stage operation in which all of the deformities are corrected simultaneously with the major goal being reduction of the talonavicular joint. Frequently, this joint is stabilized with a smooth Steinmann pin. However, the use of a pin does not appear to affect the long-term results but does make initial postoperative management easier. Satisfactory long-term results can be expected in 80% to 90% of cases following a complete release. Feet with unsatisfactory results that require additional treatment are usually secondary to extrinsic muscle imbalance rather than incomplete correction.

Postoperatively, radiographs are obtained at three to six month intervals during the first year and then yearly thereafter. Radiographic features that are indicative of satisfactory correction include: anterior-posterior talocalcaneal angle, lateral talocalcaneal angle, 0-1+ talocalcaneal overlap, and neutral position of the navicular and os calcis.

The use of tendon transfers and bone procedures, including arthrodeses, are used primarily for salvage of recurrent or incompletely corrected feet. Centralization of the tibialis anterior tendon has been particularly beneficial in young children with a dynamic pes varus, the most common residual abnormality. Triple arthrodeses are indicated in painful deformed feet in adolescence.

When to Consult

All clubfeet require orthopaedic evaluation, preferentially in the newborn nursery.

Hypermobile Pes Planus (Flexible Flatfeet)

Hypermobile or flexible flatfeet or pronated feet are common sources of concerns by parents. In general, these children are asymptomatic and have no limitations of activities. Flexible flatfeet are common in neonates and toddlers due to associated laxity in bone-ligament complexes of the feet and fat in the area of the medial longitudinal arch.

These children usually demonstrate significant improvement by six years of age. In the older child, flexible flatfeet are usually secondary to generalized ligamentous laxity, an autosomal dominant condition. Almost all children and adolescents with flexible flatfeet will be asymptomatic.

Clinical Examination

In the non-weight-bearing position, in the older child with a flexible flatfoot, the normal medial longitudinal arch is present but in the weight-bearing position, the foot becomes pronated with varying degrees of pes planus and heel valgus. Instead of weight-bearing over the lateral column of the foot, weight is shifted medially producing pronation. Subtalar motion is examined with the ankle in a neutral position and should be normal or slightly increased. Loss of subtalar motion may indicate a rigid flatfoot. Common causes of rigid flatfeet include tight tendoachilles (heelcords), tarsal coalitions, and neuromuscular abnormalities (cerebral palsy). Rigid flatfeet may be a familial trait. Evaluation of other joints, especially the elbow, hand and knees, will usually demonstrate generalized ligamentous laxity.

Radiographic Evaluation

Routine radiographs of asymptomatic flexible flatfeet is usually not indicated. Standing or weight-bearing anterior-posterior and lateral radiographs are obtained, if necessary. On the anterior-posterior radiograph there will be an increase in the talocalcaneal angle (greater than 35 degrees) due to the excessive heel valgus. The lateral view shows distortion of the normal straight line relationship between the axis of the talus and the first metatarsal with either a sag of the talonavicular or naviculocuneiform joints and flattening of the normal medial longitudinal arch.

Treatment

The treatment of flexible flatfeet is conservative. Involved children do not predictably have symptoms related to their feet. Therefore, modified shoes and orthoses do not significantly alter the clinical or radiographic appearance of the feet. It should be emphasized that the diagnosis of flexible flatfeet is usually not possible until after six years of age. Treatment is indicated only for persistent symptoms not attributable to other causes or abnormal shoe wear. Feet that are symptomatic with vigorous physical activities usually respond readily to the use of a commercially available medial longitudinal arch support. Custom-made supports are usually much more expensive and, in most cases, not any more effective. For the child with excessive heel valgus, pronation, and abnormal shoe wear unresponsive to commercial or custom arch supports, the use of a UCB (University of California-Berkeley) orthosis may be beneficial. This orthosis will hold the hindfoot in the corrected position and restore the medial longitudinal arch.

Rarely will a patient with a flexible flatfoot be encountered who has symptoms severe enough to warrant surgery. A variety of procedures have been described including naviculocuneiform arthrodesis, advancement of the tibialis posterior tendon, calcaneal osteotomies, and other arthrodeses such as the Grice subtalar fusion.

When to Consult

All symptomatic flatfeet require an orthopaedic evaluation to assess the source of the symptoms. Asymptomatic flatfeet with abnormal shoe wear unrelieved by commercially available arch supports should also be referred.

Peroneal Spastic Flatfoot

Peroneal spastic flatfoot is a relatively common foot disorder characterized by a painful, rigid valgus deformity of the midfoot and hindfoot (flatfoot) and peroneal (lateral calf) muscle spasm but without true spasticity. Peroneal spastic flatfoot is almost always synonymous with tarsal coalition, a congenital fusion or failure of segmentation between two or more tarsal bones. However, any condition that alters the normal gliding and rotatory motion of the subtalar joint may produce the clinical appearance of a peroneal spastic flatfoot. Thus, congenital malformations, arthritis or inflammatory disorders, infection, neoplasms, and trauma can be potential, although uncommon, etiologies.

The most common tarsal coalitions occur at medical talocalcaneal (subtalar) facet and between the calcaneus and navicular tarsal bones. Coalitions can either be fibrous, cartilaginous, or osseous. The incidence of tarsal coalition is approximately 1% and they appear to be inherited as a unifactorial autosomal dominant trait with nearly full penetrance. Approximately 60% of calcaneonavicular and 50% of the talocalcaneal coalitions will be bilateral.

Clinical Examination

The onset of symptoms usually occurs during the second decade of life. Although mild limitation of subtalar motion and a valgus deformity have been present since early childhood, the onset of symptoms vary with the age at which the fibrous or cartilaginous bar begins to ossify and further decrease motion. The talonavicular coalitions ossify between three and five years, the calcaneonavicular coalitions between eight and 12 years, and the middle-facet talocalcaneal coalitions between 12 and 16 years of age. The pain is typically felt laterally in the hindfoot and radiates laterally along the lateral malleolus and distal fibula (peroneal muscle spasm). Symptoms are frequently aggravated by sports or walking on uneven ground. Clinically, the foot is pronated both in the weight-bearing and non-weight-bearing position. Subtalar or mid-tarsal joint motion is diminished or absent and attempts at motion may produce pain. There is usually little or no subtalar motion and this may produce pain.

Radiographic Evaluation

The diagnosis of tarsal coalition is confirmed radiographically. Initial radiographs should include an anterior-posterior and lateral weight-bearing radiographs of the foot and an oblique radiograph. Beaking of the anterior aspect of the talus on the lateral view is suspicious for a tarsal coalition. Axial views through the posterior and middle talocalcaneal joints can be useful in the diagnosis of the middle facet talocalcaneal coalition. However, computed tomography scan is the procedure of choice in the evaluation of coalitions, especially those involving the middle facet.

Treatment

The treatment of symptomatic tarsal coalition varies according to the type of coalition, the age of the patient, the extent of the coalition, the presence or absence of degenerative osteoarthritis, and the degree of disability. The treatment may be non-operative or operative. Nonoperative treatment may consist of cast immobilization, shoe inserts, or orthotics. Operative management consists of excision of the coalition and interposition of muscle (calcaneonavicular) and of fat (middle facet talocalcaneal) to prevent hematoma formation and reossification of the coalition. Resections are very effective in relieving pain, improving subtalar motion, and allowing resumption of normal activities. However, if degenerative osteoarthritis is present, a triple arthrodesis may be necessary.

When to Consult

Any child presenting with a painful flatfoot should be referred for orthopaedic evaluation.

Bibliography

General

Anderson M., Green W.T., and Messner M.B.: Growth and Prediction of Growth in the Lower Extremity. J Bone Joint Surg, 1963; 45A:1-14.

Beltran J., Herman L.J., Burk J.M., et al.: Femoral Head Avascular Necrosis: MR Imaging With Clinical-Pathologic and Radionuclide Correlation. Radiology, 1988; 166:215-220.

Berman L. and Klenerman L.: Ultrasound Screening for Hip Abnormalities: Preliminary Findings in 1001 Neonates. Br. Med. J., 1986; 293:719-722.

Castelein R.M. and Sauter A.M.: Ultrasound Screening for Congenital Dysplasia of the Hip in Neonates: Its Value. J. Pediatr. Orthop., 1988; 8:666-670.

Dooms G.C., Fisher M.R., Hricak H., et al.: Bone Marrow Imaging: Magnetic Resonance Studies Related to Age and Sex. Radiology, 1985; 155:429-432.

Forero N., Okamura L.A., and Larson M.A.: Normal Ranges of Hip Motion in Neonates. J. Pediatr. Orthop., 1989; 9:391-395.

Hall T.R., and Kangarloo H.: Magnetic Resonance Imaging of the Musculoskeletal System in Children. Clin. Orthop., 1989; 244:119-130.

Harcke H.T., Grissom L.E., and Finkelstein M.S.: Evaluation of the Musculoskeletal System with Sonography. AJR, 1988; 150:1253-1261.

Jeanty P. and Romero R.: Obstetrical Ultrasound. New York: McGraw-Hill, 1983, pp. 183-194.

Moore S.G., Gooding C.A., Brasch R.C., et al.: Bone Marrow in Children with Acute Lymphocytic Leukemia: MR Relaxation Times. Radiology, 1986; 160:237-240.

Morin C., Harcke H.T., and MacEwen G.D.: The Infant Hip: Real-time US Assessment of Acetabular Development. Radiology, 1985; 157:673-677.

Moseley C.F.: A Straight-Line Graph for Leg Length Discrepancies. J. Bone Joint Surg., 1977; 59A:174-179.

Pritchett J.W.: Growth and Prediction of Growth in the Upper Extremity. J. Bone Joint Surg., 1988; 70A:520-525.

Scheible W., James H.E., Leopold G.R., and Hilton SW: Occult Spinal Dysraphism in Infants: Screening with High-Resolution Real-Time Ultrasound. Radiology, 1983; 146:743-746.

Todd F.N., Lamoreaux L.W., Skinner S.R., et al.: Variations in the Gait of Normal Children. A Graph Applicable to the Documentation of Abnormalities. J. Bone Joint Surg., 1989; 71A:196-204.

Unger E., Moldofsky P., Gatenby R., et al.: Diagnosis of Osteomyelitis by MR Imaging. AJR, 1988; 150:605-610.

Vanderwilde R., Staheli L.T., Chew D.E., and Malagon V.: Measurements on Radiographs of the Foot in Normal Infants and Children. J. Bone Joint Surg., 1988; 70A:407-415.

Idiopathic Scoliosis

Bradford D.S., Lonstein J.E., Ogilvie J.W., and Winter R.B.: Moe's Textbook of Scoliosis and Other Spinal Deformities, Second Edition. Philadelphia, W.B. Saunders, 1987, pp. 191-233.

Bunnell W.P.: The Natural History of Idiopathic Scoliosis. Clin Orthop, 1988; 229:20-25.

Ceballas T., Ferrer-Torrelles M., Castillo F., and Fernandez-Paredes E.: Prognosis in Infantile Idiopathic Scoliosis. J. Bone Joint Surg., 1980; 62A:863-875.

Figueiredo U.M. and James J.P.: Juvenile Idiopathic Scoliosis. J. Bone Joint Surg., 1979; 61B:36-42.

Lonstein J.E. and Carlson J.M.: The Prediction of Curve Progression in Untreated Idiopathic Scoliosis During Growth. J. Bone Joint Surg., 1984; 66A:1061-1071.

Lonstein J.E.: Natural History and School Screening for Scoliosis. Ortho. Clin. N. Am., 1988; 19:227-238.

MacEwen G.D., Bunnell W.P., and Sriram K.: Acute Neurologic Complications in the Treatment of Scoliosis (A Report of the Scoliosis Research Society). J. Bone Joint Surg., 1975; 57A:404-408.

MacLean W.E., Jr., Green N.E., Pierre C.B., and Ray D.C.: Stress and Coping with Scoliosis. Psychological Effects on Adolescents and their Families. J. Pediatr. Orthop., 1989; 9:257-261.

Nottage W., Waugh T.R., and McMaster W.C.: Radiation Exposure During Scoliosis Screening Radiology. Spine, 1981; 6:456-459.

Renshaw T.S.: Screening School Children for Scoliosis. Clin. Orthop., 1988; 229:26-33.

Scoles P.V., Salvagno R., Villalba D., and Riew D.: Relationship of Iliac Crest Maturation to Skeletal and Chronological Age. J. Pediatr. Orthop., 1988; 8:639-644.

Weinstein S.L. and Ponseti I.V.: Curve Progression in Idiopathic Scoliosis. J. Bone Joint Surg., 1983; 65A:447-455.

Winter R.B., Lonstein J.E., Drogt J., and Noren C.A.: The Effectiveness of Bracing in the Nonoperative Treatment of Idiopathic Scoliosis. <u>Spine</u>, 1986; 11:790-791.

Wyatt M.P., Barrack R.L., Mubarak S.J., et al.: Vibratory Response in Idiopathic Scoliosis. <u>J. Bone Joint Surg.</u>, 1986; 68B:714-718.

Yekutiel M., Robin G.C., and Yarom R. Proprioceptive Function in Children with Adolescent Idiopathic Scoliosis. <u>Spine</u>, 1981; 6:560-566.

Congenital Scoliosis

McMaster M.J. and Ohtsuka K.: The Natural History of Congenital Scoliosis: A Study of 251 Patients. <u>J. Bone Joint Surg.</u>, 1986; 68B:588-595.

McMaster M.J.: Occult Intraspinal Anomalies and Congenital Scoliosis. <u>J. Bone Joint Surg.</u>, 1984; 66A:588-601.

MacEwen G.D., Winter R.B., and Hardy J.H.: Evaluation of Kidney Anomalies in Congenital Scoliosis. <u>J. Bone Joint Surg.</u>, 1972; 54A:1451-1454.

Reckles L.N., Peterson H.A., Bianco A.J., and Weidman W.H.: The Association of Scoliosis and Congenital Heart Defects. <u>J. Bone Joint Surg.</u>, 1975; 57A:449-455.

Winter R.B.: <u>Congenital Deformities of the Spine</u>. New York: Thieme-Stratton, 1983.

Winter R.B., Haven J.J., Moe J.H., and Legaard S.M.: Diastematomyelia and Congenital Spine Deformities. <u>J. Bone Joint Surg.</u>, 1974; 56A:27-39.

Winter R.B., Moe J.H., and Eilers V.E.: Congenital Scoliosis - A Study of 234 Patients Treated and Untreated. J. Bone Joint Surg., 1968; 50A:1-47.

Neuromuscular Scoliosis

Cambridge W., and Drennan J.C.: Scoliosis Associated with Duchenne Muscular Dystrophy. J. Pediatr. Orthop., 1987; 7:436-440.

Daher Y.H., Lonstein J.E., Winter R.B., and Bradford D.S.: Spinal Surgery in Spinal Muscular Atrophy. J. Pediatr. Orthop., 1985; 5:391-395.

Ferguson R.I. and Allen B.L., Jr.: Consideration in the Treatment of Cerebral Palsy Patients with Spinal Deformities. Orthop. Clin. N. Amer., 1988; 19:419-425.

Kalamchi A. and Thompson G.H.: Congenital Anomalies of the Spine. In Dee R., Mango E., and Hurst L.C. (eds). Principles of Orthopaedic Practice. New York: McGraw-Hill, 1989; pp. 839-860.

Nash C.L. Spinal Deformities. In Thompson G.H., Rubin I.L., and Bilenker R.M. (eds). Comprehensive Management of Cerebral Palsy. New York: Grune and Stratton, 1983; pp. 257-272.

Osebold W.R., Mayfield J.K., Winter R.B., and Moe J.H.: Surgical Treatment of Paralytic Scoliosis Associated with Myelomeningocele. J. Bone Joint Surg., 1982; 64A:841-856.

Piggott H. The Natural History of Scoliosis in Myelodysplasia. J. Bone Joint Surg., 1980; 62B:54-58.

Rosenthal R.K., Levine D.B., and McCarver C.L.: The Occurance of Scoliosis in Cerebral Palsy. Dev. Med. Child. Neurol., 1974; 16:664-670.

Smith A.D., Koreska J., and Moseley C.F.: Progression of Scoliosis in Duchenne Muscular Dystrophy. <u>J. Bone Joint Surg.</u>, 1989; 71A:1066-1074.

Kyphosis - Scheurmann's and Congenital

Bradford D.S., Ahmed K., Moe B., et al.: The Surgical Management of Patients with Scheuermann's Disease: A Review of 24 Cases Managed by Combined Anterior and Posterior Spine Fusion. <u>J. Bone Joint Surg.</u>, 1980; 62A:705-712.

Lonstein J.E., Winter R.B., J.H. Moe, et al.: Spinal Cord Compression Due to Spine Deformity. <u>Reconstr. Surg. Traumatol.</u>, 1972; 13:58-65.

Sachs B., Bradford D., Winter R., et al.: Scheuermann's Kyphosis. Follow-up of Milwaukee Brace Treatment. <u>J. Bone Joint Surg.</u>, 1987; 69A:50-57.

Seitsalo S., Österman K., Hyvärinen H., et al.: Severe Spondylolisthesis in Children and Adolescents. <u>J. Bone Joint Surg.</u>, 1990; 72B:259-265.

Winter R.B., Moe J.H., and Wang J.F.: Congenital Kyphosis. Its Natural History and Treatment as Observed in a Study of 130 patients. <u>J. Bone Joint Surg.</u>, 1973; 55A:223-256.

Spondylosis/Spondylolisthesis

Bell D.F., Ehrlich M.G., and Zaleski D.: Brace Treatment for Symptomatic Spondylolisthesis. <u>Clin. Orthop.</u>, 1988; 236:192-198.

Fredrickson B.E., Baker D., McHolick W.J., Yuan, et al.: The Natural History of Spondylolysis and Spondylolisthesis. <u>J. Bone Joint Surg.</u>, 1990; 66A:699-707.

Hensinger R.: Spondylolysis and Spondylolisthesis in Children. In American Academy of Orthopaedic Surgeons Instructional Course Lectures. St. Louis: C.V. Mosby, 1983; 32:132-151.

Pizzutillo P.D., Hummer C.D.III: Nonoperative Treatment of Painful Adolescent Spondylolysis or Spondylolisthesis. J. Pediatr. Orthop., 1989; 9:538-540.

Saraste H.: Long-Term Clinical and Radiographical Follow-up of Spondylolysis and Spondylolisthesis. J. Pediatr. Orthop., 1987; 7:631-638.

Seitsalo S., Österman K., Hyvärinen H., et al.: Severe Spondylolisthesis in Children and Adolescents. J. Bone Joint Surg., 1990; 72B:259-265.

Disc Space Infection

Green N.E. and Edwards K.: Bone and Joint Infections in Children. Orthop. Clin. N. Amer., 1987; 18:555-576.

Scoles P.V. and Quinn T.P.: Intervertebral Discitis in Children and Adolescents. Clin. Orthop., 1982; 162:31-36.

Szaly E., Green N., and Heller R.: Magnetic Resonance Imaging in the Diagnosis of Childhood Discitis. J. Pediatr. Orthop., 1987; 7:164- 17

Wenger D.R., Bobechko W.P., and Gilday D.L.: The Spectrum of Intervertebral Disc-Space Infection in Children. J. Bone Joint Surg., 1978; 60A:100-108.

Back Pain

DeOrio J.K. and Bianco A.J., Jr.: Lumbar Disc Excision in Children and Adolescents. J. Bone Joint Surg., 1982; 64A:991-996.

Hensinger R.N.:   Back Pain in Children.   In Brandord D.S. and Hensinger R.N. (Eds). The Pediatric Spine. New York: Theime Inc., 1985; pp. 41-60.

Tachdjian M.O. and Matsen D.D.: Orthopaedic Aspects of Intraspinal Tumors in Infants and Children. J. Bone Joint Surg., 1965; 47A:223-231.

Congenital Dislocation of the Hip

Allan D.B., Gray R.H., Scott T.D., et al.: The Relationship Between Ligamentous Clicks Arising from the Newborn Hip and Congenital Dislocation. J. Bone Joint Surg., 1985; 67B:491.

Bernard A.A., O'Hara J.N., Bazin S., et al.: An Improved Screening System for the Early Detection of Congenital Dislocation of the Hip. J. Pediatr. Orthop., 1987; 7:277-282

Bialik V., Tishman J., Katzir J., and Zeltzer M.: Clinical Assessment of Hip Instability in the Newborn by an Orthopaedic Surgeon and a Pediatrician. Pediatr. Orthop., 1986; 6:703-705.

DeRosa G.P. and Feller N.: Treatment of Congenital Dislocation of the Hip. Management Before Walking Age. Clin. Orthop., 1987; 225:77-85.

Green N.E. and Griffin P.P.: Hip Dysplasia Associated with Abduction Contracture of the Contralateral Hip. J. Bone Joint Surg., 1982; 64A:1273-1281.

Grill F., Bensahel H., Candell J., et al.: The Pavlik Harness in the Treatment of the Congenitally Dislocating Hip. Report on a Multicenter Study of the European Pediatric Orthopaedic Society. J. Pediatr. Orthop., 1988; 8:1-8.

Hensinger R.D.: Congenital Dislocation of the Hip. Treatment in Infancy to Walking Age. <u>Orthop. Clin. North Am.</u>, 1987; 18:597-616.

Hummer C.D. and MacEwen G.D.: The Coexistence of Torticollis and Congenital Dislocation of the Hip. <u>J. Bone Joint Surg.</u>, 1972; 54A:1255-1256.

Iwasaki K.: Treatment of Congenital Dislocation of the Hip by the Pavlik Harness. <u>J. Bone Joint Surg.</u>, 1983; 65A:760-767.

Kalamchi A. and MacFarlane R., III.: The Pavlik Harness: Results in Patients Over Three Months of Age. <u>J. Pediatr. Orthop.</u>, 1982; 2:3-8.

Kumar S.J. and MacEwen G.D.: The Incidence of Hip Dysplasia with Metatarsus Adductus. <u>Clin. Orthop.</u>, 1982; 164:234-235.

Staheli L.T., Coleman S.S., Hensinger R.N., et al.: Congenital Hip Dysplasia. <u>In American Academy of Orthopaedic Surgeons Instructional Course Lectures</u>. St. Louis: C.V. Mosby Co., 1984; 33:340-363.

Tachdjian M.O.: <u>Congenital Dislocation of the Hip</u>. New York: Churchill Livingston, 1982.

Treadwell S.J. and Bell H.M. Efficacy of Neonatal Hip Examination. <u>J. Pediatr. Orthop.</u>, 1981; 1:61-65.

Viere R.G., Birch J.G., Herring J.A., et al.: Use of the Pavlik Harness in Congenital Dislocation of the Hip. An Analysis of Failures of Treatment. <u>J. Bone Joint Surg.</u>, 1990; 72A:238-244.

Weinstein S.: Natural History of Congenital Hip Dislocation and Hip Dysplasia. <u>Clin. Orthop.</u>, 1987; 225:62-65.

Septic Arthritis and Osteomyelitis of the Hip

Fletcher B.D., Scoles P.V., and Nelson A.D. Osteomyelitis in Children: Detection by Magnetic Resonance. <u>Radiology</u>, 1984; 150:57-60.

Green N.E. and Edwards K.: Bone and Joint Infection in Children. <u>Orthop. Clin. North Am.</u>, 1987; 18:555-576.

Griffin P.P. and Green W.T. Jr.: Hip Joint Infections in Infants and Children. <u>Orthop. Clin. North. Am.</u>, 1978; 9:123-124.

Morrissy R.T.: Bone and Joint Sepsis in Children. <u>In American Academy of Orthopaedic Surgeons Instructional Course Lectures</u>. St. Louis: C.V. Mosby Co., 1982; 31:49-61.

Scoles P.V.: Antimicrobial Therapy of Childhood Skeletal Infections. <u>J. Bone Joint. Surg</u>, 1984; 66A:1487-1492.

Shaw B.A. and Kasser J.R.: Acute Septic Arthritis in Infancy and Childhood. <u>Clin. Orthop.</u>, 1990; 257:212-225.

Whalen J.L., Fitzgerald R.H., and Morrissy R.T.: A Histological Study of Acute Hematogenous Osteomyelitis Following Physeal Injuries in Rabbits. <u>J. Bone Joint Surg.</u>, 1988; 70A:1383-1392.

Transient Mono-Articular Synovitis

Hauseisen D.C., Weiner D.S., and Weiner S.D.: The Characterization of "Transient Synovitis of the Hip" in Children. <u>J Pediatr Orthop</u>, 1986; 6:11-17.

Landin L.A., Danielsson L.G., and Wattsgard C.: Transient Synovitis of the Hip - Its Incidence, Epidemiology and Relation to Perthes Disease. <u>J. Bone Joint Surg.</u>, 1987; 69B:238-242.

Legg-Calve´-Perthes Disease

Burwell, R.G., Dangerfield, P.H., Hall, D.J., Vernon, C.L., Harrison, M.H.M.: Perthes' Disease. An Anthropometric Study Revealing Impaired and Proportional Growth. J Bone Joint Surg, 1978; 60B:461-477.

Catterall, A., Pringle, J., Byers, P.D., et al. A Review of the Morphology of Perthes' Disease. J Bone Joint Surg, 1982; 64B:269-275.

Catterall, A.: The Natural History of Perthes Disease. J Bone Joint Surg, 1971; 53B:37-62.

Chung, S.M.K.: The Arterial Supply of the Developing Proximal End of the Human Femur. J Bone Joint Surg, 1976; 58A:961-970.

Inoue, A., Freeman, M.A.R., Vernon-Roberts, B., Mizuno, S.: The Pathogenesis of Perthes' Disease. J Bone Joint Surg, 1976; 58B:453-461.

Pinto, M.R., Peterson, H.A., Berquist, T.H.: Magnetic Resonance Imaging in Early Diagnosis of Legg-Calve´-Perthes Disease. J Pediatr Orthop, 1989; 9:19-22.

Salter, R.B.: Current Concepts Review. The Present Status of Surgical Treatment of Legg-Perthes' disease. J Bone Joint Surg, 1984; 66A:961-966.

Salter, R.B., Thompson, G.H.: Legg-Calve´-Perthes Disease. The Prognostic Significance of the Subchondral Fracture and a Two-Group Classification of the Femoral Head Involvement. J Bone Joint Surg, 1984; 66A:479-489.

Scoles, P.V., Yoon, Y.S., Makley, J.T., Kalamchi, A.: Nuclear Magnetic Resonance Imaging in Legg-Calve´-Perthes Disease. J Bone Joint Surg, 1984; 66A:1357-1363.

Stulberg, S.D., Cooperman, D.R., Wallensten, R.: The Natural History of Legg-Calve´-Perthes Disease. J Bone Joint Surg, 1981; 63A:1095-1108.

Thompson, G.H., Westin, G.W.: Legg-Calve´-Perthes Disease. Results of Discontinuing Treatment in the Early Reossification Phase. Clin Orthop, 1979; 139:70-80.

Thompson, G.H., Salter, R.B.: Legg-Calve´-Perthes Disease: Current Concepts and Controversies. Orthop Clin North Am, 1987; 18:617-635.

Weinstein, S.C.: Legg-Calve´-Perthes Disease. In American Academy of Orthopaedic Surgeons Instructional Course Lectures. St. Louis: C.V. Mosby Co., 1983; 32:272-291.

Wynne-Davies, R., Gormely, J.: The Etiology of Perthes' Disease: Genetic Epidemiological and Growth Factors in 310 Edinburgh and Glasgow Patients. J Bone Joint Surg, 1978; 60B:6-14.

Slipped Captial Femoral Epiphysis

Aadalen, R.J., Weiner, D.S., Hoyt, W., Herndon, C.H.: Acute Slipped Capital Femoral Epiphysis. J Bone Joint Surg, 1974; 56A:1473-1487.

Agamanolis, D.P., Weiner, D.S., Lloyd. J.K.: Slipped Capital Femoral Epiphysis: A Pathological Study I. A Microscopy and Histochemical Study of 21 Patients. J Pediatr Orthop, 1985; 5:40-46.

Agamanolis, D.P., Weiner, D.S., Lloyd, J.K.: Slipped Capital Femoral Epiphysis. A Pathological Study. II. An Ultrastructure Study of 23 Cases. J Pediatr Orthop, 1985; 5:47-58.

Betz, R., Steel, H.H., Emper, W.D., Huss, G.K., Clancy, M.: Treatment of Slipped Capital Femoral Epiphysis. Spica Cast Immobilization. J Bone Joint Surg, 1990; 72A:587-600.

Busch, M.T., Morrissey, R.T.: Slipped Capital Femoral Epiphysis. Orthop Clin North Am, 1987; 18:637-647.

Crawford, A.H.: Slipped Capital Femoral Epiphysis. J Bone Joint Surg, 1988; 70A:1422-1427.

Eisenstein, A., Rothschild, S.: Biomechanical Abnormalities in Patients with Slipped Capital Femoral Epiphysis and Chondrolysis. J Bone Joint Surg, 1976; 58A:459-467.

Ingram, A.J., Clarke, M.S., Clarke, C.S,, Jr., Marshall, W.R.: Chondrolysis Complicating Slipped Capital Femoral Epiphysis. Clin Orthop, 1982; 165:99-109.

Ippolito, E. Mickelson, M., Ponseti, I.: A Histochemical Study of Slipped Capital Femoral Epiphysis. J Bone Joint Surg, 1981; 63A:1109-1113.

Koval, K.J., Lehman, W.B., Rose, D., Koval R.P., Grant, A., Strongwater, A.: Treatment of Slipped Capital Femoral Epiphysis with a Cannulated Screw Technique. J Bone Joint Surg, 1989; 71A:1370-1377.

Mann, D.C., Weddington, J., Richton, S.: Hormonal Studies in Patients with Slipped Capital Femoral Epiphysis Without Evidence of Endocrinopathy. J Pediatr Orthop, 1988; 8:543-545.

Melby, A., Holt, W.A., J., Weiner, D.A.: Treatment of Chronic Slipped Capital Femoral Epiphysis by Bone Graft Epiphysiodesis. J Bone Joint Surg, 1980; 62A:119-125.

O'Brien, E.T., Fahey, J.J.: Remodeling the Femoral Neck after Insight to Pain for Slipped Capital Femoral Epiphysis. <u>J Bone Joint Surg</u>, 1977; 59A:62-68.

Slipped Capital Femoral Epiphysis. <u>In American Academy of Orthopaedic Surgeons Instructional Course Lectures</u>. St. Louis: C.V. Mosby Co., 1984; 33:310-349.

Southwick, W.O.: Osteotomy of the Lesser Trochanter for Slipped Capital Femoral Epiphysis. <u>J Bone Joint Surg</u>, 1967; 49A:807-835.

Wilcox, P., Weiner, D., Leighly, B.: Maturation Factors in Slipped Capital Femoral Epiphysis. <u>J Pediatr Orthop</u>, 1988; 8:196-200.

Torsional and Angular Variations

Bunch, W.: Origin and Mechanism of Postnatal Deformities. <u>Ped Clin North Am</u>, 1977; 24:679-687.

Hubbard, D.D., Staheli, L.T., Chew, D.E., Mosca, V.S.: Medial Femoral Torsion and Osteoarthritis. <u>J Pediatr Orthop</u>, 1988; 8:540-542

Johnston, C.E., II: Infantile Tibia Vara. <u>Clin Orthop</u>, 1990; 255:13-23.

Kling, T.F., Jr., Hensinger, R.N.: Angular and Torsional Deformities of the Lower Limbs in Children. <u>Clin Orthop</u>, 1983; 176:136-147.

Kling, T.F., Jr.: Angular Deformities of the Lower Limbs in Children. <u>Orthop Clin North Am</u>, 1987; 18:513-4527.

Levine, A.M., Drennan, J.C.: Physiologic Bowing and Tibia Vara: The Metaphyseal-Diaphyseal Angle in the Measurement of Bowleg Deformities. <u>J Bone Joint Surg</u>, 1982; 64A:1158-1163.

Salenius, P., Vankka, E.: The Development of the Tibiofemoral Angle in Children. <u>J Bone Joint Surg</u>, 1975; 57A:259-261.

Smith, C.F.: Tibia Vara (Blount's Disease). Current Concepts. <u>J Bone Joint Surg</u>, 1982; 64A:630-632.

Staheli, L.T., Corbett, M., Wyss, C., King, H.: Lower Extremity Rotational Problems in Children. Normal Values to Guide Management. <u>J Bone Joint Surg</u>, 1985; 67A:39-47.

Staheli, L.T.: Rotational Problems of the Lower Extremities. <u>Orthop Clin North Am</u>, 1987; 18:503-512.

Svenvingsen, S., Terjesen, T., Auflem, M., Berg, V.: Hip Rotation and In-Toeing Gait. A Study of Normal Subjects from Four Years Until Adult Age. <u>Clin Orthop</u>, 1990; 251:177-182.

Thompson, G.H., Carter, J.R.: Late-Onset Tibia Vara (Blount's Disease): Current Concepts. <u>Clin Orthop</u>, 1990; 255:24-35.

Metatarsus Adductus

Berg, E.E. A Reappraisal of Metatarsus Adductus and Skewfoot. <u>J Bone and Joint Surg</u>, 1986; 68A:1185-1196.

Berman, A., Gartland, J.J.: Metatarsal Osteotomy for Correction of Adduction of the Forepart of the Foot in Children. <u>J Bone Joint Surg</u>, 1971; 53A:498-506.

Bleck, E.E.: Metatarsus Adductus: Classification and Relationship to Outcomes of Treatment. <u>J Pediatr Orthop</u>, 1983; 3:2-9.

Crawford, H.H. and Gabriel, K.R.: Foot and Ankle Problems. In The Pediatric Lower Extremity. <u>Orthop Clin North Am</u>, 1987; 18:649-666.

Ghali, N.N., Abberton, M.J., Silk, F.F.: The Management of Metatarsus Adductus et Supinatus. J Bone Joint Surg, 1984; 66B:376-380.

Heyman, C.H., Herndon, C.H., Strong, J.M.: Mobilization of the Tarsal, Metatarsal, and Intermetatarsal Joints for Correction of Resistant Adduction of the Forepart of the Foot in Congenital Clubfoot or Congenital Metatarsus Varus. J Bone Joint Surg, 1958; 40A: 299-309.

Jacobs, J.E.: Metatarsus Varus and Hip Dysplasia. Clin Orthop, 1960; 16:203-213.

Kendrick, R.E., Sharma, N.K., Hassler, W.L., Herndon, C.H.: Tarsometatarsal Mobilization for Resistant Adduction of the Forepart of the Foot. J Bone Joint Surg, 1970; 52A:61-70.

Rushford, G.F.: The National History of Hooked Foot. J Bone Joint Surg, 1987; 60B:530-532.

Staheli, L.T.: Torsion-Treatment Indications. Clin Orthop, 1989; 247:61-66.

Calcaneovalgus Feet

Gibson, D.H.: Torsional Variations in the Lower Limbs of Children. Applied Therapeutics, 1966; 8:236-241.

Meehan, Peter: Other Conditions of the Foot. In Pediatric Orthopaedics. Morrissy, R.T. (Ed). Philadelphia: J. B. Lippincott. 1990; pp. 997-998.

Talipes Equinovarus

Carroll, N.C., McMurtry, R., Leete, S.F. The Pathoanatomy of Congenital Clubfoot. Orthop Clin North Am, 1978; 9:225-232.

Cowell, H.R., Wein, B.K.   Genetic Aspects of Clubfoot.   Current Concepts Review. J Bone Joint Surg, 1980; 62A:1381-1384.

Crawford, A.H., Marxen, J.L., Osterfeld, D.L.:   The Cincinnati Incision: A Comprehensive Approach for Surgical Procedures of the Foot and Ankle in Childhood. J Bone Joint Surg, 1982; 64A:1355-1358.

Handelsman, J., Badalamente, M.A.:   Neuromuscular Studies in Clubfoot. J Pediatr Orthop, 1981; 1:23-31.

Kite, J.H.: Conservative Treatment of Resistant Recurrent Clubfoot. Clin Orthop, 1979; 70:93-110.

McKay, D.W. New Concepts of an Approach to Clubfoot Treatment: Section I: Principles in Morbid Anatomy. J Pediatr Orthop, 1982; 2:347-356.

McKay, D.W. New Concepts of an Approach to Clubfoot Treatment: Section II: Correction of the Clubfoot. J Pediatr Orthop, 1983; 3:10-21.

McKay, D.W. New Concepts of an Approach to Clubfoot Treatment: Section III: Evaluation of and Results. J Pediatr Orthop, 1983; 3:141-148.

Ryoppy, S., Sairanen, H.: Neonatal Operative Treatment of Clubfoot: A Preliminary Report. J Bone Joint Surg, 1983; 65B:320-325.

Simons, G.W.: The Complete Subtalar Release in Clubfeet. Ortho Clin North Am, 1987; 18:667-688.

Thompson, G.H., Richardson, A.B., Westin, G.W.   Surgical Management of Resistant Congenital Talipes Equinovarus Deformities. J Bone Joint Surg, 1982; 64A:652-665.

Turco, J.V. Resistant Congenital Clubfoot - One Stage Posteromedial Release with Internal Fixation: A Follow-up Report of 15 Years Experience. <u>J Bone Joint Surg</u> 1979; 61a:805-814.

Hypermobile Pes Planus (Flexible Flatfeet)

Bordelon, F.L.: Hypermobile Flatfoot in Children: Comprehension, Evaluation and Treatment. <u>Clin Orthop</u>, 1983; 181:7-14.

Meehan, P.L.: Flexible Flatfoot. <u>In American Acadmy of Orthopaedic Surgeons Instructional Course Lectures</u>. St. Louis: C.V. Mosby Co., 1982; Vol. 31:261-262.

Staheli, L.T., Chew, D.E., Corbett, M.: The Longitudinal Arch. <u>J Bone Joint Surg</u>, 1987; 69A:426-428.

Wenger, Dr. R., Mauldin, D., Speck, G., Morgan, D., Lieber, R.L.: Corrective Shoes and Inserts as Treatment for Flexible Flatfoot in Infants and Children. <u>J Bone and Joint Surg</u>, 1989; 71A:800-810.

Peroneal Spastic Flatfoot

Chambers, R.B., Cook, T.M., Cowell, H.R.: Surgical Reconstruction for Calcaneonavicular Coalition. Evaluation of Function and Gait. <u>J Bone and Joint Surg</u>, 1982; 64A:829-836.

Cowell, H.R.: Tarsal Coalition - Review and Update. <u>In American Academy of Orthopaedic Surgeons Instructional Course Lectures</u>. St. Louis: C.V. Mosby Co., 1982; Vol. 31:264-271.

Cowell, H. R., Elener, V.: Rigid Painful Flatfoot Secondary to Tarsal Coalition. <u>Clin Orthop</u>, 1983; 177:54-60.

Harris, R.I., Beath, T.: Etiology of Peroneal Spastic Flat Foot (Rigid Valgus Foot). <u>J Bone and Joint Surg</u>, 1948; 30B:624-634.

Herzenberg, J.E., Goldner, J.L., Martinez, S., Silverman, P.M.: Computed Tomography of Talocalcaneal Tarsal Coalition. A Clinical and Anatomical Study. Foot Ankle, 1986; 6:273-288.

Leonard, M.A.: The Inheritance of Tarsal Coalition and Its Relationship to Spastic Flat Foot. J Bone Joint Surg, 1974; 56B:520-526.

Martinez, S., Herzenberg, J.E., Apple, J.S.: Computed Tomography of the Hindfoot. Orthop Clin North Am, 1985; 16:481-496.

Mosier, K.M., Asher, M.: Tarsal Coalitions and Peroneal Spastic Flat Foot. J Bone Joint Surg, 1984; 66A:976-984.

Oestreich, A.E., Mize, W.A., Crawford, A.H., Morgan, R.C., Jr.: The "Anteater Nose": A Direct Sign of Calcaneonavicular Coalition in the Lateral Radiograph. J Pediatr Orthop, 1987; 7:709-711.

Olney, B.W., Asher, M.A.: Excision of Symptomatic Coalition of the Middle Facet of the Talocalcaneal Joint. J Bone Joint Surg, 1987; 69A:539-544.

Pineda, C., Resnick, D., Greenway, G.: Diagnosis of Tarsal Coalition with Computed Tomography. Clin Orthop, 1986; 208:282-288.

Sarno, R.C., Carter, B.L., Bankoff, M.F., Semine, M.C.: Computed Tomography in Tarsal Coalition. J Comput Assist Tomog, 1984; 8:1155-1160.

Scranton, P.E., Jr.: Treatment of Symptomatic Talocalcaneal Coalition. J Bone Joint Surg, 1987; 69A:533-539.

Stoskpopf, C.A., Hernandez, R.J., Kelikian, A., Tachdjian, M.O., Dias, L.S.: Evaluation of Tarsal Coalition by Computed Tomography. J Pediatr Orthop, 1984; 4:365-369.

Swiontkowski, M.F., Scranton, P.E., Hansen, S.: Tarsal Coalitions: Long-Term Results of Surgical Treatment. <u>J Pediatr Orthop</u>, 1983; 3:287-292.

9

LUMPS AND BUMPS

By Ronald P. Williams, M.D., Ph.D.
and John T. Makley, M.D.

The primary management of patients with neoplasms in the skeleton and in the soft tissues of the extremities is a problem that has historically been poorly handled. The relative rarity of these tumors prevents primary care physicians from being thoroughly familiar with their management but is not an excuse for failure to suspect their presence. Management of these problems without forethought to the consequences can result in loss of the limb or shortening of the patient's life span by increasing the risk of metastases. Enneking has estimated that as many as two-thirds of soft tissue tumors and one-fourth of bone lesions are not referred to the orthopaedic oncologist until after one or more recurrences. The hazard of this approach is that with each recurrence the risk of subsequent metastases doubles and chances of survival diminishes.

Because of their rarity, soft tissue tumors are often mistakenly diagnosed as a "pulled muscle," "thrombophlebitis," or a "hematoma" and "watched" as they continue to enlarge. This chapter emphasizes the common pitfalls in the diagnosis and early management of lesions in the bones and soft tissues of the extremities and provides a systematic approach to evaluating these perplexing problems.

Initial Evaluation

As in any patient evaluation, the history and physical examination provide the most important clues to the diagnosis. The initial presentation, such as a painless or painful soft tissue mass, an incidental radiographic finding, or a spontaneous fracture, is important. Any pain associated with the lesion should be characterized by the intensity, persistence, and length of time the pain has been present. Activities that augment the pain should be noted.

Any family history of cancer or heritable conditions, such as neurofibromatosis or multiple exostoses, that predispose the patient to musculoskeletal sarcomas should be recorded. Previous treatment with chemotherapy or radiation should cause concern because of the association of these treatments with the development of a secondary sarcoma. As a general rule, sarcomas grow relentlessly over a period of two or three months up to one year. Therefore, a mass that rapidly enlarges over a period of a few weeks is more likely to be a benign tumor such as fibromatosis or nodular fasciitis or an inflammatory lesion. Similarly, a mass that has not enlarged over several years is probably benign. However, there are exceptions to both of these rules, and any lesions must be suspected of being malignant until there is adequate proof that it is benign.

Soft Tissue Lumps

The historical description of a soft tissue mass should include how the patient first became aware of the mass, any antecedent trauma, any change in size of the mass, and any pain associated with it. The pain should be carefully characterized by the length of time it has been present, its intensity and persistence, and any factors that augment or diminish it. Associated systemic symptoms such as fever, weight loss, malaise, cough, etc. should be noted.

The physical description should localize the mass and carefully outline the boundaries. The texture and mobility of the mass and any warmth, skin changes (such as dimpling, discoloration, or venous dilatation), muscle atrophy, nerve or vessel involvement, joint motion limitation, or regional lymph node involvement should be recorded. Examination of the lungs and abdomen are also important to evaluate for metastatic disease.

Radiographs should be obtained for all soft tissue lesions. Of greatest diagnostic value is the location of the mass, the presence and pattern of distribution of any calcification or ossification within the mass, and the reaction of the adjacent bone to the tumor.

Calcifications occur in only a small portion of soft tissue tumors but, when present, can help to narrow the differential diagnosis. The pattern of calcification within the mass can help to differentiate such problems as myositis ossificans or tumoral calcinosis from true neoplasms (see Fig. 9-1). Soft tissue neoplasms, which characteristically contain calcifications, include vascular tumors (benign and malignant), synovial sarcoma, ancient schwannomas, and old lipomas. A periosteal reaction, such as a Codman's triangle adjacent to a soft tissue mass, indicates only that the mass is stimulating the periosteum. This is a non-specific finding that may reflect either a stress fracture, infection, or tumor. A more aggressive periosteal pattern such as "onion skinning" or "hair-on-end" appearance suggests a tumor aggressively invading the periosteum and is typical of Ewing's sarcoma or malignant lymphoma (see Fig. 9-2).

Initial laboratory evaluation is necessary to differentiate between the broad categories of infection (inflammation), tumor, and metabolic disease. This should include a complete blood count and erythrocyte sedimentation rate. Although these studies are non-specific, an elevated white cell count and sedimentation rate may suggest inflammation instead of primary tumor. Anemia and an abnormal white cell count may also suggest more extensive disease associated with a tumor mass such as acute leukemia or Ewing's sarcoma in a child or a leukemoid reaction related to extensive metastatic disease in an adult. The serum chemistry profile can provide evidence of occult problems, such as elevated liver enzymes suggesting liver metastases.

Evaluation of the serum electrolytes, calcium, phosphate and alkaline phosphatase levels, along with analysis of the urine pH and electrolytes, can help to differentiate between metabolic problems such as chronic renal failure, renal tubular acidosis or milk alkali syndrome, which may be associated with a calcified soft tissue mass, from other benign calcified soft tissue masses such as tumoral calcinosis or myositis ossificans.

Figure 9-1. Myositis ossificans, a benign tumor of the shoulder. Note the well circumscribed, uniform calcification in the soft tissue with no adjacent periosteal reaction.

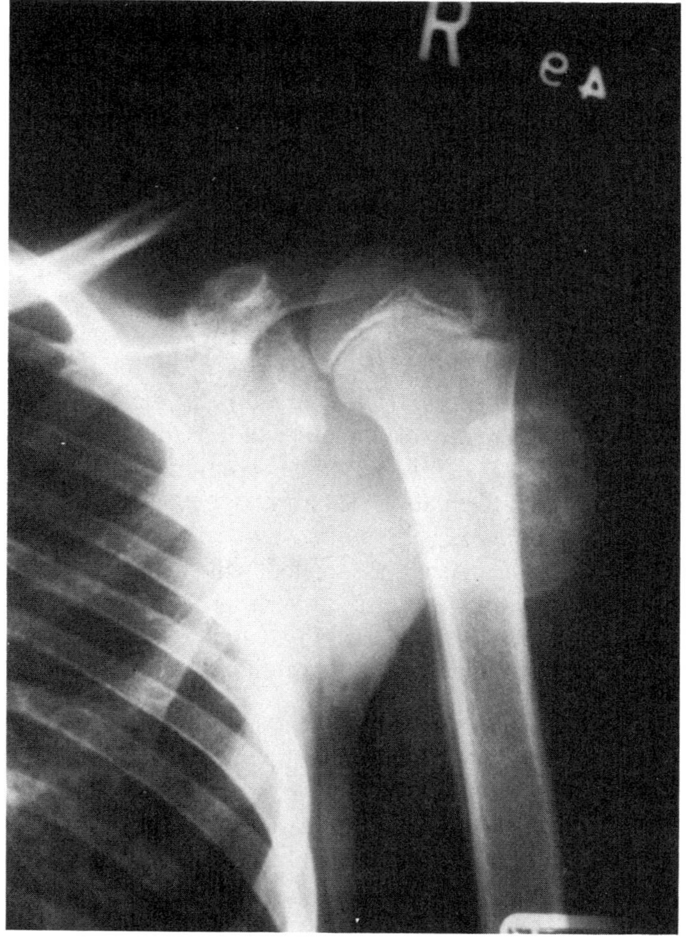

Figure 9-2. Osteosarcoma of the humerus with multiple radiographic features suggesting malignancy. Note the mixed osteolytic and blastic regions with cortical destruction and periosteal reaction.

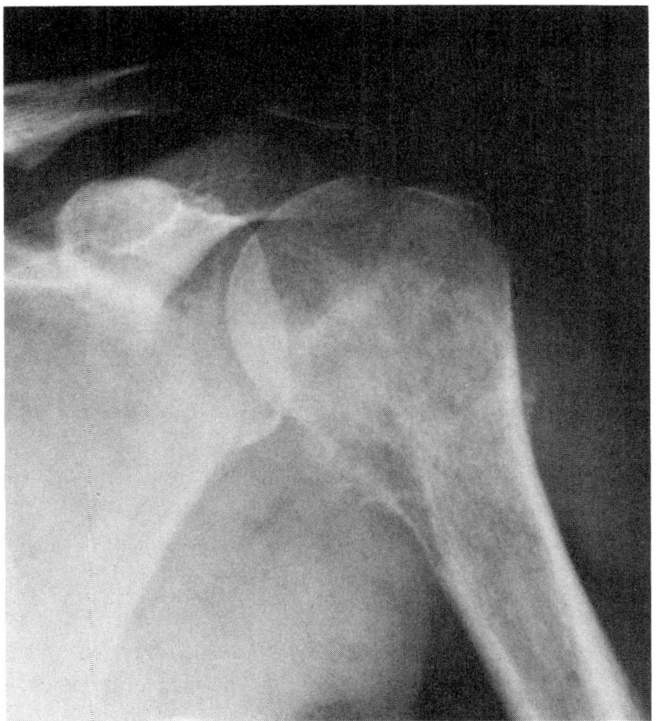

The selection of further staging studies and biopsy should be left to the surgeon responsible for the definitive care of the patient. This insures that the staging evaluation can be done efficiently and cost effectively.

Bone Bumps

The evaluation of bone lesions depends primarily on the medical history. An unusual-appearing radiograph of an asymptomatic patient usually reflects a benign process. Conversely, any bony lesion that is associated with pain warrants further investigation. A detailed description of the character of the pain and any association with activity or radicular pattern should be noted. Persistent, deep "boring" pain that interferes with the patient's sleep or activity suggests a malignant lesion in the bone. In the middle-aged or older patient, a history of cancer, especially of the breast, kidney, prostate, lung or thyroid, should alert the physician to the possibility of bone metastases. Any specific risk factors such as smoking, previous radiation or chemotherapy, or a family history of breast cancer or other heritable disorders such as multiple osteochondromas or enchondromas, are important. Any evidence of metabolic disease, especially chronic renal failure, malabsorption syndromes, or liver disease, should be examined carefully to differentiate osteomalacia or secondary hyperparathyroidism from osteoporosis as a cause of osteopenia or osteolytic lesions. All patients presenting with "pathologic" fractures through an area of abnormal bone should be evaluated before the fracture is surgically fixed to prevent inadvertent spread of primary sarcoma.

The physical signs of a bone lesion are usually non-specific and may consist of nothing more than localized point tenderness or a palpable mass. However, a comprehensive physical examination is necessary to find evidence of carcinoma in a patient suspected of having a metastatic bone lesion. The examination should include the head and neck (especially oropharynx and thyroid), breasts, abdomen, and pelvis, including a rectal examination of the prostate and a test of the stool for occult blood.

Screening radiographs often provide a clue to the specific diagnosis. For example, bone islands (osteomas), non-ossifying fibromas (fibrous cortical defects), enchondromas, and osteochondromas in an asymptomatic patient can be diagnosed on the basis of their radiographic appearance. The "popcorn" calcification of a cartilaginous lesion in a long bone of a middle-aged person with bone pain is almost pathognomonic of a chondrosarcoma, whereas a cartilaginous lesion in the digit of a child is just as certainly an enchondroma. Similarly, the "ground glass" appearance of fibrous dysplasia, the "fallen leaf" sign of a unicameral bone cyst, the course trabeculations and "flame"-shaped erosion of Paget's disease, and the "soap bubble" dilatation of the cortex by aneurysmal bone cyst and adamantinoma are well-described radiographic patterns that can be easily recognized.

The laboratory studies needed for the evaluation of patients with bony lesions are similar to those for soft tissue masses. Primary tumors of bone generally will not produce any specific biochemical abnormalities. However, the laboratory data can help to differentiate between the broad categories of metabolic bone
disease, infection, and bone marrow tumors (leukemia, lymphoma, or myeloma), Paget's disease, or carcinoma metastatic to bone.

In the child, the differential diagnosis of an aggressive-appearing lesion in the bone will often be between osteomyelitis, Ewing's sarcoma, and osteosarcoma. There are no specific laboratory tests to distinguish these entities. However, the differential white cell count and erythrocyte sedimentation rate can be useful in differentiating these diseases. In the case of Ewing's sarcoma, the sedimentation rate may be of prognostic significance. In osteosarcoma, the alkaline phosphatase level may be of prognostic value.

In the adult with bone pain, abnormalities in the serum calcium and phosphate levels will usually reflect a significant metabolic disease. Although primary hyperparathyroidism is rare, secondary hyperparathyroidism in patients with chronic renal disease or other metabolic illnesses is fairly common. Carcinoma metastatic to bone or bone marrow tumors (lymphoma or myeloma) can produce significant hypercalcemia. A markedly elevated alkaline phosphatase level with a normal serum calcium and phosphate may suggest active Paget's disease.

Prostatic acid phosphatase is a useful screen for prostate cancer, as is serum and urine protein electrophoresis from myeloma, if these diseases are suspected on the basis of the initial evaluation. Other serologic studies such as carcinoembryonic antigen (CEA), alpha-fetoprotein, or beta-human are not useful in the initial evaluation of these patients.

Mammography is a useful screening examination in a patient with a suspicious breast mass. If the patient has hematuria, then an intravenous pyelogram, sonogram, or abdominal CT scan is necessary to evaluate the patient for a renal cell carcinoma. Other studies, such as upper and lower gastrointestinal studies, renal arteriography, proctoscopy, and angiography, are not useful screening examinations for evaluating patients for possible metastatic carcinoma. A total body bone scan is useful to locate occult lesions in patients with suspected bone metastases. This is a sensitive screening tool for most tumors except multiple myeloma, which may have "cold" lesions. In this case, a skeletal survey is necessary to screen for additional bony metastases. A thyroid scan is only useful if the patient has a suggestive history such as previous treatment of thyroid carcinoma or radiation of the neck.

In a patient with a history of carcinoma and bone pain with a radiographically localized lesion, the diagnosis of metastatic carcinoma can be confirmed by needle aspiration cytology or needle biopsy under CT control.

When a metastatic lesion in the bone is found, it is recommended that an orthopedist be consulted early in the clinical course to assess the need for prophylactic fixation. Early fixation is often recommended to prevent complications of a pathologic fracture and to alleviate pain. Even in patients with advanced disease, resection of the destroyed bone and reconstruction may be useful to maintain mobility and improve quality of life.

Staging Studies

The selection of further staging studies to assess a lesion suspected of being a primary sarcoma should be left to the surgeon responsible for the definitive care of the patient. If the patient has a non-tender mass that appears to be a ganglion or lipoma, needle aspiration, CT scan, or MRI scan should confirm the diagnosis, and the patient can be reassured or the mass excised. However, comprehensive evaluation is mandatory for most other lesions because primary sarcomas have a non-specific presentation. An accurate staging evaluation requires direct communication between the physician who has examined the patient, the radiologist who has assisted in interpreting the studies, and the pathologist reviewing the biopsy materials. Embarking on part of the staging studies before the patient is referred to an oncologist often results in multiple tests being performed that are unnecessary or must be repeated because of imprecise or incomplete information. More invasive tests, such as arteriograms, are performed at some risk to the patient. Ordering these tests without a specific need for information obtained is unnecessarily risking complications for the patient and liability for the physician.

The Biopsy

An accurate staging evaluation of the local lesion must precede the biopsy. Tissue disruption by surgical dissection prevents precise imaging of the boundaries of the tumor. Consultation with the radiologist and surgical pathologist prior to the biopsy can avoid major misunderstandings that can lead to a delayed or inaccurate diagnosis. A comprehensive systematic routine for processing the biopsy tissue should be established preoperatively. This routine may include fine needle aspiration cytology, frozen sections to confirm adequacy of biopsy, preservation of tissue for histochemical markers, formalin fixation for routine histology and special stains, glutaraldehyde fixation for electron microscopy, and multiple cultures for bacteria, fungi, and acid-fast bacilli. Although some of these tests may be of low yield in the routine evaluation of a tumor, many confusing cases of infection or tumor will be correctly diagnosed only by this comprehensive evaluation.

The diagnostic tissue sample can be obtained by either needle or open biopsy. Needle biopsy has the advantage of being performed without a major surgical procedure. However, it is difficult to insure that the specimen obtained by needle biopsy is adequate for a definitive diagnosis. Fine needle aspiration can provide a provisional differentiation of sarcomas from metastatic carcinoma or infection but requires specialized training by the pathologist for accurate interpretation. The needle tract must be presumed to be contaminated by tumor cells and is impossible to visualize three to five days after the biopsy. However, communication between the surgical oncologist and the person performing the biopsy should ensure that the needle tract is placed within the area of definitive resection.

An open biopsy requires careful planning so that the surgeon is sure that adequate tissue for diagnosis is obtained. The biopsy tract should be longitudinally oriented and placed so that it can be easily excised at the time of definitive surgery. This requires that the surgeon performing the biopsy must have an intimate understanding of the planned definitive surgery. In addition, meticulous hemostasis, minimal soft tissue dissection, avoidance of neurovascular bundles, and appropriate wound closure are all integral parts of the surgical biopsy. An incisional biopsy is the method of choice for most suspected soft tissue or bone sarcomas. However, in cases of suspected sarcomas where the diagnosis can be specified on the basis of the staging evaluation (such as chondrosarcoma) or where the tumor is positioned in an expendable compartment (such as the head of the fibula or medial thigh), an excisional biopsy allows a wide resection of the tumor without contamination of any remaining tissue planes. These situations are unusual, and more often a hasty decision to excise a mass results in a marginal excision of a tumor. This causes a high risk of local recurrence and may prevent the oncologist from salvaging the limb.

The incisional biopsy of a bone tumor must be performed so that it minimizes the risk of pathologic fracture and prevents postoperative bone bleeding. It is preferable to biopsy the soft tissue component of a tumor, if one is present, to prevent creating a defect in the bone. When bone biopsy is necessary, it should be performed through a round or oval hole on the convex side of the bone, if possible, to minimize the risk of fracture. The surgical approach to the bone must also be performed so that the dissection tract can be excised at the time of definitive surgery. Bleeding from the bone can be controlled by placing methacrylate cement into the bony defect. This extremity must be adequately immobilized after a bone biopsy to prevent a pathologic fracture. This can result in a large hematoma and spread of the tumor into the surrounding tissues. The other potential complications of a biopsy include uncontrolled bleeding and infection that may threaten the life or limb of the patient. Thus, it is recommended that the biopsy be left to the hands of the surgeon responsible for the definitive care of the patient.

The patient who presents to the emergency room with a pathologic fracture without a history of carcinoma should at least cause the surgeon to suspect the possibility of a primary bone sarcoma. Surgical fixation of the fracture is not an emergency and should be postponed until the search for the primary tumor is complete. Inadvertent immediate internal fixation of a primary bone tumor results in contamination of a large area and may necessitate a radical amputation for adequate local tumor control.

Communication with the Patient and Consultant

Prompt, direct communication with the consultant is the most expedient way to insure efficient, complete patient care. A phone call to the consultant, after the patient has been examined and screening studies reviewed, provides the consultant with a synopsis of the problem and allows for the opportunity to elicit critical information from the referring physician to assess the urgency of care. This also gives the consultant an opportunity to assist the primary physician in providing appropriate screening studies and preliminary advice to the patients.

Communication with the patient at this point is critical in developing rapport between the consultant and the patient and family. The primary physician should not prognosticate for the consultant or outline a specific treatment plan for the patient when the definitive diagnosis is unknown. At this time the patient is frightened and anxious to know what will happen. Prompt, systematic diagnosis is the best way to resolve the problem for the patient. The patient should be assured that the primary physician will continue to provide future care as necessary and assist in arranging for long-term treatment (such as radiation therapy or chemotherapy) as needed. Finally, the physician should be aware that patients with primary sarcomas will require prolonged follow-up and should be alert for any evidence to suggest recurrences of the lesion.

Bibliography

Enneking, W.F.: "The Clinical Presentation and Management." In Musculoskeletal Tumor Surgery, Vol. 1. New York: Churchill Livingstone, 1983, pp. 123-140.

Enneking, W.F.: "Surgical Planning." 169-183.

Enneking, W.F.: "Metastatic Carcinoma." 1541-1559.

Enneking, W.F., "Surgical Technique." 185-213.

Enzinger, F.M.,Weiss, S.W.: "General Considerations." In Soft Tissue Tumors, St. Louis: Mosby, 1983, pp. 1-13.

Patts, J.T., Jr.: "Disorders of Parathyroid Glands." In Principles of Internal Medicine, Ninth Edition. Isselbeckher, K., Adams, R., Braunwoald, E., Petersclor, R., and Wilson, J. (eds) New York: McGraw-Hill, 1980, pp. 1832-1843.

Simon, M.A., Bartucci, E.J.: "The Search for the Primary Tumor in Patients with Skeletal Metastases of Unknown Origin." Cancer 1986; 58:1088-1095.

Simon, M.A., Karlik, M.B.: "Skeletal Metastases of Unknown Origin: Diagnostic Strategy for Orthopaedic Surgeons." Clin. Orthop., 1982;166:96-103.

10

ORTHOPAEDIC EMERGENCIES

By Daniel R. Cooperman, M.D.

An orthopaedic emergency exists when immediate action is required to ease great pain or prevent a patient's prognosis from worsening. Trauma and infection cause many emergencies. In this chapter both trauma and infection will be discussed in general terms and specific examples of each will be highlighted, stressing the role of the physician who does not have subspecialty training in orthopaedic surgery. Additionally, we will underline the concerns of the orthopaedic surgeon with respect to orthopaedic emergencies.

Trauma

Dislocations

When two sides at a joint are no longer in contact, the joint is dislocated. Great force is required to cause an acute dislocation and this force usually causes more than just displacement of the joint. It frequently causes damage to surrounding nerves and blood vessels as well as to ligaments, joint capsules, and articular cartilage. A complete clinical inventory of neurovascular function is necessary before any form of treatment is initiated in an acute dislocation. For example, in acute hip dislocations sciatic nerve injury is frequent. If a manipulation and reduction is carried out prior to the evaluation of sciatic integrity, confusion would result if the post reduction physical examination demonstrated a sciatic deficit. At that point, it would be difficult to evaluate how the sciatic nerve injury occurred. The nerve could have been injured by the dislocation and was non-functional prior to reduction. Or the previously normal nerve could have been injured by the manipulation needed to reduce the hip. Or a normal nerve may have become entrapped in the hip socket during reduction. The appropriate course of action for scenario one and two would be observation while scenario three would require immediate surgical exploration, to maximize the chances for recovery.

Adequate x-ray evaluation of dislocations is necessary prior to reduction to identify possible obstacles to reduction. Also, accompanying fractures that would make manipulation ineffective or inadvisable need to be identified. Some shoulder dislocations are accompanied by fractures of the proximal humerus. Forceful manipulation of non-displaced fractures of the proximal humerus can cause wide displacement of the fragments. When patients have non-displaced fractures of the proximal humerus and dislocations, it is frequently advisable to reduce the dislocations in the operating room under general anesthesia where complete muscle relaxation is possible. In the absence of fractures of the proximal humerus, it is usually safe to reduce shoulder dislocations in the emergency room under analgesia.

We will discuss some dislocations seen in a busy office practice, including shoulder and patellar dislocations. We will also discuss some dislocations commonly encountered in the emergency room that have serious neurovascular consequences, including knee dislocation and hip dislocation.

Shoulder Dislocation

Shoulder dislocation is frequently due to indirect injury to the shoulder. In other words, forces are applied to the arm in such a way that the shoulder becomes dislocated. Dislocation can be divided into the traumatic type and the atraumatic type. Traumatic dislocations are quite common while atraumatic are uncommon. Atraumatic dislocations can be further subdivided into voluntary dislocation and congenital dislocation. Patients with congenital dislocations frequently have very compromised anatomy that predisposes them to multiple shoulder dislocations. Such patients can be very difficult to treat. Patients with voluntary shoulder dislocations frequently have psychiatric problems that make their treatment extremely difficult. Since these atraumatic dislocations are not commonly encountered than in office practice, we will limit our discussion here to traumatic dislocation.

An evaluation of acute shoulder dislocation begins with a patient presenting with an episode of trauma and severe pain about the shoulder. The patient will not move the involved arm, and if the patient's shirt is removed, there is usually asymmetry between the shoulders. Over 95% of dislocations occur with the humeral head exiting the glenoid anteriorly.

A good history is important. We must know if the patient is presenting with a first time dislocation or a recurrent one. This information will help establish a prognosis for re-dislocation following closed reduction. How large was the injuring force? This will identify the true traumatic dislocation versus a dislocation with predisposing anatomic abnormality. How long ago was the dislocation? Within the first few hours, dislocations are relatively easy to reduce. After six to eight hours, muscle spasm makes dislocations very difficult to reduce. Is there numbness or tingling? Thirty percent of anterior shoulder dislocations are associated with partial or complete axillary nerve dysfunction. A history of tingling in the shoulder can frequently identify these patients.

On physical examination, a unilateral anterior shoulder dislocation victim presents with marked asymmetry at the shoulders. On the dislocated side, the arm is held still; the acromion, coracoid, and glenoid stand out; and the humeral head may be palpated in the axilla. Axillary and musculocutaneous nerve function should be tested. Testing sensation for both nerves is relatively straightforward (see Fig. 10-1). Testing motor function in the deltoid is quite difficult prior to reduction of the dislocation due to pain.

It is important to get x-rays of the dislocated shoulder prior to reduction. These x-rays are extremely helpful in determining treatment.

Figure 10-1. Left shoulder dislocation is shown. Note the sensory distribution of the axillary nerve in the deltoid region and the musculocutaneous nerve on the forearm. These nerves are often injured in anterior shoulder dislocations. The prominence just proximal to the axillary nerve sensory region is the acromion of the scapula. It becomes quite visible following anterior shoulder dislocation.

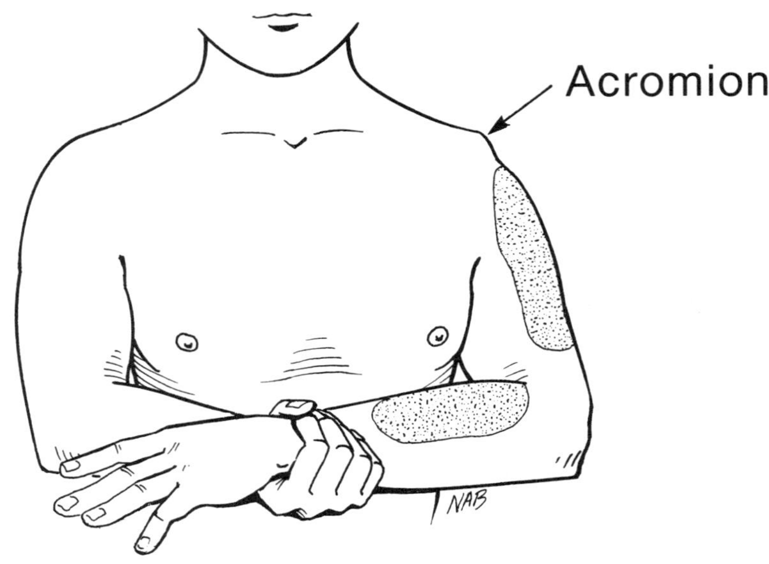

A patient with an anterior shoulder dislocation accompanied by a non-displaced fracture of the anatomic or surgical neck of the humerus is at great risk for complications relating to reduction. The patient with a fractured humerus may experience wide displacement of fracture fragments with the moderate forces involved in reduction under sedation. The patient is much better served by closed reduction in an operating room under general anesthesia or open reduction. Consequently, a patient with an anterior shoulder dislocation should receive a screening x-ray to determine if a fracture accompanies the dislocation.

Treatment of Anterior Shoulder Dislocation

In general, treatment of anterior shoulder dislocations is closed reduction and immobilization. Younger patients are immobilized for long periods of time: a 20-year-old patient would be immobilized for three to six weeks, a 40-year-old patient for one to three weeks, and a 60-year-old patient for one week or less. In general, younger patients are at higher risk for recurrent dislocations, and older patients are at higher risk for post- reduction stiffness.

Complications Associated with Anterior Dislocation of the Shoulder

There are a number of bony injuries associated with shoulder dislocations. These include humeral head fracture, fracture of the anterior lip of the glenoid, fracture of the tuberosity of the humerus, and fracture of the acromion or coracoid. There are also soft tissue injuries associated with shoulder dislocation. These include rotator cuff tears, axillary nerve injuries, and vascular injuries. Vascular injuries are uncommon and occur almost exclusively in patients with arterial sclerosis. There are fewer than 200 cases reported in the English literature. Nerve injury is common and is seen in 20% to 30% of patients with anterior shoulder dislocation.

Analysis of patients with anterior shoulder dislocation and axillary nerve dysfunction have shown that essentially all axillary nerve injuries spontaneously resolve within three to six months. It is important to know if the axillary nerve is intact, however. Patients with axillary nerve injuries frequently have difficulty with physical therapy post-reduction. In addition, it is nice to know whether the axillary nerve injury preceded the reduction or followed manipulation.

Posterior Shoulder Dislocation

Posterior dislocations of the shoulder are uncommon. Fewer than 1% of patients with shoulder dislocations will have a posterior dislocation. These can be either traumatic or atraumatic. Traumatic dislocations are frequently associated with indirect trauma to the shoulder, commonly electroshock therapy or seizures. The diagnosis is frequently missed since on inspection there is no obvious deformity. Range of motion is limited, however. The patient presents with the arm fixed in adduction and internal rotation. External rotation is painful as is shoulder abduction. This type of presentation associated with a history of epilepsy or electroshock therapy should lead the physician to recommend x-ray.

Standard anterior-posterior x-rays are very difficult to interpret in posterior shoulder dislocation. The diagnosis is frequently missed as the pathological relationship between the humerus and the glenoid is very subtle (see Fig. 10-2). An axillary x-ray is necessary to confirm or disprove the diagnosis of posterior shoulder dislocation. If posterior shoulder dislocation is diagnosed, closed reduction should be attempted followed by immobilization.

Patellar Dislocation

In most cases of patellar dislocation, the patella is displaced lateral to the lateral femoral condyle. It is more common to see patellar dislocation in "predisposed" knees than in normal knees. The anatomy of the quadriceps mechanism can lead to predisposition for lateral instability of the patella. The vastus lateralis is a powerful muscle on the lateral side of the patella. During knee extension, it produces a lateral moment. Under normal circumstances, this is well opposed by the vastus medialis with its medial pull and further aided by the triangular shape of the patella, which fits snugly into the groove between the femoral condyles. Certain factors can upset this balance. In patients presenting with valgus knees, the tibial tubercle becomes more laterally placed. This favors lateral displacement of the patella. When this is combined with a hypoplastic patella (which is flat in the anterior-posterior plane rather than triangular) or a hypoplastic lateral femoral condyle, the scene is set for the typical traumatic patellar dislocation in the "predisposed" knee.

Figure 10-2. (A) A normal shoulder. (B) A posterior shoulder dislocation. The articular surface of the humerus points posterior to the glenoid and the greater tuberosity faces anterior. The soft tissue contour of the shoulder is maintained, however. The anterior-posterior x-ray demonstrates only a subtle widening of the distance between the humerus and the glenoid. As the dislocated head is pointing posterior, the arm is internally rotated. This accounts for the physical examination sign of decreased external rotation in posterior shoulder dislocations. (C) An anterior shoulder dislocation with typical inferior displacement of the humeral head. Compare the soft tissue contours of the shoulder in (B) and (C). Note that the shoulder contour looks normal in a posterior shoulder dislocation. In an anterior shoulder dislocation, the humeral head migrates inferiorly. This elongates the deltoid and allows the acromion process of the scapula to stand out starkly.

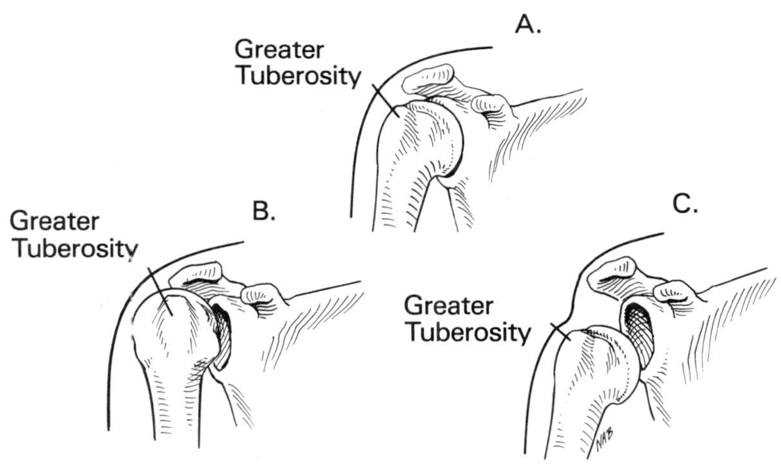

Patients frequently state that their knee pops or gives way. The patient may describe an episode of running or cutting where they have sudden knee pain and fall to the ground. Occasionally, they can feel the patella as a lateral mass and their companions will reduce the patella by simply extending the knee. In an acute situation, the patient will have a swollen knee that is quite tender. Tenderness occurs along the medial border of the patella where the medial retinaculum can be torn as the patella goes laterally. The Fairbank's test is classically quite positive. In this test, the patella is pushed laterally, which causes the patient to object strongly. This test has been called the patellar anxiety test, the panic test, the grab test, and the "don't do that again" test. Fractures can occur at the lateral femoral condyle and the articular surface of the patella. X-rays are always necessary to determine whether osteochondral fracture has occurred. X-rays should be obtained both pre-reduction and post-reduction since pre-reduction x-rays are the best time to identify loose bony fragments in the joint.

Treatment revolves around closed reduction and immobilization. If pre-reduction x-rays demonstrate large osteochondral fractures, open reduction and pinning of these fractures is probably necessary. If there are no osteochondral fractures demonstrated, closed reduction followed by immobilization is the treatment of choice. Immobilization in a cylinder cast for up to six weeks is typical treatment. Quadriceps strengthening should be started immediately after closed reduction. Nonoperative treatment is successful in the treatment of patellar dislocation 80% to 85% of the time. 15% to 20% of patients develop recurrent patellar subluxation or dislocation. Patients with recurrent patellar dislocations have bony architecture that favors dislocation. In the setting of recurrent symptomatic dislocation, these problems can be addressed surgically.

Knee Dislocation

A knee dislocation is an uncommon but devastating injury. It is especially important to be aware of knee dislocations as there is a high incidence of accompanying popliteal artery and peroneal nerve injury. The popliteal artery is very susceptible to injury because it is fixed both above and below the knee joint by muscular and fascial arcades. The common peroneal and tibial nerves are less tightly tethered but are still injured frequently.

The patient with a knee dislocation is usually the victim of major trauma, although occasionally knee dislocation occurs as an athletic injury. The dislocation can occur in any direction. The tibia can go anterior, posterior, medial or lateral with respect to the femur.

It is critically important to monitor blood flow distal to the knee. Good pulses assure that the popliteal artery is functioning. Capillary refill is not a reliable sign of an intact vascular tree. If good pulses are present, they must be monitored in a serial fashion. If they are absent, arteriograms are necessary to evaluate flow.

Numbness in a distribution of the common peroneal nerve or the tibial nerve may expose nerve injury in need of evaluation. More importantly, if a patient develops numbness in the leg that does not appear to be related to dermatomes and myotomes but is more global, it may be the result of a compartment syndrome secondary to arterial disruption. Consequently, it is extremely important to do good sequential physical examinations on patients with suspected knee dislocation.

Patients with dislocated knees and numb, pulseless feet require immediate reduction prior to x-ray. After a brief physical examination and the administration of analgesia, the knee is manipulated, splinted, and re-evaluated. If neurovascular recovery occurs, the patient is sent to x-ray. An anterior-posterior and lateral x-ray will provide almost all the information necessary to formulate the orthopaedic treatment plan. If blood flow does not return, immediate evaluation by the vascular surgery team is essential.

Treatment can be operative or non-operative. In the presence of ligament avulsions with attached pieces of bone dangling from the avulsed ligament, most orthopaedic surgeons would consider open reduction. If ligaments are torn off bone with a piece of bone attached, they can be replaced anatomically and provide excellent function. If ligaments are torn in their substance, early surgery is certainly not necessary. It is very unrewarding to reanastomose midsubstance tears of ligaments.

Many patients have both stiffness and instability following a knee dislocation due to massive disruption of soft tissues. Few patients will return to athletic activities and many will develop painful arthritis.

Hip Dislocation

Hip dislocations are often encountered in the emergency room. Patients typically are individuals involved in motor vehicle accidents who did not use seat belts. At least 50% of the patients have associated fractures. A thorough evaluation of a patient with a hip dislocation is necessary before treatment is begun.

Patients will present with asymmetry of the two limbs. Depending on the direction of the dislocation, the limb may be shortened and externally rotated or internally rotated in adduction. Additionally, injuries of the sciatic nerve are quite common. This nerve must always be evaluated prior to any type of manipulation of the hip joint.

A simple anterior-posterior of the pelvis is sufficient for making the diagnosis of a hip dislocation. After this, a CT scan is frequently needed to determine if there are associated problems, which can include acetabular fractures, femoral head and neck fractures, and especially the presence of osteocartilaginous debris in the hip joint. A CT scan is frequently obtained both prior to and following reduction. Treatment revolves around closed reduction. If a closed reduction can be accomplished, a patient is usually kept in bed until comfortable and then gradually mobilized. Weight bearing is generally forbidden for at least six weeks.

The most common complications of hip dislocation are sciatic nerve injury (see Fig. 10-3) and avascular necrosis. Sciatic nerve injury is present in at least 10% of patients with posterior hip dislocation. In the presence of a hip dislocation, sciatic nerve function must be monitored both pre-reduction and post-reduction. If the sciatic nerve is functioning properly pre-reduction and it is not functioning post-reduction, a number of possibilities exist. The sciatic nerve may have become trapped in the joint or it may be impaled on the spike of bone. Under either of these circumstances, open reduction is necessary to evaluate and treat the problem. If the sciatic nerve is non-functional prior to reduction, no formal nerve exploration should be undertaken. The vast majority of these injuries are stretch injuries and there is no available treatment. If nerve dysfunction is still present six months after the injury, secondary muscle and bony procedures may be indicated.

Figure 10-3. A typical posterior hip dislocation. As the femoral head dislocates from the acetabulum it frequently impacts the sciatic nerve causing nerve dysfunction.

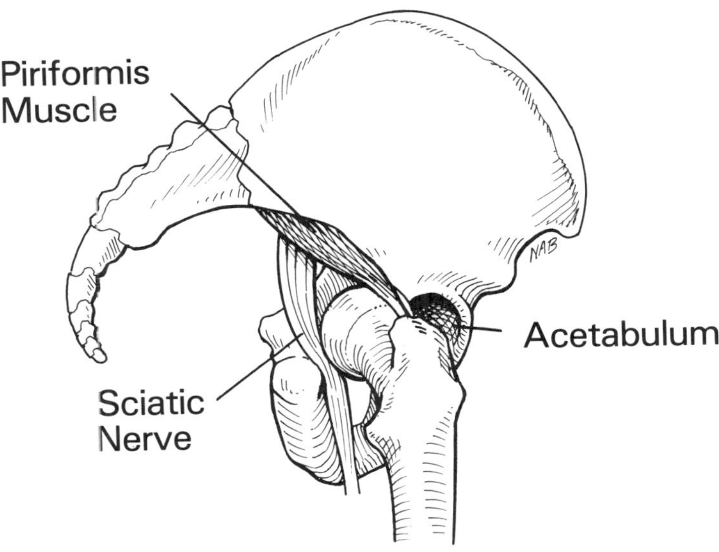

Avascular necrosis of the femoral head is a common sequela to hip dislocation. From 6% to 40% of patients will experience avascular necrosis, depending on the violence involved in the dislocation. It occurs because the blood supply to the femoral head is easily disrupted. Patients who have hip dislocation in the absence of pelvic or femoral fractures generally do well if their femoral head is reduced within 12 hours of injury. In this setting, avascular necrosis is seldom seen. If patients have associated pelvic fractures, the incidence of avascular necrosis climbs as does the incidence of post-traumatic arthritis because greater violence causes these injuries. It may take two to five years for avascular necrosis to become obvious on plain x-rays. Because of this, hip dislocation patients should be followed for many years. Avascular necrosis can be either symptomatic or asymptomatic. Patients with symptomatic avascular necrosis will need total hip replacement whereas patients with asymptomatic avascular necrosis will frequently do well with more conservative treatment.

Fractures

Fractures can occur under many circumstances. Most commonly, fractures occur when normal bone is rapidly loaded beyond its strength. Less commonly, we see fractures due to repetitive low load stressing of normal bone (stress fractures) or moderate stressing of diseased bone (pathologic fractures). Most fractures are emergencies. Additionally, any fracture associated with a skin laceration requires special attention. If there is a chance that a bone may have penetrated the skin, the patient's risk for catastrophic infection is quite high. Consequently, these patients need extremely urgent treatment.

The diagnosis of fracture may be made on physical examination when a bone is deformed and the site of deformity is painful. There is frequently crepitus, swelling, and ecchymosis at the typical fracture site. Following the clinical diagnosis of fracture, a splint should be applied. Under most circumstances, the patient should be splinted "as they lay" with no attempt made to straighten the bone. Splinting will certainly make a patient more comfortable because the splint will prevent the bone ends from shifting. In addition, splinting reduces the chance that a sharp bone end will penetrate the skin or damage a nerve or blood vessel. Ice and elevation are also important to minimize swelling. Swelling will interfere with reduction and circulation. After splinting the patient should be sent for radiologic evaluation. An important exception to this approach involves fractures with vascular compromise distal to the fracture site. As muscles and nerves are quite sensitive to anoxia, an ischemic limb requires special measures. These limbs are frequently reduced before splinting or x-ray. The risks of reducing a deformity without x-rays are great but they are justified if the limb distal to the deformity is numb and cold. Blood flow must be re-established within six hours of disruption to have any hope of useful function in the limb.

Wrist Fractures

Fractures at the wrist are usually due to indirect trauma. A patient will fall on an outstretched hand and in this way sustain their injury. In 1814, Abraham Colles described what he felt was a distal radius fracture that occurred an inch to an inch and a half above the wrist joint. The forearm was considerably deformed. He noted fullness on the flexor side of the wrist and a hollowed-out dorsal surface. He noted that reduction was relatively easy to accomplish, but he also noted that when the surgeon removed his hands, the deformity recurred. It was his experience that putting splints and bandages on the wrist did not lead to permanent correction as the fracture fragments would shorten up while in the splints. He also mentions, "One consolation only remains, that the limb at some remote period again will enjoy perfect freedom in all its motions and be completely exempt from pain: the deformity, however, will remain undiminished throughout life."

Colles touched on points that are certainly relevant today. First of all, the diagnosis of distal radius fracture can frequently be made on the basis of history and physical. The mechanism of injury tends to be a fall on the outstretched hand. The deformity occurs with dorsal displacement of the hand and distal radius with respect to the forearm. Post-menorrheal women with osteoporosis are most likely to incur this injury. The mechanism of injury causes compaction of the honeycomb-like cancellous bone of the distal radius, especially on the dorsal surface of the bone. Following reduction of the fracture, there is a large empty space dorsally where the crushed bone ends are disimpacted. The fracture frequently collapses into this space during the course of healing. As Colles also noted, in distal radius fractures, function is usually quite good even if deformity is present.

Treatment methods and duration will be determined by the amount of joint involvement present and the amount of displacement of fracture fragments. Usually fractures that do not involve the wrist joint are treated non-surgically with a reduction under analgesia or anesthesia followed by a short arm or long arm cast. Fractures that involve the wrist joint are not true Colles fractures, since the fracture he described did not involve the joint. When the fracture involves the joint surface, anatomical reduction must be obtained and held. If the radial-carpal joint or the radial-ulnar joint is displaced, there is a high probability that secondary arthritis will occur. This justifies aggressive treatment of displaced intra-articular fractures leading to the use of internal and external fixation in these cases.

The treatment of distal radius fractures should be prompt, but is usually not urgent. During the first few hours, reduction is the easiest. After a week, the organization of clot causes the fracture fragments to be less mobile, but reduction is not greatly impeded.

Complications

Acute vascular injuries are unusual in distal radius fractures. Arterial avulsions that would put the hand at risk are not encountered in the typical patient who falls and sustains a distal radius fracture. Nerve injuries are common however. Median nerve injuries are most common followed by ulnar and then radial nerve injuries. The majority of median and ulnar nerve injuries are due to stretching of these nerves at the time of impact. It is possible, however, for bone to pierce the median or ulnar nerves, and in addition, swelling within the carpal tunnel or the flexor surface of the wrist can cause nerve compression. This is a reversible cause of nerve dysfunction and, frequently, reduction of the fracture relieves the dysfunction. If reduction does not alleviate the dysfunction, surgery may be indicated.   Late problems with distal radius fractures are related to the fracture configuration. If the fractures do not involve the wrist joint, function will usually be good even if cosmesis is not. The incidence of post-traumatic arthritis is related to the integrity of the joint surface post reduction and the amount of damage the initial fracture causes on the joint surface. The surgeon can control the articular surface with external or internal fixation, if necessary. In general, the better the articular surface realigns, the better the outcome is in the long run. Of course, wrist cartilage damage that occurs at the moment of injury cannot be repaired.

Ankle Fractures

Injuries about the ankle are common in active adults. The primary care physician's first responsibility is to determine whether a patient has an ankle sprain or an ankle fracture. This process begins with careful physical examination. The most common type of ankle sprain occurs when a patient tears ligaments running from the fibula to the lateral side of the talus. This anterior talofibular ligament is frequently ruptured in its substance. A patient presenting with a typical ankle sprain has swelling and ecchymosis on the lateral side of the foot with remarkable point tenderness distal to the tip of the fibula. This patient should not have significant point tenderness along the fibula. In addition, tenderness on the medial malleolus is not encountered. Occasionally, patients with severe ankle sprains may have tenderness at the anterior talofibular ligament and in addition around the posterior aspect of the ankle all the way to the medial side of the ankle joint. This type of massive sprain is difficult to differentiate from a fracture. Patients with ankle fractures will have marked point tenderness over the bone. The most common ankle fractures occur at the distal fibula. They are associated with ecchymosis, swelling, crepitus, and exquisite point tenderness. Fractures of the posterior tibia and the medial side of the tibia are also common. These fractures also are accompanied by swelling, ecchymosis, and point tenderness. Maisonneuve described an ankle injury associated with a fibular fracture at the proximal third of the fibula. Consequently, when patients have ankle dysfunction, the entire fibula is palpated.

When an ankle fracture is suspected on the basis of physical examination, the patient should be immediately splinted, iced and elevated. Neurovascular function should be checked and then x-rays should be taken to determine the course of treatment.

Most ankle sprains are treated non-surgically. Mild sprains are treated with protected weight bearing and active range of motion exercises. Very severe sprains are frequently treated with a period of immobilization followed by protected weight bearing and active range of motion. The goal of treatment in ankle sprains is to regain a pain-free range of motion.

The goal of treatment in ankle fractures is to re-establish a normal ankle mortise. To do this, the medial malleolus, distal tibia, fibula, and talus must be aligned anatomically. After an anatomic union has occurred, range of motion exercises should begin, and strengthening exercises are begun to return as much mobility as possible to the ankle joint.

Complications

Malunion is a serious complication following ankle fractures. A malunion has occurred if there is an abnormal relationship between the tibia, the talus, and the fibula. Because of the precise fit of these three bones, malunion is not well tolerated, and it will lead to degenerative joint disease.

Acute neurovascular injuries following ankle fractures are quite rare. A serious and often encountered problem is reflex sympathetic dystrophy or Sudeck's atrophy. This process of unknown etiology is reflected by burning pain in the affected lower extremity, trophic changes in the skin, vascular disturbances, and profound osteoporosis. This process may present while a patient is still in a cast for treatment of ankle fracture. Early aggressive treatment is important in Sudeck's atrophy. The treatment begins with physical therapy and may require nerve blocks and other invasive modalities.

Hip Fractures

Fractures about the hip are frequently encountered in emergency rooms. The vast majority of these injuries occur in older people who have osteoporotic bone. A common mechanism of injury is a fall in the home. There are two distinct types of hip fractures. The first type is a fracture of the femoral neck within the capsule of the hip joint. The second type of hip fracture is an intertrochanteric fracture, which is extracapsular fracture, in other words, a fracture distal to the capsule of the hip joint. As intracapsular fractures of the hip joints are often associated with vascular problems and extracapsular fractures are not, we will discuss them separately.

Femoral Neck Fractures (Intracapsular Fractures of the Hip Joint)

Femoral neck fractures are common in the elderly. The prognosis for recovery of good hip function is almost entirely related to the integrity of the blood supply to the femoral head. When it is not damaged, patients do well. When it is damaged, avascular necrosis of the femoral head occurs. This usually leads to rapid arthritis and very poor function.

The femoral head receives its blood supply from three sources -the ligamentum teres, the vessels running within the bone of the femoral neck into the femoral head, and the vessels running along the surface of the femoral neck in the subsynovial space that penetrate directly into the femoral head. The vessels that run along the femoral neck in the subsynovial space are the most important ones supplying the femoral head (see Fig. 10-4). In femoral neck fractures with minimal displacement, the subsynovial vessels are not badly damaged. Avascular necrosis of the femoral head is very uncommon in this setting. When the fracture is severe with wide displacement of fracture fragments, many subsynovial vessels are torn and avascular necrosis occurs in 50% of cases.

Patients with femoral neck fractures usually present with pain in the hip. On physical examination, these patients may present with their femur in anatomic alignment or they may present with some shortening and external rotation. These patients do not have as much deformity as patients with intertrochanteric fractures. In the femoral neck fracture, there is frequently some intact hip joint capsule that runs from the acetabulum to the femoral shaft. As the fracture is interposed between the insertion of the capsule onto the femur and the pelvis, this capsule lends support to the hip joint. Patients with suspected femoral neck fractures benefit from immediate splinting with Buck's traction or sandbags for pain control. Also, this immobilization may prevent further damage to the blood supply during evaluation. Anterior-posterior and lateral x-rays will determine the extent of femoral damage.

Figure 10-4. A majority of blood flow to the femoral head comes from subsynovial vessels. These branch off the main extracapsular vessels, pierce the hip joint capsule and run along the femoral neck. Fractures through the femoral neck can disrupt this circulation.

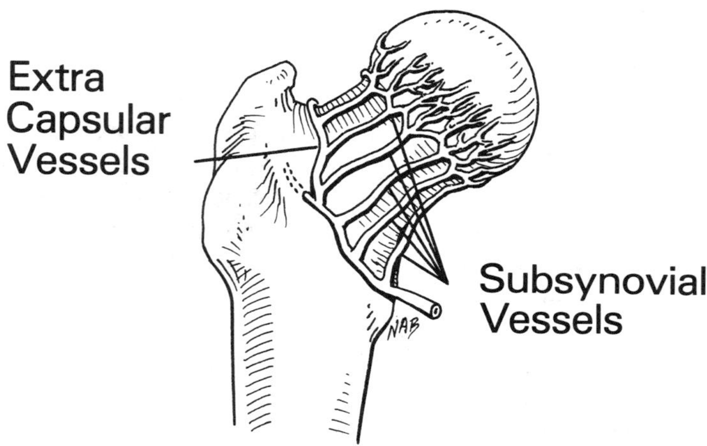

Treatment of femoral neck fractures is dependent on fracture type. Patients with minimally displaced fractures of the impacted type can be treated operatively or non-operatively (see Fig. 10-5). Patients with impacted minimally displaced femoral neck fractures who are comfortable, cooperative and agile can be treated non-surgically with non-weight-bearing for eight to 12 weeks. In addition, patients who are poor candidates for surgery due to systemic illness may also be treated in this fashion. These patients who undertake a non-operative course avoid the risks of surgery and accept the risk that their minimally displaced impacted fracture will displace during healing. If this were to happen, the patient's prognosis for complications such as avascular necrosis would increase considerably. Many physicians believe that all non-displaced or minimally displaced femoral neck fractures that present within a few days of injury (see Figs. 10-5A,B) should be treated with percutaneous internal fixation using threaded pins or other types of internal fixation devices. Following surgery, these patients are at very low risk for further displacement of fracture fragments. Patients with displaced femoral neck fractures (see Figs. 10-5C,D) present a treatment dilemma. It is clear that displaced femoral neck fractures have a poor prognosis for vascular survival. It has been estimated that 50% of patients will have avascular necrosis even with anatomic reduction of fracture fragments and ideal internal fixation. Many of these patients who develop avascular necrosis will have symptomatic disease with femoral head collapse and arthritis. For this reason, older patients with displaced hip fractures are often offered prosthetic replacement. This may take the form of a hemiarthroplasty such as a unipolar Austin-Moore or bipolar prosthesis or may take the form of a total hip arthroplasty. These options will provide a patient with very good function although function may not be as good as patients who have successful healing of their femoral neck fractures. In general, indications for hemiarthroplasty include patients with a quite advanced physiologic age who will make few demands on their hip and patients with pathologic fractures of the femoral head and neck who are unlikely to heal their fractures. Patients with certain neurologic conditions such as Parkinson's disease or spastic hemiplegia heal poorly and do best with prosthetic replacement. By and large, the contraindication for hemiarthroplasty and indication for total hip replacement is acetabular disease.

Open reduction and pinning of displaced fractures is usually offered to young patients. These patients will usually remain non-weight-bearing on crutches for at least six to 12 weeks. If they develop symptomatic avascular necrosis postoperatively, a prosthetic replacement is then performed. If they do not develop avascular necrosis and 50% will not, they are better serviced by their natural hip. If open reduction is attempted, it should be done within the first 24 hours post-injury to maximize the chances of success. If surgery is delayed past the one week mark, the prognosis for femoral head vascular recovery is very poor. Clinical studies demonstrate this need for urgent surgery. Vascular studies show that many displaced fractures have some intact subsynovial vessels. When the fracture fragments are displaced, the vessels can be kinked and blood flow sluggish. When reduction is obtained, blood flow is maximized. This is probably the explanation for the time window that exists in the treatment of displaced femoral neck fractures.

Figure 10-5. (A) A valgus impacted (Garden I) fracture. The medial lateral and inferior femoral neck is intact. This is a relatively stable fracture because the fracture impacts on itself superiorly. Avascular necrosis is not commonly encountered. (B) A Garden II fracture with fracture line running through the entire femoral neck with no displacement of fracture fragments. These fractures need internal fixation as there is no impaction of fracture fragments. Avascular necrosis is not commonly encountered. (C) A Garden III fracture. A Garden III fracture has only a narrow bridge of intact bone at the superior femoral neck. There is considerable disruption of subsynovial blood vessels as the fracture displaces into varus. Avascular necrosis is common. (D) A Garden IV fracture. A Garden IV fracture has complete separation of the femoral head from the femoral neck. The blood supply to the femoral head is massively disrupted and avascular necrosis is quite likely.

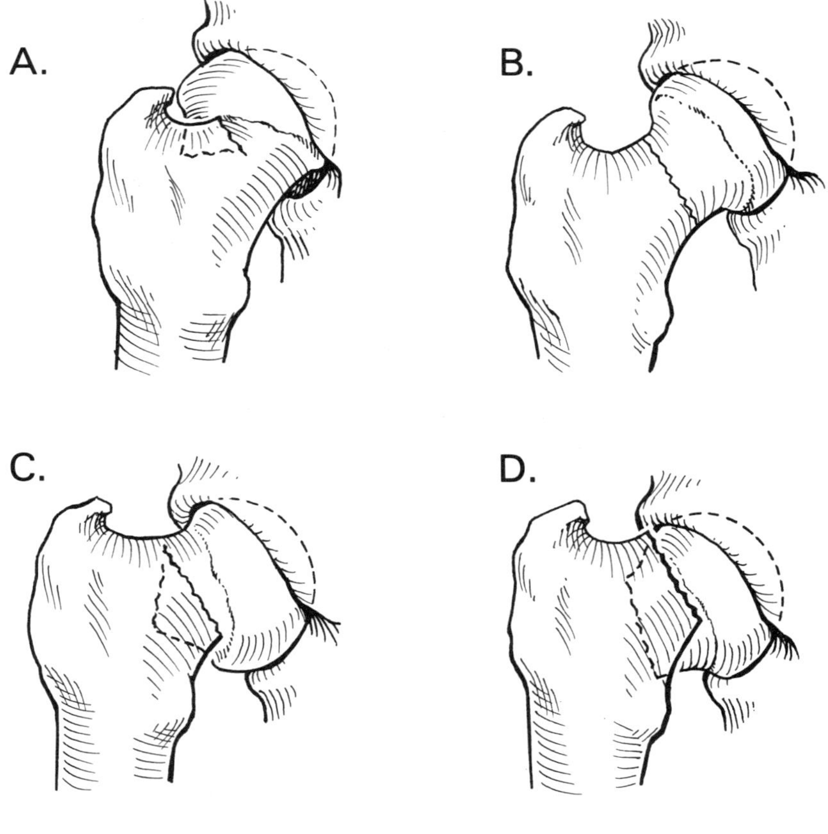

Complications

Thromboembolism is a feared complication in the treatment of hip disease. By and large, all patients with hip fractures are treated with anti-embolism measures. Many orthopaedists will use aspirin prophylaxis for patients without a history of thromboembolism and Coumadin or Heparin for patients with a previous history of thromboembolism.

The most common local complications of femoral neck fractures are avascular necrosis and nonunion. Non-union or a failure of the bone ends to heal occurs in 10% to 20% of displaced fractures. This is related to a number of special features of femoral neck fractures. First, there is no periosteum present at the site of femoral neck fracture as the fracture is intracapsular. Without periosteum, it is impossible to have peripheral callus. All fracture healing must occur within the medullary canal. If there is poor apposition of fracture fragments or marked avascularity, union will not occur. A nonunion of a femoral neck fracture will usually make function painful and difficult, if not impossible.

Another problem in treating patients with femoral neck fractures is determining the likelihood that the femoral head will develop avascular necrosis and whether it will be symptomatic if it does occur. If we knew in every instance which femoral head would collapse and become symptomatic, we would do primary arthroplasties on all of these patients. There is no test at this time that will provide that information with accuracy. Consequently, a large number of patients who have femoral neck fractures will have internal fixation of their fractures with pins or a sliding nail device. Some of these patients will develop avascular necrosis and need a second operation, a total hip arthroplasty, for pain control. At this time, the degree of fracture fragment displacement is our best guide in predicting outcome in femoral neck fractures; the more displaced the fracture fragments, the worse the prognosis.

Intertrochanteric Hip Fractures

Intertrochanteric hip fractures are common in the elderly. This is an extracapsular fracture (see Fig. 10-6). The blood supply to the femoral head and neck is not at risk because the important intracapsular, subsynovial vessels are not involved. Therefore, fracture healing almost always occurs without the complication of avascular necrosis or non-union. These fractures are more common in women than in men. This is thought due to the increased incidence of osteoporosis in elderly women. In general, these fractures occur secondary to a fall. On physical examination, the patient presents with marked shortening and external rotation of the lower extremity. They should be placed in Buck's traction or immobilized with sand bags when they go to x-ray. This will result in some pain control.

The diagnosis of intertrochanteric hip fracture can be made easily on an anterior-posterior and lateral x-ray. It is generally agreed that treatment should be carried out as soon as the patient is medically stable and this will hopefully be within the first 48 to 72 hours after fracture.

Figure 10-6. Intertrochanteric fractures of the two-(A), three-(B), and four-(C) part variety. Note the lesser and greater trochanter are fractured off in the four-part fracture. The four-part fracture may be quite unstable.

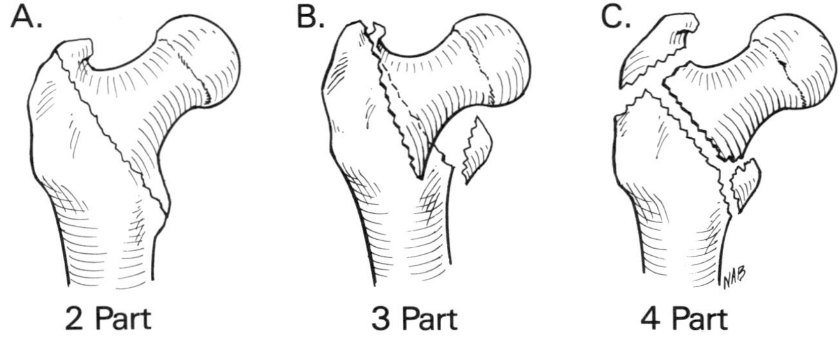

Treatment is usually operative. Non-operative treatment should be reserved for either the terminal patient or patients who are comfortable and non-ambulatory. Operative pinning is indicated in almost all other situations. It will realign the leg, control pain and allow mobilization of the patient. A small subset of the population benefits from immediate prosthetic replacement. These patients are usually quite old physiologically with severely comminuted intertrochanteric fractures. Prosthetic replacement allows early full weight bearing on the injured extremity.

Complications

10% to 15% of the patients who present with intertrochanteric fractures will die during the six months following their fracture secondary to heart failure, renal failure, and respiratory compromise or thromboembolism. It is widely believed that during the first month after fracture, the risk of death is 10 to 20 times that of appropriately matched controls who have not had fractures. During the second month following fracture, the risk of dying is five to 10 times that of patients who do not have hip fractures. After a patient has survived two months, that patient returns to the risk pool of other individuals of the same age.

The most common local complications are wound infections in 5% to 10% of patients and loss of fixation. Loss of fixation is seen in very osteopenic individuals. In these patients the metal internal fixation devices cut out of the relatively soft bone and fractures can re-deform the proximal femur. The treatment of this complication is highly varied but usually results in the need for prosthetic replacement.

Complicated Trauma

Management of Open Fractures

An open fracture is one that communicates with the outside world through an opening in the skin. Any laceration that extends down to a fracture qualifies as an open fracture. Any bone that punctures the skin qualifies as an open fracture. The ultimate outcome of an open fracture is related to the severity of the violence that produced it and the amount of contamination it received. All open fractures are orthopaedic emergencies due to the high rate of catastrophic infections.

Most orthopaedists divide open fractures into three specific types with the most severe type having three subgroups. The most common and benign fracture is the type I injury where the skin wound is less that one centimeter long. This is frequently caused by a spike of bone exiting through the skin and then typically retracking back underneath it. With optimal care, the infection rate is less than 2%. Type II injuries have larger lacerations associated with them, minimal to moderate soft tissue damage, and essentially no loss of skin or muscle. With optimal treatment, the infection rate is under 10% for these injuries. Type III fractures have massive soft tissue damage with lacerations usually greater than 10 centimeter in length. In type III-A injuries, there is sufficient soft tissue to eventually cover the bone. No skin grafting or skin flaps are necessary. The infection rate for these patients is 10% to 15%. In type III-B injuries, there is sufficient loss of soft tissues so that sophisticated soft tissue coverage procedures are necessary to eventually cover the bone. The rate of infections in these injuries is up to 50%, and the amputation rate is 10%. In type III-C injuries, vascular injuries exist that mandate vascular repair to save the limb. In these injuries, the infection rate is at least 50%, and the amputation rate is about 50%
All open fractures are treated in a similar fashion. The general principles surrounding the treatment of open fractures include evaluation for other life threatening injuries, culture of the open wound, antibiotics and tetanus prophylaxis, wound debridement, and stabilization of the bones followed by delayed wound coverage.

Certain types of open fractures are notorious for specific infections. Open fractures caused by farm accidents are often associated with gas gangrene caused by <u>Clostridium perfringens</u>. Open fractures sustained in injuries in fresh water lakes and rivers are associated with infections of <u>Pseudomonas aeruginosa</u> and <u>Aeromonas hydrophila</u>. These associations should be considered when antibiotics are chosen.

Antibiotics are used in the treatment of all open fractures. During the first 12 to 24 hours, an open fracture is considered contaminated but not infected. The contaminated tissues are debrided from the area surgically. The antibiotics support the debridement. Wound cultures from the emergency room and the initial surgical debridement are checked and antibiotics are adjusted. If the wound is infected, further antibiotics alone are unlikely to cure the patient, since the infection is probably centered in damaged tissues with a poor blood supply. The debridements should continue until the wound is clean. Then the wound is closed.

The management of the soft tissues in open fractures revolves around debridement of devitalized tissue. For the one-centimeter, type I wounds, the soft tissues are usually intact. There is little disruption of blood supply. Most of these wounds are left open for a few days and then re-evaluated. Skin closure within the first week of injury is common. In the larger type II and type III wounds, repeated trips to the operating room for debridement is the rule. During these repeated debridements, devitalized tissue can be identified and removed. It is extremely difficult, at initial presentation, to identify all soft tissues that will eventually be nonviable. This decision is easier to make if the wound is followed over time through repeated trips to the operating room and repeated debridements.

Generally speaking, there are no open fractures that should be closed on the day of injury. It is safest to leave wounds open and to close the wounds some time during the first week after injury. The techniques used to stabilize fractures will be determined by the severity of injury. In the one-centimeter, type I wounds, techniques similar to those used for closed fractures should be used. The fractures under type I wounds can be treated with casts or internal fixation devices. External fixation devices such as external fixators are used occasionally. In the type II or type III wounds, casts are seldom used. It is very difficult to manage severe soft tissue injuries if they are underneath casts, and the type II and type III wounds are frequently accompanied by fractures that are very comminuted. Comminuted fractures do not maintain their length in casts. Because of this, external fixators are often used in open, comminuted fractures. Pins are placed in good strong bone above and below the fracture site and then these pins are attached to external rods. Fractures are usually treated in the external fixators until the soft tissue wounds are completely healed and the bones are stable enough so that a cast can be applied.

Occasionally, patients will present with traumatic amputations of their extremities. Under certain circumstances, extremities can be reimplanted. Occasionally, patients will present with open fractures and immediate amputation is recommended. It is difficult for some to understand why a fracture can be considered severe enough to require immediate amputation when there is a feeling in the community that most patients with complete amputations can have their limbs reimplanted. The experience with open fractures suggests that patients with severe injuries to the lower extremity that share certain specific characteristics often do better with immediate amputation. These are patients with type III-C fractures and complete tibial nerve loss or patients with massively contaminated type III-C wounds. Some in the medical community feel that immediate amputation represents a failure on the part of the treating team to try and save the limb. Others believe that a prolonged attempt to save a limb that has a poor prognosis for useful function represents a failure to present a decision for amputation in a reasonable light.

Compartment Syndromes

A compartment syndrome is an orthopaedic emergency. A compartment syndrome exists when pressure rises within a closed space, small vessels collapse, and ischemia to nerves and muscles result (See fig. 10-7). When nerves are rendered ischemic, nerve function becomes compromised within 30 minutes, and permanent damage occurs in 12 to 24 hours. When muscle is rendered ischemic, permanent damage can occur within four hours. Because of the sensitivity of peripheral nerve and muscular structures to anoxia, compartment syndromes must be rapidly diagnosed and treated.

The diagnosis of a compartment syndrome revolves around the "four P's" - pain, pallor, paralysis, and pulselessness. These are the hallmarks of a compartment syndrome. It is unnecessary for all four to be present to establish the diagnosis of compartment syndrome.

Pain is the most common sign of a compartment syndrome. The pain tends to be unrelenting, throbbing, deep, and difficult to localize. It is difficult to get a good analgesic response to this type of pain. Unfortunately, patients with compartment syndromes frequently are patients with associated injuries such as fractures or crushing injuries to the extremities, and pain is also a part of their other condition.

Pallor is sometimes seen. A pallorous or mottled limb can be encountered when compartment pressures rise and profusion rates fall in the compartments of a limb. We would hope to make a diagnosis of a compartment syndrome before the limb becomes cyanotic.

Paralysis also occurs in compartment syndromes. This tends to be a relatively late finding. Bradley noted that patients with anterior

Figure 10-7. This cross section of the tibia demonstrates the muscle compartments of the lower leg. The fascia is the dark line that surrounds the muscles firmly fixing the muscles to the tibia and fibula. This arrangement is excellent for leverage, but the thick fascial envelope that anchors these muscles compartments to the tibia and fibula are not elastic. Consequently, if the muscles within the compartments swell or if blood or edema fluid fills the compartments, pressure rises.

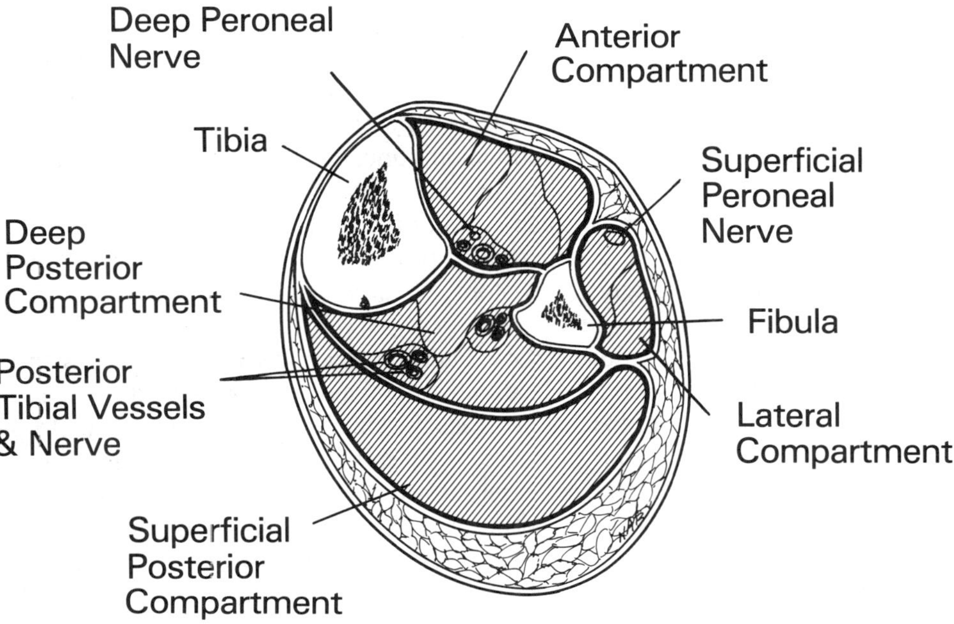

compartment syndromes and foot drop recovered normal function only 13% of the time.

Pulselessness is also a very late sign of compartment syndrome for it is possible to have palpable pulses and a compartment syndrome. It is common to have Doppler-able pulses in compartment syndromes. Arterial flow within relatively large vessels can occur even when profusion of capillary beds has ceased. A pulseless limb would be one that was extremely compromised.

There are usually two events that occur simultaneously as compartment syndromes are building. The first event is the collapse of arteriolar blood flow. Small arterioles running through the compartments exist in the environment of low surrounding pressure. If the pressure surrounding the arterioles increases, the arterioles may stop flowing. The second area of concern is the capillary beds. The capillary beds are relatively low pressure areas. When they are placed in a high pressure environment they collapse. Anoxia in soft tissues results when these two circulations collapse.

The muscles respond to anoxia with the liberation of histamine-like substances that dilate capillary beds and increase endothelial permeability. This results in considerable intramuscular transudation of plasma, which increases intracompartmental pressure and further decreases microcirculatory flow within the compartment. The measured weight of the compartments can actually increase by 30% to 50% due to these effects. As the compartment pressure approaches the diastolic pressure, microcirculatory flow stops. Within hours, there is irreversible necrosis of muscle and nerve.

Mattson suggests a long list of conditions that may be associated with compartment syndromes. He divides them up into two groups. One group includes conditions that decrease the size of compartments, thereby increasing compartment pressure. In this group he includes tight dressings and casts, localized external pressure, and the surgical closure of fascial defects. The other group includes a long list of conditions that increase compartmental contents. The most commonly encountered condition is bleeding. This can be the result of a vascular injury or a bleeding disorder such as hemophilia. Conditions that increase capillary permeability may also increase compartment pressure. Within this group would be burns, intra-arterial injection of drugs and many types of orthopaedic surgery. Excessive exercise may also do this as seen in seizures or just extremely vigorous volitional exercise.

The normal intracompartmental pressure is very low, less than a few millimeters of mercury. It can be measured directly with simple measuring tools described by Whitesides and others. When signs or symptoms of compartment pressure are encountered, direct measurement of intracompartmental pressures should be undertaken. When the pressures climb within 30 mm Hg of diastolic pressure, treatment is vital. If the patient has any circumferential bandages in place, such as a cast, they should be removed, since they can decrease the volume of compartments. If removing the cast decreases intracompartmental pressures sufficiently to get the patient out of the danger zone, the patient should be observed. If the pressure is still elevated, surgical compartment releases are undertaken. All constricting structures such as fascia and skin are surgically incised. Because of this, skin incisions can be large and may be left open for up to a week. It is usually possible to close the incisions without skin grafting. Occasionally, skin grafting is necessary when edema is slow to resolve.

Childhood Skeletal Infections

In 1874, Thomas Smith reported 21 cases of acute septic arthritis. The mortality rate was over 50%, and the surviving patients were all crippled. Since the advent of modern medical and surgical treatment, few patients die from bone and joint infections. With timely diagnosis and appropriate surgical and antibiotic therapy, most patients have excellent outcomes and only a few develop chronic infection, permanent deformity, and significant functional losses.

Osteomyelitis

Pathology and Etiology

Osseous infections occur by three mechanisms: (1) hematogenous seeding of bony sites following septicemia or bacteremia, (2) direct inoculation of bone by a puncture wound or open fracture, and (3) contiguous spread from an adjacent focus of infection. In neonates and children, most bone infections are hematogenous in origin and most often involve the metaphysis. The anatomic arrangement of metaphyseal vessels and the dynamics of blood flow in the region permit bacteria to lodge and proliferate (see Fig. 10-8). Bacterial and inflammatory exudates increase metaphyseal pressure and compromise circulation. Without treatment, decompression occurs via the haversian system to the cortex and then to the subperiosteal space. The continued subperiosteal accumulation of purulent material strips periosteum from the bone. As the periosteum supplies blood to the cortex, this stripping interrupts cortical blood flow (see Fig. 10-9). As a result, large areas of bone become devascularized (sequestra) and serve as sites of chronic infection. Draining cutaneous sinuses may arise when pus ruptures through overlying soft tissues and skin. Occasionally, infection may spread into an adjacent joint space, causing secondary septic arthritis. Destruction of the growth plate may occur either by direct spread of infection or by compromise of blood flow, resulting in permanent shortening or angular deformity of the limb. Children under 12 months of age are at particularly high risk for epiphyseal and growth plate destruction because these children have transepiphyseal vessels that connect the metaphysis and epiphysis (see Fig. 10-9). These vessels allow bacteria to cross from the metaphysis to the epiphysis with ease.

The etiologic agents responsible for neonatal osteomyelitis over the last four decades have varied. Hemolytic streptococci predominated before the 1940s. Between 1940 and the mid-1960s, almost 85% of the osseous infections in neonates were caused by <u>Staphylococcus aureus</u>. In the early 1970s, <u>Streptococcus agalactiae</u> (group B streptococci) emerged as an important neonatal pathogen, and it has become the major cause of both neonatal septicemia and osteomyelitis. Today more than 50% of bone infections in newborns are caused by this organism. <u>Staphylococcus aureus</u> and the enteric aerobic bacilli are less frequently responsible.

The pathogens responsible for bone infections in older children and adults have remained constant over the past four decades. <u>S. aureus</u> has been recovered from 80% of these patients with osteomyelitis and, together with group A streptococci and <u>S. pneumoniae</u>, account for 95%

Figure 10-8. (A) During the first year of life, nutrient vessels communicate with the epiphyseal vessels. These nutrient vessels pierce the growth plate. Infections during the first year of life frequently cross the growth plate and can destroy it because of this communication between epiphyseal and metaphyseal vessels. (B) This is the typical arrangement of the blood supply to the growing bone after 12 months of age. The nutrient artery carries blood to the metaphysis of the bone. It does not penetrate the growth plate. The epiphysis has a special system of epiphyseal vessels. The nutrient vessel takes a 180 degree turn at the growth plate, and this leads to sluggish flow. Infection is common in this area of sluggish flow.

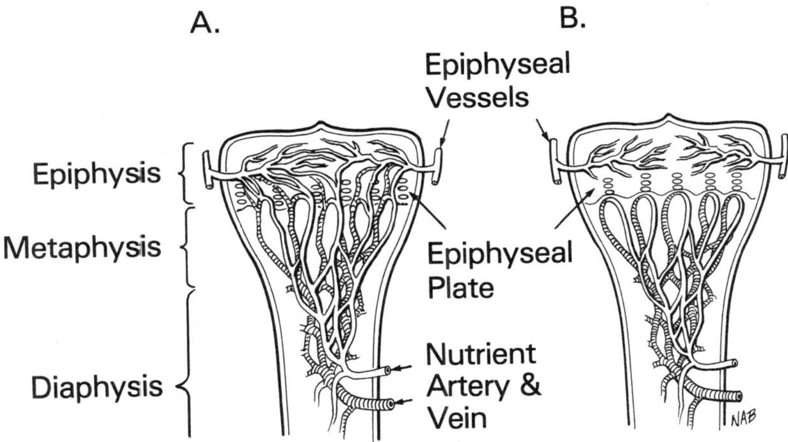

Figure 10-9. (A) Cortical bone derives its blood supply from the periosteum. The blood flows through the haversian canals within the cortical bone. The cancellous bone within the firm cortical shell derives its blood supply from the nutrient artery (see Fig. 10-8). (B) A small infection shaded in grey is present in the cancellous bone of the metaphysis. (C) As the infection enlarges, purulent exudates increase the pressure within the metaphysis. This increased pressure is decompressed through the haversian systems of the cortical bone into the subperiosteal space. As this space fills with purulent exudate, the periosteum is lifted off the cortical bone. This ruptures the periosteal vessels that nourish the cortical bone. In this way, the cortical bone becomes avascular and sequestrum form.

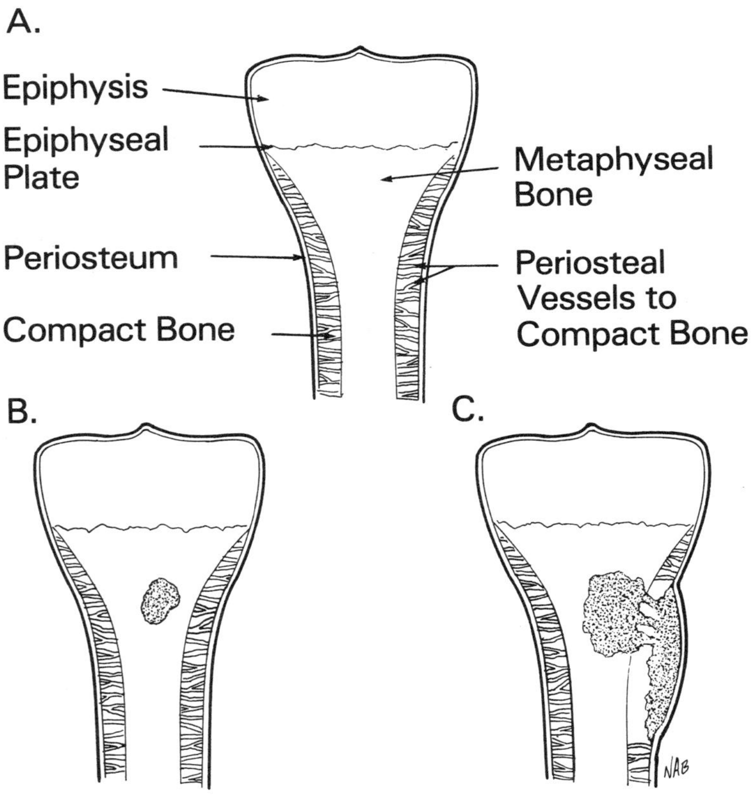

of all bony infections. Other organisms can cause osteomyelitis in special circumstances. Patients with sickle hemoglobinopathies have a propensity for salmonella infection. Pseudomonas osteomyelitis may occur in heroin addicts or after puncture wounds of the foot. Hemophilus influenzae type b, a common cause of septic arthritis in infants, is rarely a cause of osteomyelitis. Anaerobic organisms have been implicated in bony infections arising from an intraoral focus and following human and animal bites.

Diagnosis

The clinical manifestations of osteomyelitis in children vary with age. Osteomyelitis in neonates usually presents with limitation of spontaneous movement, so-called pseudo-paralysis of the involved extremity. Localized tenderness, erythema, and swelling may be noted. Associated septic arthritis occurs in 50% of cases. Less commonly, neonatal osteomyelitis presents as septicemia. Older children with acute hematogenous osteomyelitis characteristically present with localized pain, tenderness to palpation, fever, erythema, and swelling. Pain on attempted active or passive motion of the involved extremity is common, and point tenderness overlying the site of infection is the best localizing sign. Early in the course of the disease, roentgenograms and bone scans may be normal; however, changes develop later with continued destruction of bone. Aspirates of subperiosteal pus or metaphyseal fluid yield a pathogen in 70% of cases. The point of maximal bone tenderness on physical examination is the most appropriate location for needle aspiration. The skin overlying the affected region should be prepared with an antiseptic solution and draped with sterile towels. Following infiltration of the area with local anesthetic, an 18-gauge spinal needle, with stilette in place, is passed through the skin to the bone. The subperiosteal space should be aspirated first. If the tap is dry, the needle should then be twisted through the bony cortex into the metaphysis and metaphyseal fluid aspirated. Recovered material should be immediately cultured and gram-stained. The responsible organism may also be recovered from other sources. Blood cultures are positive in 60% of children with osteomyelitis. In traumatic osteomyelitis, cultures from the wound site often yield the pathogen. When osteomyelitis complicates meningitis, the organism may be recovered from the cerebrospinal fluid. Indirect demonstration of bacterial antigens by counter-immunoelectrophoresis, latex agglutination, or enzyme-linked immunosorbent assay may be valuable in the absence of positive cultures, although such tests are currently employed infrequently.

Therapy

Initial Antibiotic Therapy

Treatment must not be delayed in children with suspected musculoskeletal infection. Antimicrobial therapy should be initiated, usually with a combination of agents, as soon as a tentative diagnosis is established and cultures have been obtained. Later, treatment can be altered appropriately according to drug sensitivities. For neonates, optimal coverage is provided by a penicillinase-resistant penicillin coupled with an aminoglycoside. The newer third-generation cephalosporins have been successfully used in the treatment of osteomyelitis caused by enteric bacilli; however, these agents should not be used alone as initial treatment, since their activity against group B streptococci is inadequate. When these drugs are used as part of the initial therapeutic regimen, a penicillinase-resistant penicillin should be used concomitantly.

In older children, optimal initial therapy may be provided by a penicillinase-resistant penicillin, provided the child is not at risk for a gram-negative infection. For children under two years, especially those with associated septic arthritis, chloramphenicol may be added.

Drug therapy is more complex for children with underlying disease states. Chloramphenicol should be used when salmonella is suspected. If pseudomonas or enteric bacilli are likely pathogens, initial therapy should consist of a broad-spectrum penicillin (for example, carbenicillin, ticarcillin, or piperacillin) combined with an aminoglycoside. A newer third- generation cephalosporin (for example, cefotaxime or moxalactam) may be used, but experience with these is limited. Anaerobic infections resulting from human bites, animal bites, or intraoral infections may be treated initially with penicillin G or a second-generation cephalosporin, such as cefazolin or cefoxitin.

Initial Surgical Therapy

Primary surgical treatment depends on the results of bone aspiration. If grossly purulent material is recovered from either the subperiosteal space or the metaphysis, an abscess has formed. In these cases, surgical drainage is necessary to decompress the abscess. This facilitates blood flow and the subsequent delivery of antibiotics. Also, surgical drainage allows for evaluation of foreign material and evacuation of sequestered, dead bone. When pus is not removed at the time of initial aspiration, the patient's infection is in a cellulitic phase, not an abscess phase. Any recovered material is sent for culture and blood cultures, and antibiotics are started. The affected limb should be immobilized with splints or in balanced suspension for comfort. Such patients must be carefully followed during the early phases of treatment. Surgical intervention may become necessary if adequate clinical response is not obtained after 48 hours of medical therapy.

Appropriate antimicrobial therapy for bony infections requires the administration of an effective drug, for an effective period of time, by an effective route. In most cases, sensitivities of the bacterial pathogen permit selection of a single effective antimicrobial agent. The drug used for long-term therapy should be bactericidal against the pathogen, have readily achievable serum concentration, and possess little toxicity. Chloramphenicol, with its inherent dose-dependent marrow suppression, and aminoglycosides, with their renal and auditory toxicities, should be avoided for prolonged therapy. In the future, agents such as cefotaxime and moxalactam may replace these more toxic drugs. Duration of antimicrobial therapy is controversial. Several studies have demonstrated unacceptable failure rates in children treated for less than three weeks. Recent studies recommend a minimum of four to six weeks of antimicrobial therapy. The extent of initial bone destruction, the rapidity of initial response to treatment, the extent of necessary surgical debridement, and the rate of return of laboratory parameters such as white count and sedimentation rate to normal may be used to gauge duration of treatment.

Initial drug therapy should be given by the intravenous route. This may be maintained throughout treatment. A number of studies, however, have shown that, under certain circumstances, oral therapy can supplant much of the intravenous treatment. Composite recommendations suggest that the following criteria must be fulfilled in order for oral therapy to be successful: (1) isolation of a bacterial pathogen that is sensitive to oral agent, (2) administration of the drug in a fashion that ensures peak serum bactericidal titers greater than 1:8 and trough titers greater than 1:2, (3) clinical improvement during the first five to seven days of intravenous therapy, and (4) patient compliance with the drug course, usually ensured by hospitalization. The importance of monitoring the serum bactericidal titers cannot be overemphasized. Total daily dosages and frequency of drug administration often must be changed to ensure adequate bactericidal titers.

Chronic Osteomyelitis

The therapy of chronic osteomyelitis differs significantly from the treatment of acute bony infection. Debridement, excision of the sinus tract, removal of infected sequestra, thorough curettage, and multiple bone grafting are often necessary. The recommended duration of antimicrobial therapy is often six months. Parenteral therapy is often maintained for months. Even with this regimen, 20% of patients with chronic osteomyelitis continue to have relapses requiring repeat hospitalization and long courses of therapy.

Infectious Arthritis

Pathophysiology and Etiology

The mechanisms responsible for joint infections parallel those of bone infection: hematogenous seeding of the joint following bacteremia or septicemia, contiguous spread from an adjacent locus of infection, and traumatic penetration of the joint space. Regardless of source, the ensuing inflammatory response results in synovial hypertrophy and altered capillary permeability. Purulent fluid accumulates and fibrinous clots may coat joint surfaces. Diffusion of nutrients across the articular cartilage is interrupted, and normal lubrication processes are altered. Lysosomal enzymes, released in neutrophil degeneration, attack the mucopolysaccharide components of articular cartilage. Hypertrophic granulation tissue forms a pannus that erodes underlying joint surfaces, and extension of infection to subchondral bone is possible. Fibrous, and later, bony ankylosis of opposing bone surfaces may develop. Increased intra-articular pressure may occlude vessels that supply the secondary ossification center and germinal layers of the physis in children, resulting in avascular necrosis. Rupture of pus through the synovial membrane into surrounding tissues produces soft tissue abscesses that may later develop into chronic draining sinuses.

Neonatal pyogenic arthritis is often secondary to osseous infection, and therefore the bacterial agents responsible for the joint infections are similar to those previously described for neonatal osteomyelitis. Less frequently, septic arthritis occurs as a primary entity; the Enterobacteriaceae family, species of Pseudomonas, and <u>N. gonorrhoeae</u> may be isolated in the latter cases.

Although <u>S. aureus</u> is the major bacterial cause of pyogenic infections in older infants and children, <u>Hemophilus influenzae</u> type b predominates in children under two years of age. Less often, <u>Streptococcus pyogenes</u> or <u>S. pneumoniae</u> are recovered. Salmonella species occasionally cause joint infections in children with sickle hemoglobinopathies, and enteric gram-negative bacilli have been implicated in joint infections among the immunocompromised. <u>N. gonorrhoeae</u> is a common cause of septic arthritis in sexually active adolescents and adults.

Diagnosis

The clinical presentation of neonatal septic arthritis is similar to that described for neonatal osteomyelitis. Often a joint effusion may be noted on physical or radiographic examination. Infectious arthritis in older infants and children is usually monoarticular and most often presents acutely with localized pain, fever, limitation of spontaneous motion, and effusion. The knee is the most common site followed by the hip, ankle, elbow, and wrist. The shoulder and sacroiliac joints are less often involved. While the small joints of the hands and feet are unusual locations for hematogenous joint infection, they are often the site of infection following puncture wound or other trauma. Gonococcal periarthritis typically involves the extensor surfaces of the hands and feet, while the monoarticular form of the disease affects the large, weight-bearing joints of the lower extremities.

The definitive diagnosis of pyogenic arthritis requires aspiration of the affected joint. The causative agent can be recovered in 60% of the cases. The procedure should be performed under sterile conditions by an experienced physician, since repeated attempts to penetrate the joint may further damage the joint surface and damage the underlying bone. Following culture and gram-staining of the fluid, determinations of the cellular content, glucose concentration, and protein content should be obtained. Infected synovial fluid typically contains more than 50,000 cells per cubic millimeter (primarily polymorphonuclear leukocytes), a glucose concentration of less than 40 mg/dl, or less than 30% of the serum concentration, and an elevated protein concentration. In children with pyogenic arthritis, blood cultures are positive in 40% of the cases. Patients with gonococcal periarthritis typically have sterile synovial fluid in the face of bacteremia; however, the organism can be recovered from the synovial fluid in the monoarticular form of the disease. Urethral, cervical, rectal, and pharyngeal cultures frequently demonstrate Neisseria species when cultures from other sources are sterile. Demonstration of bacterial antigens in the serum or urine is valuable when all bacterial cultures are sterile. This is particularly useful in <u>H. influenzae</u> septic arthritis.

Therapy

Initial Treatment

Septic arthritis is a medical and surgical emergency. Irreversible joint damage may occur unless intra-articular pus is evacuated and effective antimicrobial therapy started as soon as the diagnosis is established.

The age of the patient and the organism demonstrated on gram stain dictate the initial selection of antimicrobial agents. In newborns and immunocompromised children, the presence of gram negative bacilli in the synovial fluid mandates the initial use of a broad spectrum penicillin plus an aminoglycoside. For children with sickle hemoglobinopathies, chloramphenicol should replace the aminoglycoside to provide coverage against ampicillin-resistant strains of Salmonella. Similarly, in children under two years of age, the presence of gram negative bacilli in the synovial fluid suggests H. influenzae and requires the use of chloramphenicol, alone or in combination with ampicillin, to provide adequate antibacterial activity. Cefuroxime is also used in this situation.

If gram positive cocci appear on the smear of the synovial fluid, the selection of initial antimicrobial therapy is markedly simplified. A semisynthetic, penicillinase-resistant penicillin provides adequate antimicrobial activity against the aerobic gram positive pathogens associated with septic arthritis from the neonate to the adolescent. Vancomycin or a cephalosporin may be substituted in the non-neonates with suspected penicillin allergy.

In those cases in which an organism is not observed on gram stain, combinations of drugs should be selected to cover the most likely pathogens. Thus, a penicillinase-resistant penicillin together with an aminoglycoside or chloramphenicol will provide adequate protection. Agents like cefotaxime or moxalactam may replace chloramphenicol and aminoglycosides in the future.

Joint decompression is an essential component of successful therapy of pyogenic arthritis. Opinions vary, however, on the most effective methods, specifically surgical drainage versus repeated aspiration. Primary decompression is usually accomplished at the time of initial joint aspiration. This may be sufficient in joints such as the knee, ankle, and elbow, which are easily aspirated and in which blood flow to intra-articular epiphyses is not at risk. Needle aspiration is not sufficient for definitive decompression of the hip; increases in intra-articular pressure may occlude blood flow to the femoral head and cause irreversible damage. Immediate surgical drainage is mandatory for septic arthritis of the hip (see Fig. 10-10).

Repeat aspiration of joints other than the hip may be appropriate if initial systemic response to antibiotics is good. The morbidity of careful aspirations is certainly less than that of arthrotomy in the knee, ankle, and elbow, but persistent infection after repeated aspiration is probably more harmful than primary arthrotomy. Poorly executed needle aspirations may permanently damage articular surfaces and inoculate underlying bone.

Like the therapy of osteomyelitis, effective antimicrobial therapy of pyogenic arthritis is a function of agent, route, and duration of drug administration. Once the pathogen has been isolated and the sensitivities are known, a single agent may be used. Initial therapy should be intravenous; intra-articular installation of antimicrobial agents is unnecessary since adequate drug concentrations are achieved in synovial fluid by the parenteral route, and since damage may result to the cartilage surfaces from the injections. After adequate initial clinical response to parenteral agents has occurred, oral therapy may be initiated if the same criteria needed for oral treatment of osteomyelitis are met. Joint infections caused by H. influenzae require two to three weeks of therapy, while infections by other agents or those complicated by osteomyelitis may require four or more weeks. The treatment of gonococcal arthritis differs significantly from the treatment of arthritis due to other pathogens. Penicillin G, ampicillin, amoxicillin, tetracycline, and erythromycin have all been used successfully in the therapy of gonococcal arthritis in seven to 10 day courses. Other than diagnostic arthrocentesis, surgical intervention is usually not necessary in this disease.

Figure 10-10. A hip infection can increase pressure within the hip joint through proliferation of purulent exudate. As pressure rises, the subsynovial vessels are collapsed, and the epiphysis is at risk to undergo avascular necrosis. If the capsule is surgically opened, the pressure is relieved, and the epiphyseal blood flow is restored.

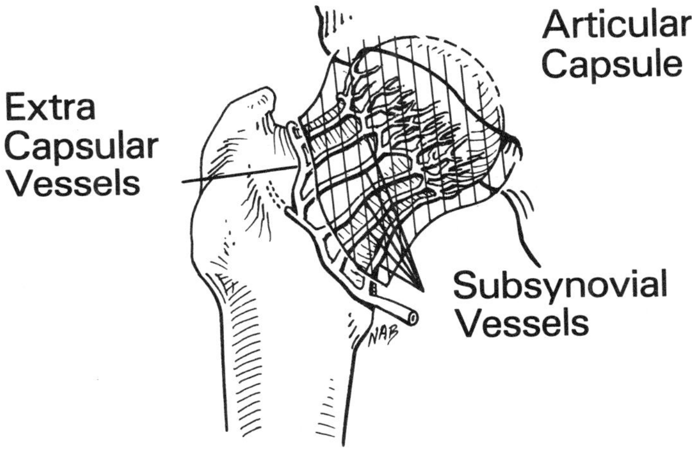

Bibliography

Trauma

Crenshaw, A.H.: <u>Campbell's Operative Orthopedics</u>. St. Louis: C.V. Mosby, 1987.

D'Ambrosia, R.D.: <u>Musculoskeletal Disorders.</u> Philadelphia: J.B. Lippincott, 1977.

Evarts, C.M.: <u>Surgery of the Musculoskeletal System</u>. New York: Churchill Livingstone, 1983.

Rockwood, C.A., Jr, Green, D.P.: <u>Fractures in Adults</u>. Philadelphia: J.B. Lippincott, 1984.

Salter, R.B.: <u>Textbook of Disorders and Injuries of the Musculoskeletal System</u>. Baltimore: Williams and Wilkins, 1970.

Dislocations

Shoulder

Rockwood, C.A., Jr.: Subluxations and Dislocations about the Shoulder. In Rockwood, C.A., Jr., Green D.P. (eds): <u>Fractures in Adults</u>. Philadelphia: J.B. Lippincott, 1984.

Patella

Merchant, A.C., Mercer, R.L., Jacobsen, R.H., Cool, C.R.: Roentgenographic Analysis of Patellofemoral Congruence. <u>J. Bone Joint Surg.</u>,1974; 56A: 1391-1396.

Knee

Green, N.E., Allen, B.L.: Vascular Injuries Associated with Dislocation of the Knee. <u>J. Bone Joint Surg.</u>, 1977; 59A: 236-239.

Taylor, A.R., Arden, G.P., Rainey, M.A.: Traumatic Dislocation of the Knee. A Report of 43 Cases with Special Reference to Conservative Treatment. <u>J. Bone Joint Surg.</u>, 1972; 54B: 96-102.

Hip

Coventry, M.B.: The Treatment of Fracture-Dislocation of the Hip by Total Hip Arthroplasty, <u>J. Bone Joint Surg.</u>, 1974; 56A: 1128-1134.

Epstein, H.C.: Traumatic Dislocations of the Hip. <u>Clin. Orthop.</u>, 1973; 92: 116-142.

Fractures

Wrist

Frykman, G.: Fracture of the Distal Radius including Sequelae - Shoulder-Hand-Finger Syndrome, Disturbance in the Distal Radio-Ulnar Joint and Impairment of Nerve Function: A Clinical and Experimental Study. <u>Acta. Orthop. Scand.</u>, 1967; 108 [Suppl]: 1-155.

Knirk, J.L., Jupiter, J.B.: Intra-articular Fractures of the Distal End of the Radius in Young Adults. <u>J. Bone Joint Surg.</u>, 1986;68A: 647.

Ankle

Lauge-Hansen, N.: Fractures of the Ankle. II. Combined Experimental-Surgical and Experimental-Roentgenologic Investigations. <u>Arch. Surg.</u>, 1958; 60: 957-985.

Phillips, W.A., Schwartz, H.S., Keller, G.S., et al.: A Prospective, Randomized Study of the Management of Severe Ankle Fractures. J. Bone Joint Surg., 1987; 67A: 67.

Hip

Hirsch, C., Frankel, V.H.: Analysis of Forces Producing Fractures of the Proximal End of the Femur. J. Bone Joint Surg., 1960; 42B: 633-640.

Keller, C.C., Laros, G.S.: Indications for Open Reduction of Femoral Neck Fractures. Clin. Orthop., 1980; 152: 131-137.

Laros, G.S., Spiegel, P.G.: Rigid Internal Fixation of Fractures. Editorial Comments. Clin. Orthop., 1979; 138:2-4.

Meyers, M.H.: The Role of Posterior Bone Grafts (Muscle-Pedicle) in Femoral Neck Fractures. Clin. Orthop., 1988; 152:143-146.

Open Fractures

Gustilo, R.B., Simpson, L., Nixon, R., Ruiz, A.: Analysis of 511 Open Fractures. Clin. Orthop., 1969; 66:148-154.

Gustilo, R.B., Anderson, J.T.: Prevention of Infection in the Treatment of One Thousand and Twenty-five Open Fractures of Long Bones. J. Bone Joint Surg., 1976; 58A:453.

Gustilo, R.B., Merkow, R.R., Templeman, D.: The Management of Open Fractures. J. Bone Joint Surg., 1990; 72A, 299.

Compartment Syndromes

Garfin, S., Mubarak, S., Evang, K., et al.: Quantification of Intracompartmental Pressure and Volume Under Plaster Casts. J. Bone Joint Surg., 1981; 63A: 449-453.

Matsen, F.A., III: Compartmental Syndrome: A Unified Concept. <u>Clin. Orthop.</u>, 1975; 113:8-14.

Mubarak, S.J., Owen, C.A., Hargens, A.R., Garetto, L.P., Akeson, W.H.: Acute Compartment Syndromes: Diagnosis and Treatment with the Aid of Wick Catheter. <u>J. Bone Joint Surg.</u>, 1978; 60A:1091-1095.

Whitesides, T.E., Jr., Haney, T.C., Marimoto, K., Harada, H.: Tissue Pressure Measurements as a Determinant for the Need of Fasciotomy. <u>Clin. Orthop.</u>, 1975; 113: 43.

Septic Arthritis/Osteomyelitis

Green, N.E., Edwards, K.: Bone and Joint Infections in Children. <u>Orthop. Clin. North. Am.</u>, 1987; 18:555-576,

Griffin, P.P., Green, N.T.: Hip Joint Infections in Infants and Children. <u>Orthop. Clin. North Am.</u>, 1978; 9:123-134.

Lunseth, P., Heiple, K.: Prognosis in Septic Arthritis of the Hip in Children. <u>Clin. Orthop.</u>, 1979; 139:81-85.

Morrissey, R.T.: Bone and Joint Sepsis in Children. <u>In American Academy of Orthopaedic Surgeons Instructional Course Lectures</u>. St. Louis: C.V. Mosby Co., 1982;49-61.

Scoles, P.V., Aronoff, S.C.: Antimicrobial Therapy of Childhood Skeletal Infections. Current Concepts Review. <u>J. Bone Joint Surg.</u> 1984; 66A:1487-1492.

INDEX

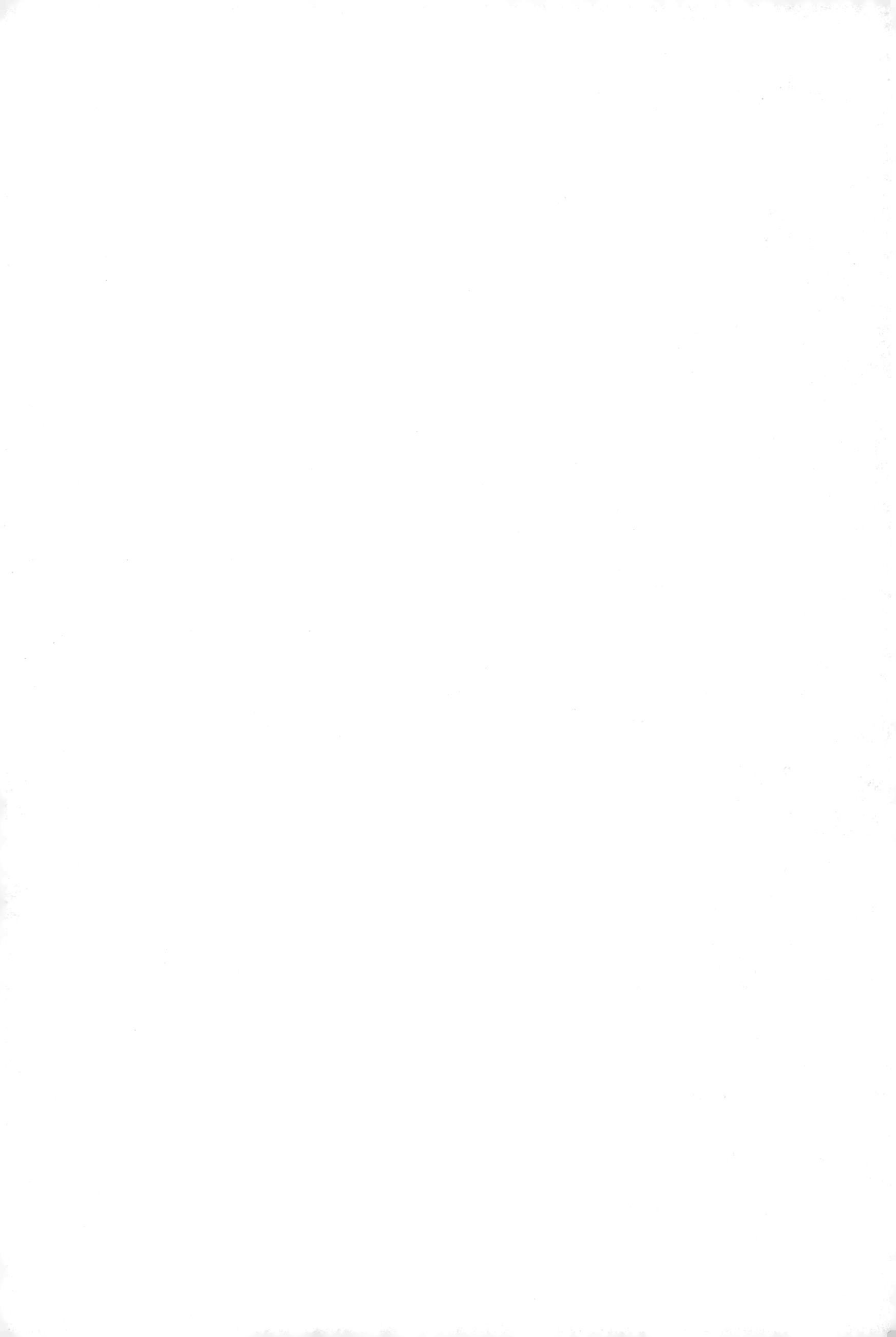

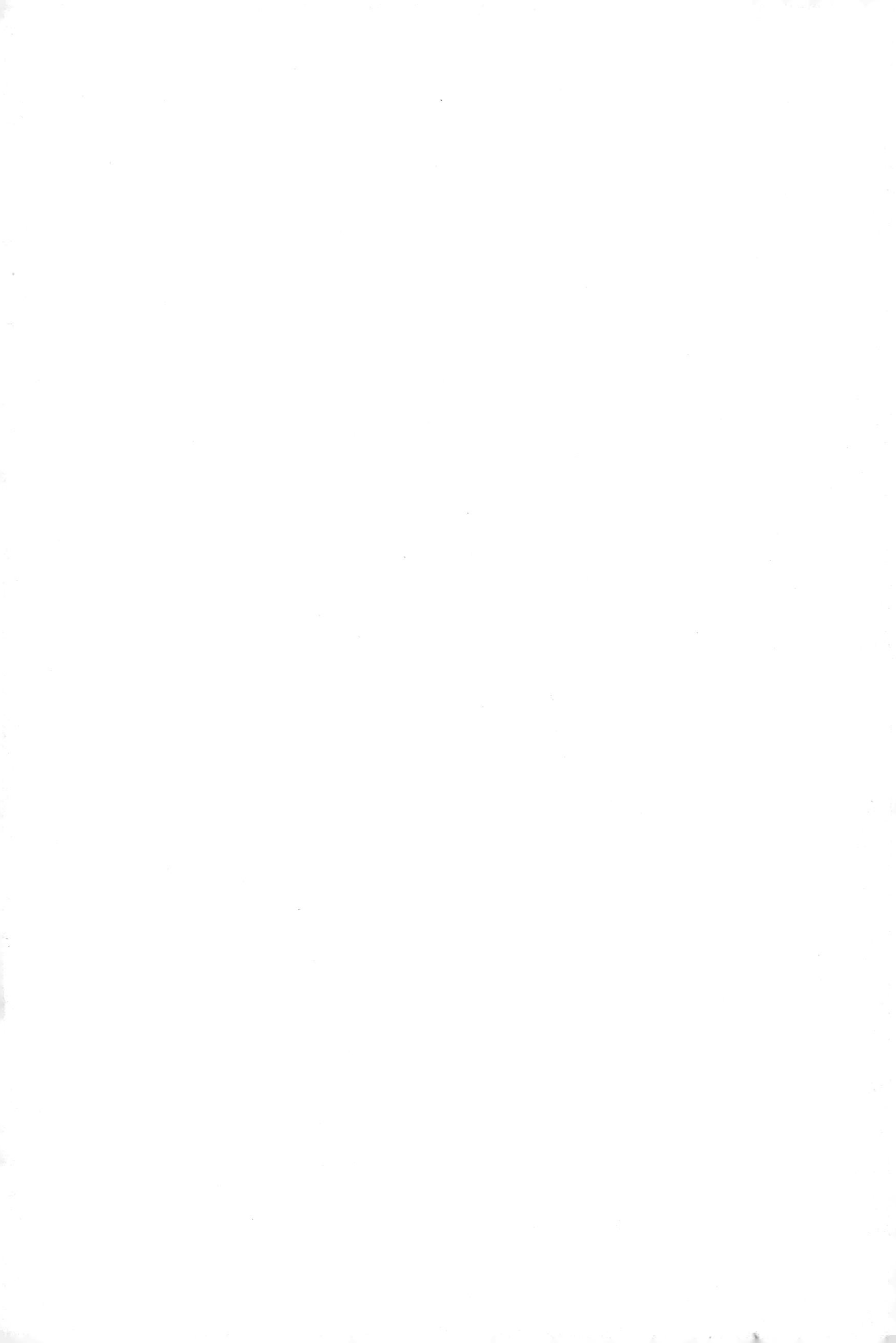